Handbook of STRESS MEDICINE *and* HEALTH

Second Edition

Handbook of STRESS MEDICINE *and* HEALTH

Second Edition

Edited by
CARY L. COOPER
Professor of Organizational Psychology and Health
Lancaster University
Lancaster, U.K.

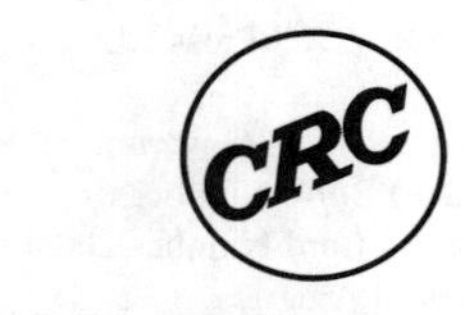

CRC PRESS
Boca Raton London New York Washington, D.C.

Library of Congress Cataloging-in-Publication Data

Handbook of stress medicine and health / edited by Cary L. Cooper.—2nd ed.
p. cm.
Includes bibliographical references and index.
ISBN 0-8493-1820-3
1. Stress (Physiology) 2. Stress (Psychology). 3. Health. I. Cooper, Cary L.
[DNLM: 1. Stress, Psychological—complications. 2. Disease—etiology. 3. Health. 4. Life Change Events. 5. Social Support. WM 172 H23694 2004]
QP82.2S8H363 2004
616.9'8—dc22 2004051937

Direct all inquiries to CRC Press LLC, 2000 N.W. Corporate Blvd., Boca Raton, Florida 33431.

Visit the CRC Press Web site at www.crcpress.com

International Standard Book Number 0-8493-1820-3
Library of Congress Card Number 2004051937
Printed in the United States of America 1 2 3 4 5 6 7 8 9 0
Printed on acid-free paper

Preface

Hippocrates once proclaimed that "the nature of the body can only be understood as a whole, for this is the great error of our day in the treatment of the human body, that physicians separate the soul from the body." Even today, centuries later, we still have some physicians who have trouble appreciating that there are direct links between the psychosocial and physical worlds of the individual, and how these linking relationships reflect themselves in health and in the disease process. Changes did begin to take place, however, at the turn of the 20th century, with physicians like Sir William Osler, who explored the relationship between angina pectoris and "a hectic pace of life." The idea that environmental forces could actually cause disease rather than just short-term ill effects was also seen in the work of Walter Cannon in the 1930s, when he studied the effects of fight-or-flight reactions of animals and people under stress. Cannon observed that when his subjects experienced situations of cold, lack of oxygen, and excitement, he could detect physiological changes such as adrenalin secretions.

From these beginnings, Hans Selye developed, in the 1940s, his three-stage process of stress-related illnesses: the alarm reaction, resistance, and exhaustion. Since Selye's seminal work showing the direct connection between the personality and environment and ill health, research on the impact of the psychosocial factors has grown from strength to strength (Cooper and Dewe, 2004). This has taken place not only in the medical sciences but also in the physical and social sciences, in diverse disciplines like cardiology, oncology, psychology, psychiatry, medical sociology, psychosomatic medicine, social work, and so on. Much of this research is coming together in interdisciplinary studies involving medics, psychologists, occupational health physicians, and the like, helping to create a field of study that this volume and the previous one (Cooper, 1996) hope to christen "stress medicine." Indeed, there is already the journal *Stress and Health* (formerly *Stress Medicine*), which has over the last few years published articles from all the diverse disciplines mentioned above. It is the intention of this volume, therefore, to develop the field further by bringing together some of the most distinguished scholars in the various disciplines and to explore a range of psychosocial factors that contribute to many of today's major illnesses and what can be done to prevent and manage them.

This book is divided into four sections. The first section is the Introduction, which lays the context of stress in society and its links to ill health. The second section comprises several chapters that explore the relationship of stress to a number of health outcomes: heart disease, cancer, mental ill health, burnout, and problems with the endocrine and immune systems. The section starts with a generic theory of stress and health, providing an overview for the following chapters. In examining the critical research in a specific field, we also, for some of the health outcomes, provide the practice implications of the basic research. The third section is in two parts: the link between *stress and personality* and the impact and relationship between *social support and health* (i.e., heart disease, HIV, and disease and ill health prevention). The final section is composed of chapters dealing with stress and its ill health consequences. They explore the emotional processing of traumatic events, gender differences in coping, the handling of stress with families and in chronic disease, and the handling of workplace stress and control at work.

All of these chapters are written by active and distinguished researchers and scholars in the field, from a wide range of countries: the United States, Sweden, Denmark, Australia, Canada, and the Netherlands. We hope that this volume will help to encourage further interdisciplinary and cross-cultural research in the newly emerging field of stress medicine, so that we can better understand what William Shakespeare was alluding to in *Love's Labour's Lost* (V.ii 14–18):

> He made her melancholy, sad, and heavy;
> and so she died; had she been light like you,
> of such a merry, nimble, stirring spirit,
> she might ha'been a grandam ere she died;
> and so may you; for a light heart lives long.

REFERENCES

Cooper, C. L. *Handbook of Stress, Medicine and Health*. Boca Raton, Florida: CRC Press, 1996.

Cooper, C. L. and Dewe, P. *A Brief History of Stress*. Boston: Blackwell Publishing, 2004.

Cary L. Cooper

Editor

Cary L. Cooper is Professor of Organizational Psychology and Health at Lancaster University Management School, and Pro Vice Chancellor (External Relations) at Lancaster University. He is formerly Deputy Vice Chancellor (External Relations) of the University of Manchester Institute of Science and Technology (UMIST). The author of more than 100 books (on occupational stress, women at work, and industrial and organizational psychology), Professor Cooper has written more than 400 scholarly articles for academic journals and is a frequent contributor to national newspapers, TV and radio. He is currently founding editor of the *Journal of Organizational Behavior* and co-editor of the medical journal *Stress & Health* (formerly *Stress Medicine*). He is a Fellow of the British Psychological Society, The Royal Society of Arts, The Royal Society of Medicine, The Royal Society of Health, and an Academician of the Academy for the Social Sciences. Professor Cooper is the President of the British Academy of Management, a Companion of the Chartered Management Institute and one of the first U.K.-based Fellows of the (American) Academy of Management (having also won the 1998 Distinguished Service Award for his contribution to management science from the Academy of Management). In 2001, Professor Cary was awarded a CBE in the Queen's Birthday Honours List for his contribution to organizational health. He holds Honorary Doctorates from Aston University (DSc), Heriot-Watt University (DLitt), Middlesex University (Doc. Univ), and Wolverhampton University (DBA).

Professor Cooper is the editor (jointly with Professor Chris Argyris of Harvard Business School) of the international scholarly *Blackwell Encyclopedia of Management* (12-volume set) and of *Who's Who in the Management Sciences*. He has been an adviser to the World Health Organization and ILO, and has published a major report for the EU's European Foundation for the Improvement of Living and Work Conditions on "Stress Prevention in the Workplace."

Professor Cooper is also the President of the Institute of Welfare Officers, Vice President of the British Association of Counselling, an Ambassador of The Samaritans and Patron of the National Phobic Society.

Contributors

Julian Barling
Queen's University
Kingston, Ontario

Terry A. Beehr
Department of Psychology
Central Michigan University
Mt. Pleasant, Michigan

Ellen Boesen
Department of Psychosocial Cancer Research
Institute of Cancer Epidemiology
Danish Cancer Society
Copenhagen, Denmark

Nathan A. Bowling
Department of Psychology
Central Michigan University
Mt. Pleasant, Michigan

John G. Bruhn
Northern Arizona University
Flagstaff, Arizona

G. Burrows
Department of Psychiatry (Austin Health)
University of Melbourne
Melbourne, Australia

Edith Chen
Department of Psychology
University of British Columbia
Vancouver, British Columbia

George P. Chrousos
First Department of Pediatrics
Ag. Sophia Children's Hospital
Athens University Medical School
Athens, Greece
and
Pediatric and Reproductive Endocrinology Branch
National Institutes of Health
Bethesda, Maryland

Cary L. Cooper
Lancaster University Management School
Lancaster University
Lancaster, United Kingdom

Suzanne Oksbjerg Dalton
Institute of Cancer Epidemiology
Danish Cancer Society
Copenhagen, Denmark

Kathryne E. Dupré
Memorial University of Newfoundland
St. Johns, Newfoundland

Ashley Frize
Department of Clinical Health Psychology
Clarence Wing
St. Mary's Hospital, London
London, United Kingdom

John Green
Department of Clinical Health Psychology
Clarence Wing
St. Mary's Hospital, London
London, United Kingdom

Christoffer Johansen
Department of Psychosocial Cancer Research
Institute of Cancer Epidemiology
Danish Cancer Society
Copenhagen, Denmark

David Kissane
Memorial-Sloan-Kettering Cancer Center
New York, New York

Michiel Kompier
Department of Work and Organizational Psychology
University of Nijmegen
Nijmegen, The Netherlands

Ioannis Kyrou
First Department of Pediatrics
Ag. Sophia Children's Hospital
Athens University Medical School
Athens, Greece
and
Pediatric and Reproductive Endocrinology Branch
National Institutes of Health
Bethesda, Maryland

Pittu Laungani
Manchester University
Manchester, United Kingdom

Manon Mireille LeBlanc
Queen's University
Kingston, Ontario

Michael P. Leiter
Centre for Organizational Research and Development
Acadia University
Wolfville, Nova Scotia

Lennart Levi
University of Stockholm
Stockholm, Sweden

Marilyn Macik-Frey
Goolsby Leadership Academy
University of Texas at Arlington
Arlington, Texas

Christina Maslach
Psychology Department
University of California, Berkeley
Berkeley, California

Joseph E. McGrath
University of Illinois
Urbana-Champaign, Illinois

Gregory E. Miller
Department of Psychology
University of British Columbia
Vancouver, British Columbia

Rama Murali
Department of Psychology
University of British Columbia
Vancouver, British Columbia

Debra Nelson
Department of Management
College of Business Administration
Oklahoma State University
Stillwater, Oklahoma

James Pennebaker
University of Texas at Austin
Austin, Texas

James Campbell Quick
Goolsby Leadership Academy
University of Texas at Arlington
Arlington, Texas

Jonathan D. Quick
Management Sciences for Health
Boston, Massachusetts

Lone Ross
Department of Psychosocial Cancer Research
Institute of Cancer Epidemiology
Danish Cancer Society
Copenhagen, Denmark

Norbert K. Semmer
University of Berne
Berne, Switzerland

Bret L. Simmons
College of Business Administration
North Dakota State University
Fargo, North Dakota

Richard Slatcher
University of Texas at Austin
Austin, Texas

R.O. Stanley
Department of Psychiatry (Austin Health)
University of Melbourne
Melbourne, Australia

Cinnamon Stetler
Department of Psychology
University of British Columbia
Vancouver, British Columbia

Töres Theorell
National Institute for Psychosocial Medicine
Stockholm, Sweden

Constantine Tsigos
Hellenic National Diabetes Center
Athens, Greece

Introduction: Spice of Life or Kiss of Death?

Lennart Levi

WHY *STRESS*?

According to the *American Heritage Dictionary of the English Language* (1993), the word *stress* is derived from middle English *stresse* (hardship, distress), from Old French *estresse* (narrowness), from Vulgar Latin *strictia*, from Latin *strictus* (tight, narrow), and from the past principle of *stringere* (to draw tight, to tighten).

In biological and health sciences, however, the concept derives from everyday clinical practice. Some 80 years ago, a young student sat in the lecture theater at the University of Prague and listened to his very first lecture in internal medicine (Levi, 1985). It so happened that on that day, by way of an introduction, the students were shown several instances of the earliest stages of various infectious diseases. As each patient was brought into the lecture room, the professor carefully questioned and examined him. It turned out that each of these patients felt and looked ill, had a coated tongue, and complained of more or less diffuse aches and pains in the joints and of intestinal disturbances with loss of appetite. Most of them also had fever (sometimes with mental confusion), an enlarged spleen or liver, inflamed tonsils, and so forth. All this was quite evident, but the professor attached very little significance to any of it, focusing instead on "typical features" of each disease.

The young student, Hans Selye, subsequently originator of the biological concept of stress, listened to his professor and thought that every disorder certainly had such typical features — so far very inconspicuous to his untrained eye — that of course must be considered. But the different diseases also had features in common, which would be just as interesting. For want of a better name, he called this the "syndrome of just being sick" (Selye, 1964).

Ten years passed. Selye had moved from Prague to Montreal, where, at the McGill University, he tried to identify a new ovarian hormone in extracts of cattle ovaries. When injected into experimental animals, all the extracts, no matter how prepared, produced the same syndrome characterized by a triad of enlargement of the adrenal cortex, gastrointestinal ulcers, and involution of the thymus and lymph nodes. Although at first Selye ascribed all these changes to some new ovarian hormone in his extract, he soon discovered that extracts of other organs produced the same changes. Could this be due to a "tissue hormone"?

As a further control, he now injected not any organ extract but toxic substances of various kinds, like formalin, and was surprised to find the same triad once again.

The experimental animals reacted in a typical way to each type of injection, but there were also features that were common to all types. Selye turned to one of his tutors and asked him what could be the cause of this peculiar stereotypy, this generality in the organism's way of reacting to such different stimuli. The senior scientist gave his young colleague a sad look and interpreted his findings as a result of impurities in all the extracts.

At that point, Selye suddenly remembered his classroom impression of the "syndrome of just being sick." In a flash he realized that what he had produced with his extracts and toxic agents was an experimental replica of this condition. This model was then employed in the analysis of the stress syndrome using the adrenal enlargement, gastrointestinal ulcers, and thymicolymphatic involution as objective indices of stress.

Based on his observations, Selye published his first brief article in *Nature* (Selye, 1936) on a syndrome that was produced by widely differing noxious agents. The article is about 35 column-centimeters long and does not mention the word *stress*. However, it describes for the first time this generality, this stereotypy, in the organism's tendency to react to widely differing chemical and other stimuli. It was later found that if the experimental animals were exposed to cold, heat, x-rays, noise, pain, bleeding, or muscular work, the same stereotypy occurred (Selye, 1967).

WHAT IS STRESS?

Selye now sought a suitable name for the newly discovered phenomenon and chose an analogy from physics. Here, *stress* is defined as an applied force or system of forces that tends to strain or deform a body. What happens in the body in question, for example, the tensions in the girders of a bridge when a train, column of trucks, or number of cars cross the bridge, is called strain. The tensions vary from case to case but *strain* is common to all these cases. It was the corresponding biological stereotypy that Selye wanted to describe, and when he sought an analogy from engineering, he believed "the tensions in the girders of the bridge" were called *stress*. This is not so. They are called *strain*. But Selye, who was born in the Austro-Hungarian double monarchy, was educated in Prague, and emigrated to Montreal, misunderstood the English terminology and called the phenomenon *stress*, thereby spoiling the analogy with everyday and technological language and — much to his own regret — causing a great deal of subsequent confusion.

What, then, is stress? According to Selye, it is the lowest common denominator in the organism's reactions to every conceivable kind of strain, challenge, and demand, or in other words, the stereotypy, the general features in the organism's reaction to all kinds of stresses and strains. Stress is thus an abstraction. It is very difficult to observe stress, in this sense, since Selye does not base the definition on the entire reaction but only on its nonspecific features, those that are common to all types of loads and demands. Another way to define and describe the phenomenon stress is by referring to what Selye used to call "the rate of wear and tear in the organism" (Selye, 1971).

Many attempts have been made since 1936 to abandon the concept of stress. Yet it is alive and flourishing all over the world, as shown by an in-depth report issued by the American National Academy of Sciences, "Stress and Human Health" (Elliot & Eisdorfer, 1982), a summary of teamwork by about 100 leading scientists. Other reports include Kalimo et al. (1987), Karasek & Theorell (1990), Kompier & Levi (1994), a major report from the International Labour Organization (1992), and a guidance from the European Commission (Levi & Levi, 2000).

WHAT CAUSES STRESS?

Stress is caused by a multitude of demands (stressors), such as an inadequate fit between what we need and what we are capable of, and what our environment offers and what it demands of us. We need a certain amount of responsibility, but our job offers less or demands more. We need a certain amount of work, but get either none at all — unemployment — or too much.

Another cause of stress lies in role conflicts. We all play several roles. We are husbands or wives, parents to our children, children to our parents, brothers and sisters, friends and bosses, peers and subordinates — all at the same time. And the ingredients of conflict are easy to find in trying to fill these multiple and sometimes conflicting roles.

Is stress harmful? The answer is yes and no. It all depends on the context. To use a metaphor, a car stops at a traffic light and its driver steps on the gas. In response, the engine races, leading to increased wear and deposition of soot on the valves, without the car moving from the spot. On the other hand, stepping on the gas while driving on a motorway can be sensible and productive.

Stress in the biological sense cannot be eliminated. Without it, the process of life would cease, for the absence of stress means death. What needs to be avoided is unnecessary and noxious stress in the engineering sense. The relevant questions are: How great is it? Is it appropriate to the needs of the situation?

Our sense of control over what is happening to us is critical. When we feel in control, stress becomes the spice of life, a challenge instead of a threat. When we lack this crucial sense of control, stress can spell crisis — bad news for us, our health, and our community. Our decision latitude, our influence over various aspects of our own lives, is a strong determinant of whether stress becomes a spice of life or a kiss of death (Levi, 1992; Levi & Levi, 2000).

When we are exposed to stressors — such as a lack of control over our lives combined with excessive demands, unsatisfied needs, unfulfilled expectations, over-stimulation, understimulation, or role conflicts — most of us experience dysphoric emotional reactions, such as anxiety, depression, uneasiness, apathy, alienation, and hypochondriasis.

Stress also causes behavioral reactions. Some of us start smoking or overeating. We seek comfort in alcohol or take unnecessary risks at work or in traffic. Aggressive, violent, or other types of antisocial behavior can be the outlet chosen. Many commit suicide — or try to. Many of these reactions lead to disease and premature death.

We also react physiologically. Take, for example, the employee who has been unjustly criticized by his or her supervisor. The employee's typical reactions are increased blood pressure, increased or irregular heart rate, muscular tension with subsequent pain in the neck, head, and shoulders, dryness of throat and mouth, and overproduction of acid gastric juice. When long-lasting, intensive, or frequently recurring, some of these reactions can lead, for example, to hypertension, myocardial infarction, or stroke.

Although everyone can experience these reactions, those with type A neuroendocrinologically mediated behavior are particularly at risk. These are people leading highly competitive, hard-driving ways of life, combining hostility, speed, impatience, and obsessive concern with doing more and more in less and less time, with no opportunity or ability for unwinding and recuperation.

But these reactions can be buffered. Much depends not only on what we are exposed to but also on how we cope with the situation. We can change our environment, we can flee from our problems, we can ask for help, we can accept things as they are, or we can bury our heads in the sand by changing our appraisal of our environment (denial). Whatever our choice, it influences our stress reactions. Coping can thus mean either altering the situation or (without doing this) altering one's perception of, or adaptation to, the situation. Both approaches affect health and well-being.

HEALTH EFFECTS

The relationships between exposures to stressors, on the one hand, and the outcome in terms of morbidity and mortality, on the other hand, have been studied by integrating the concepts and methods of psychophysiology and epidemiology. In this way, dissatisfaction, health-related behaviors, and physiological stress reactions can be associated with various characteristics of our social environment, as well as with general and specific mental and physical ill health.

Disturbances in bodily functions commonly found in people exposed to stressful situations include muscular symptoms such as tension and pain; gastrointestinal symptoms such as dyspepsia, indigestion, vomiting, heartburn, constipation, and irritable colon; cardiovascular symptoms such as palpitation, arrhythmia, and inframammary pain; respiratory symptoms such as dyspnea and hyperventilation; central nervous system symptoms such as depressive reactions, insomnia, weakness, faintness, and headaches; and sexual dysfunctions such as dysmenorrhea, frigidity, and impotence. Not only do these symptoms cause the patient much distress and suffering, but they also entail very high cost to the community and very considerable losses in work time and productivity for the employer.

How much "say" an employee has in his or her job is a critical factor. In a study on 1600 Swedish men, heart disease symptoms were most common (with 20% of the workers affected) among those who described their work as both psychologically demanding and having a low degree of decision-making latitude (Karasek & Theorell, 1990). By contrast, workers who reported low psychological demands and a high level of skill discretion had no symptoms of heart disease. Their jobs were associated with a much better state of health than that of the average worker.

A number of studies in different countries have shown a relationship between exposure to environmental stressors (such as high psychological demands combined with low decision-making latitude and low level of social support) and morbidity and mortality (Karasek & Theorell, 1990). Although correlation is not causation, the evidence is strong enough to justify measures to prevent or reduce stress, at least if applied in an experimental manner and if properly evaluated (Kompier & Levi, 1994; Levi & Levi, 2000).

STRESS MANAGEMENT

There are three basic paths to consider:

1. Eliminate or modify the stress-producing situation or remove the individual from it; find "the right shoe for the right foot," or allow the person concerned to adjust the shoe to fit his or her foot.
2. Adjust the shoe — that is, change the social situation — to fit the individual's foot.
3. Strengthen the person's resilience to stress, for example, through physical exercise, meditation and relaxation techniques, and social support.

Stress management has traditionally focused on individual approaches, usually by counseling individuals or small groups on ways to adapt to, or cope with, various stressors and their consequences. More recently, approaches have started to encourage the individual to adjust his environment to his abilities and needs, improving the person–environment fit, and to advise decision makers and administrators to allow or even promote such adjustments.

Four general categories of approaches and strategies can be applied in any community:

- Improve content and organization of life conditions to control psychosocial risk factors.
- Monitor changes in social situation, people's health, and their interrelationship, with proper feedback to all concerned.
- Increase awareness, inform, train, and educate.
- Broaden goals and strategies of health services.

Most important, we must create, for ourselves and others, those occupational and other situations that give our lives meaning, content, and structure, as well as identity, self-esteem, companions, friends, and material means. If we succeed, we will be productive without being destructive.

A HOLISTIC APPROACH

In all industrialized and most developing countries, rapid, fundamental changes are taking place in such basic social structures as the way children are reared, the types of environments in which people work, the way work is organized and conducted, and the mechanisms for taking care of the old and the sick. These changes are influenced by and influence phenomena such as urbanization, mechanization and automation, environmental pollution, uneven distribution of resources, and shortages of work and housing. At the same time, increases in communication, education, and advertising have resulted in greater public awareness and expectations.

Singly and interacting with one another, various aspects of these phenomena are of great significance in promoting health and in causing disease. These structural problems have not been dealt with adequately in the context and scope of physical and psychosocial environmental planning, health care, and stress research.

An exception to this rule is provided in the Swedish Public Health Service Bill (1985, p. 11), in which the government declared that "our health is determined in large measure by our living conditions and lifestyle." The bill goes on to state that "the health risks in contemporary society take the form of, for instance, work, traffic, and living environments that are physically and socially deficient, unemployment, abuse of alcohol and drugs, consumption of tobacco, unsuitable dietary habits, as well as psychological and social strains associated with our relationship — and lack of relationship — with our fellow beings.... These health risks ... are now a major determinant of our possibilities of living a healthy life. This is true of practically all the health risks which give rise to today's most common diseases, e.g., cardiovascular disorders, mental ill health, tumors and allergies, as well as accidents."

As seen by the Swedish government, therefore, "care must start from a holistic approach.... By a holistic approach we mean that people's symptoms and illnesses, their causes and consequences, are appraised in both a medical and a psychological and social perspective."

An estimate made in a World Health Organization teleconference on October 12, 1990, indicates that such "diseases of lifestyle" are the cause of 70 to 80% of premature deaths in industrialized countries. This insight was expressed about one decade earlier by the secretary of health, education and welfare of the U.S. (Califano, 1979) in three summarizing sentences about these "modern killers":

- We are killing ourselves by our own careless habits.
- We are killing ourselves by carelessly polluting the environment.
- We are killing ourselves by permitting harmful social conditions to persist.

Environments and lifestyles are now changing more rapidly than ever. Many of these changes are well intended, but still carry negative side effects. Others are unintentional and can also lead to unforeseeable noxious effects. Some of the changes are planned and intentional, and their noxious effects are easily foreseeable, as in the case of exploitation of other people. Or, eventually, problems are created, not by the change, but by the lack of change, for example, by permitting harmful conditions to persist (Levi, 1993).

Rather than describing a smooth curve, these interactions tend to be discontinuous, besides being intertwined and uncontrolled. Their effects in terms of health and well-being are often dramatic and destructive. The Club of Rome correctly conceives such problems as an untidy tangle of interrelated issues (the "problematique world"). The interactions between the different "threads" are many and varied but only dimly understood.

Against this background, a fundamental issue is whether governments, with the support of scientists and planners in all sectors and disciplines and of an informed community, will be able (and willing) to use the new opportunities offered by advanced technologies to analyze deliberately and consciously this untidy tangle, to try to shape a better society and working life. Or will they passively attempt mere adjustment, postfactum, as a matter of current expediency (King, 1986)?

FROM RESEARCH TO LEGISLATION AND IMPLEMENTATION

The Swedish government chose the former approach as related to one of the key components of the "living conditions" mentioned in its Public Health Service Bill (see above), namely, the work environment. It appointed and issued its terms of reference for a Swedish Commission on the Work Environment, against a background of the government's concern about recent trends in work-related morbidity, long-term absence due to sickness, and premature retirement. The commission, in close collaboration with the scientific community, reviewed available evidence and presented its final report in June 1990. The report proposed amendments to the Swedish Work Environment Act.

Based on these formulations, the resulting amended Swedish Work Environment Act now states the following concerning the characteristics of the work environment:

- Working conditions shall be adapted to people's differing physical and psychological circumstances.
- The employee shall be enabled to participate in the arrangement of his own job situation as well as in work on changes and developments that affect his own job.
- Technology, work organization, and job content shall be arranged so that the employee is not exposed to physical or mental loads that can cause ill health or accidents.
- The matters to be considered in this context shall include forms of remuneration and the scheduling of working hours.
- Rigorously controlled or "tied" work, where the worker may not leave his post for a phone call or even a bathroom break, shall be avoided or restricted.
- It shall be the aim for work to afford opportunities for variety, social contacts, and cooperation as well as continuity between individual tasks.
- It shall be the aim for working conditions to afford opportunities for personal and occupational development as well as for self-determination and occupational responsibility.

These objectives can be promoted using a stick (liability to penalty) or a carrot (financial incentives to management). Sweden has chosen to give priority to the latter approach.

The Swedish Work Environment Act was also based on the EU Framework Directive, according to which employers have a "duty to ensure the safety and health of workers in every aspect related to the work." The directive's principles of prevention include "avoiding risks," "combating the risks at source," and "adapting the work to the individual." In addition, the directive indicates employers' duty to develop "a coherent overall prevention policy." The European Commission's Guidance (Levi, 2000; Levi & Levi, 2002) aims at providing a basis for such endeavors.

Based on surveillance at individual workplaces and monitoring at national and regional levels, work-related stress should be prevented or counteracted by job redesign (e.g., by empowering the employees, by avoiding both over- and underload), by improving social support, and by providing reasonable reward for the effort invested by workers, as integral parts of the overall management system. And, of course, it should also be prevented or counteracted by adjusting occupational physical, chemical, and psychosocial settings to the workers' abilities, needs, and reasonable expectations — all in line with the requirements of the EU Framework Directive and Article 152 of the Treaty of Amsterdam, according to which "a high level of human health protection shall be ensured in the definition and implementation of all Community policies and activities."

The British government (Secretary of State for Health, 1998, 1999) developed similar ideas several steps further in its Green Paper, "Our Healthier Nation: A Contract for Health," and its White Paper, "Saving Lives: Our Healthier Nation." Four years later, the Swedish government (Ministry of Social Affairs, 2003) presented its Public Health Objectives Bill, which was subsequently approved by the Swedish Parliament. It is based on an intersectional structure approach, comprising 11 major goal areas to promote coherence in public health work.

The overall approach of the EU guidance on work-related stress was further endorsed in the Swedish EU presidency conclusions (2001), which said that "employment not only involves focusing on more jobs, but also on better jobs. Increased efforts should be made to promote a good working environment for all, including equal opportunities for the disabled, gender equality, good and flexible work organization permitting better reconciliation of working and personal life, lifelong learning, health and safety at work, employee involvement and diversity in working life."

The subsequent Belgian EU presidency initiated another European conference, in Brussels, on October 25–27, 2001, on "coping with stress- and depression-related problems in Europe." Based on its conclusions, the European Council of Health Ministers in its "Conclusions" (2001) invited the EU member states to "give special attention to the increasing problem of work-related stress and depression."

In its report *Mental Health in Europe*, the World Health Organization (2001) similarly emphasized that "mental health problems and stress-related disorders are the biggest overall cause of early death in Europe. Finding ways to reduce this burden is a priority." And, soon after, the executive board of the World Health Organization (2002) resolved that "mental health problems are of major importance to all societies and to all age groups and are significant contributors to the burden of disease and the loss of quality of life; they are common to all countries, cause human suffering and disability, increase risk of social exclusion, increase mortality, and have huge economic and social costs."

HEALTH PROMOTION AND STRESS-RELATED DISEASE PREVENTION

Theoretically, environment- and lifestyle-related disease can be prevented at any of the links in the pathogenic chain. Thus, environmental stressors might be removed, modified, or avoided by adjusting, for example, the work environment, organization, and content. Preventive variables that interact might be promoted (e.g., by improving social networks or expanding coping abilities). Emotional, behavioral, and physiological pathogenic mechanisms might be interrupted (e.g., by blocking adrenergic beta-receptors, antismoking campaigns, psychotherapeutic counseling, tranquilizers). Precursors of disease might be treated so that they do not progress to overt disease.

Briefly, an overall program for research and environmental and health action should aim at being:

- Systems oriented, addressing health-related interactions in the person–environment ecosystem (e.g., family, school, work, hospital, and old people's homes)
- Interdisciplinary, covering and integrating medical, physiological, emotional, behavioral, social, and economic aspects
- Oriented to problem solving, including epidemiological identification of health problems and their environmental and lifestyle correlates, followed by longitudinal interdisciplinary field studies of exposures, reactions, and health outcomes, and then by subsequent experimental evaluation under real-life conditions of presumably health-promoting and disease-preventing interventions
- Health oriented (not merely disease oriented), trying to identify what constitutes and promotes good health and counteracts ill health)
- Intersectoral, promoting and evaluating environmental and health actions administered in other sectors (e.g., employment, housing, nutrition, traffic, and education)
- Participatory, interacting closely with potential caregivers, receivers, planners, and policymakers
- International, facilitating transcultural, collaborative, and complementary projects with centers in other countries

To safeguard individual rights, prevent the perpetuation of harmful or useless measures, limit losses to the community's purse, and advance knowledge of the future, any of these or other actions must be evaluated when implemented. Such evaluation is the modern, humane substitute for nature's slow and cruel survival of the fittest and is a means of enabling man to adapt with minimal trauma to a rapidly changing environment and to control some of its changes (Kagan & Levi, 1975; Levi, 1979, 1992).

REFERENCES

American Heritage Dictionary of the English Language (p. 1343). Boston: American Heritage & Houghton Mifflin, 1993.

Califano, J.A., Jr. The secretary's foreword. In: *Healthy People: The Surgeon General's Report on Health Promotion and Disease Prevention* (p. vii). Washington, D.C.: U.S. Department of Health, Education, and Welfare, 1979.

Elliott, G.R. and Eisdorfer, C. (Eds.). *Research on Stress and Human Health.* National Academy of Sciences, Institute of Medicine, report. New York: Springer, 1982.

European Council of Health Ministers. Council conclusions adopted on November 15, 2001. In: *EU Presidency, European Commission and World Health Organization* (pp. 94–95). Final Report. Brussels: EU Presidency, 2001.

International Labour Organization (ILO). *Preventing Stress at Work. Conditions of Work Digest 2.* Geneva: International Labour Organization, 1992.

Kagan, A. and Levi, L. Health and environment: psychosocial stimuli: a review. In: Levi, L. (Ed.), *Society, Stress and Disease*, Vol. 2, *Childhood and Adolescence* (pp. 241–260). London: Oxford University Press, 1975.

Kalimo, R., El-Batawi, M.A. and Cooper, C.L. (Eds.). *Psychosocial Factors at Work and Their Relation to Health.* Geneva: World Health Organization, 1987.

Karasek, R. and Theorell, T. *Healthy Work: Stress, Productivity, and the Reconstruction of Working Life.* New York: Basic Books, 1990.

King, A. The great transition. *World Academy of Art and Science Newsletter* (pp. 1–6). July 1986.

Kompier, M. and Levi, L. *Stress at Work, Causes, Effects, and Prevention.* Dublin: European Foundation, 1994.

Levi, L. Stress: definitions, concepts and significance. *Cardiovasc. Inf.*, 1, 10, 1985.

Levi, L. Work stress. *Eur. Bull. Environ. Health*, 1, 9, 1992.

Levi, L. Conditions of life, life-styles, and health in a highly developed country. *Psychiatr. Neurol. Jpn.*, 95, 259, 1993.

Levi, L. The European Commission's Guidance on work-related stress: from words to action. *TUTB Newsletter* (pp. 12–17). September 19–20, 2002.

Levi, L. (Ed.). Psychosocial factors in preventive medicine. In: *Healthy People: The Surgeon General's Report on Health Promotion and Disease Prevention.* Background papers (pp. 207–252). Washington, D.C.: U.S. Department of Health, Education, and Welfare, 1979.

Ministry of Social Affairs. Public Health Objectives Bill, No. 2002/03:35. Stockholm: Author, 2003.

Levi, L. and Levi, I. *Guidance on Work-Related Stress: Spice of Life or Kiss of Death?* Luxembourg: European Commission, 2000.

Secretary of State for Health. Our Healthier Nation: A Contract for Health. Green Paper; and Saving Lives: Our Healthier Nation. White Paper. London: The Stationary Office, 1998 and 1999.

Selye, H. A syndrome produced by diverse noxious agents. *Nature*, 138, 32, 1936.

Selye, H. *From Dream to Discovery* (p. 51). New York: McGraw-Hill, 1964.

Selye, H. *In Vivo. The Case for Supramolecular Biology.* New York: Liveright, 1967.

Selye, H. The evolution of the stress concept: stress and cardiovascular disease. In: Levi, L. (Ed.), *Society, Stress and Disease*, Vol. 1, *The Psychosocial Environment and Psychosomatic Diseases* (pp. 299–311). London: Oxford University Press, 1971.

Swedish EU Presidency: Modernizing the European Social Model. Improving Quality of Life. Presidency Conclusions, Stockholm European Council, 23–24 March, 2001. Stockholm: Swedish Govrnment, 2001.
World Health Organization. Mental Health in Europes. Copenhagen: WHO, 2001.
World Health Organization. Strengthening Mental Health. Resolution of the WHO Executive Board. Geneva, Switzerland: WHO, January, 2001.

Contents

1 Conceptual Issues in Research on Stress and Health

Norbert K. Semmer, Joseph E. McGrath, and Terry A. Beehr

CONTENTS

0-8493-1820-3/05/$0.00+$1.50

Our aim in this chapter is to identify and discuss a number of basic conceptual issues that are embedded in theory and research on stress. The first two sections examine some key conceptual issues in regard to the definition of stress, and in regard to models of the stress and coping process, respectively. In the third section, we discuss issues that have to do with the special role of the individual, who is the subject of the stress, in that complex stress process. We close the chapter by discussing several recent/current theoretical developments that seem potentially promising for shedding light on many of these issues.

Note that all three authors come to the stress and health area via training in psychology and via interests in stress and health in work and organizational settings. Those experiences doubtless shade our understandings of conceptual issues and how they might be dealt with.

CONCEPTUAL ISSUES REGARDING THE NATURE OF STRESS

Definitional Issues: Stress as Stimulus, Response, and Transaction

Conceptual issues in treatments of stress start with its basic definition. Researchers in this area often make a distinction between (1) stimulus concepts, (2) response concepts, and (3) transactional concepts (Lazarus & Folkman, 1984; Sonnentag & Frese, 2003). *Stimulus* concepts define stress as the occurrence of certain kinds of stimuli (e.g., life events — Dohrenwend & Dohrenwend, 1974). Of course, this makes sense only if these stimuli are associated with some kind of stress reaction (however that is defined). The assumption that there are stimuli that lead to a stress reaction in each and every individual can, however, not be upheld, except perhaps for very extreme, life-threatening situations. If, on the other hand, individual differences are taken into account, a stimulus can be established as a stressor for a given individual only after a stress reaction has appeared. This, of course, is circular. *Response* concepts define stress as a response by the focal person (as, for instance, in the alarm reaction postulated by Selye, e.g., 1993). Such a concept poses similar problems, as do stimulus concepts, but, so to speak, from the other side: anything that elicits a stress reaction in a given individual has to be classified as a stressor for that person. This, again, can only be done after the fact, which implies circularity. Furthermore, since some persons, such as people with psychiatric symptoms, can react with stress symptoms to very minor situations (or, at least for the outsider, to no apparent triggering event), such an approach could lead to designating as stressors almost anything that can happen, including the most innocuous situations. This is, indeed, reflected in Selye's definition of stress as the "result of any demand upon the body" (Selye, 1993, p. 7).

Based on such considerations, both stimulus and response concepts of stress have often been dismissed (e.g., Lazarus & Folkman, 1986). The solution that is typically offered is a *transactional* approach, which defines the core element of stress neither in the environment nor in the response but in the *relationship* between the two. Thus, Lazarus & Folkman (1986, p. 63) define stress as "a relationship with the environment that the person appraises as significant for his or her well-being and in which the demands tax or exceed available coping resources."

In our view, this controversy is a spurious one. Nobody doubts that the experience of stress involves a transaction between people and their environment, and *models* of stress should include both these parts. Models, however, should be distinguished from definitions. Models make assumptions about mechanisms and relationships, and in that sense, the concept of transaction is a perfectly reasonable part of a stress model. Definitions, by contrast, state under what circumstances one acknowledges that a phenomenon in question is present or not. Based on the definition by Lazarus and Folkman, cited above, one might conclude that stress is present whenever (and only whenever) one or (more likely) several conditions are present: an individual (1) expresses verbally that he or she is stressed, or overtaxed, or emits some similar statement that is judged to be equivalent; (2) shows observable signs indicating such a state, as when the person appears nervous or anxious, starts stuttering, reacts defensively, has his or her face turn red, runs away, or the like; or (3) shows physiological signs indicating such a state, such as rising heart rate, blood pressure, hormone levels, etc. Of course, it is debatable to what extent any of these indicators, or any combination of them, can be taken as valid expressions of stress, but that is not the issue here. The issue is that whichever of those indicators, or whichever combination of them, one accepts as evidence of the occurrence of stress, that phenomenon is being inferred from a reaction by the person, which is taken as an indicator of the person's appraisal of the situation as both relevant and overtaxing. This, of course, is what stress researchers typically do in their empirical endeavors. So, the field converges, in practice, on a response definition of stress. In our view, this is perfectly reasonable: when certain conditions are fulfilled, an individual is in a state of stress. What triggered that response is of no concern for the issue of what *defines* stress. It is, of course, important with regard to the issue of *modeling* the stress process.

This, of course, leaves the problem of circularity: Is it possible to identify factors in the environment that can be classified as stressors, given the enormous interindividual differences typically found? We think yes — but such a definition must not specify that a stressor leads to stress *for each and every individual on all occasions.* Rather, stressors can be defined probabilistically, that is, in terms of an increased likelihood of stress reactions, similar to the concept of risk factors in epidemiology. We will come back to this issue when we discuss the individual and social meaning of stress below in the section entitled "In the Eye of the Beholder? Social and Individual Meaning."

Valence of the Stress Experience: Negative vs. Neutral Definition

Stress as Negative vs. Positive Experience

A second definitional controversy that runs through the stress field is the issue of negative vs. neutral concepts of stress. Selye defines stress as the reaction of the organism to any demand (Selye, 1993, p. 7), thus implying that the demand might be perceived qualitatively as positive or negative, attractive or unattractive, pleasant or unpleasant. Only intensity is important in this concept, whereas it is neutral with regard to the quality of the experience involved. Selye's legacy within the stress field is still strong, especially in the medical and biological sciences (cf. Sapolsky, 1998). His "neutral" definition of stress also characterized the development of research on critical life events (Dohrenwend & Dohrenwend, 1974). Yet it was exactly the latter research tradition that, some exceptions notwithstanding (cf. Rahe, 1974), repeatedly produced results showing that the relationships between life events and illness were mainly due to the negative events (e.g., Holahan et al., 1999; McLean & Link, 1994; Paykel, 1974; Sarason et al., 1979; Vinokur & Selzer, 1975). Overall, an emphasis on adversity has characterized the field conceptually (see Dohrenwend, 2000), and Selye (e.g., 1975) has introduced the concepts of "eustress" and "distress." It might be added that, in spite of the usual statements that stressors can be either positive or negative, the stress field tends to focus empirically on negative events or conditions — both with regard to stressors measured in the field (cf. Cohen et al., 1997; Sonnentag & Frese, 2003; Spector & Jex, 1998) and with regard to the experimental procedures that are used to induce stress in laboratory studies (e.g., Kirschbaum et al., 1993). This emphasis seems quite independent of the stress definitions being used (cf. Semmer, 1992). So overall, it seems fair to say that studies on stress are, for the most part, studies on distress. In fact, the "salutogenic" approach accuses stress research exactly of this overemphasis on the negative and urges a stronger focus on positive aspects, both in terms of resources and in terms of outcomes (Antonovsky, 1991; Nelson & Simmons, 2003; Seligman & Csikszentmihalyi, 2000).

The aversive emotional experiences that are at the core of stressful encounters center around common themes with regard to the meaning of the situation. Lazarus (e.g., 1999) suggests the themes of "harm/loss, threat, and challenge." These are cited in much of the literature on stress. In fact, they seem to be so much taken for granted in the psychological stress literature that some inconsistencies are hardly ever discussed. These inconsistencies refer to the concept of challenge.

Challenge and Stress

Challenge is included among "stress appraisals" because it includes the appraisal that "difficulties stand in the way of gain"; but at the same time, it includes the appraisal that these difficulties "can be overcome with verve, persistence, and self-confidence" (Lazarus, 1999, p. 33). Thus, challenge has some elements in common with threat. Both are anticipatory in character, and both imply the possibility of an undesired outcome. In threat, however, avoiding this undesired outcome is the dominant focus. By contrast, attainment of success is the focus in challenge appraisals.* This difference can seem small, yet research in the area of motivation suggests that it can imply quite drastic differences. It has long been recognized that approach and avoidance motivation are fundamentally different from one another (McClelland, 1987; Higgins et al., 1999; Kanfer & Heggestad, 1997). From this perspective, appraisal of threat should be associated with avoidance behavior, or a "prevention focus" (Higgins et al., 1999), whereas challenge should be associated with approach behavior, or a "promotion focus." To the extent that concern about failure is dominant, as in the case of threat appraisals, emotions such as fear or worry should therefore be prevalent. By contrast, to the extent that a focus on success is dominant, as in challenge appraisals, emotions such as cheerfulness and joy should be dominant. This is exactly how challenge has been described: "*challenge* is somewhat like Selye's eustress in that people who feel challenged enthusiastically pit themselves against obstacles, feel expansive — even joyous — about the struggle that will ensue" (Lazarus, 1999, p. 76). Jerusalem and Schwarzer (1992) conducted a unique study in which they investigated the development of stress-related appraisals over time. Participants were presented with a series of problem-solving tasks. They received feedback and were asked to answer questions about their appraisal of challenge, loss, and threat after each task. Failure feedback had a pronounced effect on participants who were low in self-efficacy: challenge appraisals declined, whereas appraisals of threat and loss increased. Overall, threat and loss showed a similar course of development, though at different levels of magnitude, whereas the development of challenge was in the opposite direction. It does not seem appropriate, therefore, to simply subsume challenge under the rubric of stress in the same way as one would the categories of threat and harm/loss (see Dienstbier, 1992, for a similar position).

From this perspective, it comes as no surprise that for an individual to define a potentially stressful situation as "challenge" is among the techniques that are considered protective against the potentially negative consequences of stress. For instance, challenge is one of the components of the so-called "hardy personality" (Ouelette, 1993; see Beehr & Bowling, this volume; Semmer, 2003), and Dienstbier (1992) regards an appraisal of a situation as challenging rather than stressful as a sign of "toughness," associated with a quick rise in catecholamines when demands have to be met, followed by quick recovery when the situation is over.

Of course, during situations defined as challenge, the focus of one's appraisal can change rather quickly as the prospects for success or failure vary. So, challenge situations certainly are *partially* stress situations. Yet, they are also partially situations of joy and pride, which distinguishes them from predominantly stressful situations,

* Note that we are talking about the *probability* of success vs. failure here. Another possibility for ambiguity can be the *meaning* of success and failure, in that success can well contain costs, and failure can imply some possible gains (see footnote 2).

where, as argued above, aversive elements are dominant. To the extent that an individual succeeds in focusing on the gain aspect, the stressfulness of the situation should lessen — which is what concepts like hardiness suggest. Thus one could question whether challenge is a true stress situation.

Challenge and true stress situations* should also vary considerably with regard to outcomes. If a stress situation is successfully resolved, the resulting situation is characterized by the avoidance of a negative outcome. By contrast, if a challenge situation is successfully resolved, the resulting situation is characterized by a substantial gain. In line with what Higgins et al. (1999) postulate about promotion vs. prevention focus, this should result predominantly in relief (quiescence) in the first case, but in pride and joy in the second case.

To the extent that these considerations are valid, they have quite substantial consequences for research as well as for practical applications. With regard to research, they imply that we should focus much more on the situational aspects of stress and challenge, as they unfold over time (see Jerusalem & Schwarzer, 1992). The rise of situation-based studies and of multilevel methodology that allows us to disentangle the situational and habitual aspects of stress are quite promising in that respect (e.g., Bolger et al., 2003; Klumb & Perrez, in press; Semmer et al., in press). In terms of practical applications, helping people to see potentially stressful situations as challenges should be a good possibility for stress prevention, as, for instance, the hardiness concept would suggest.†

Potential Misunderstandings about Implications of a Negative Definition of Stress

Advocating a definition of stress as implying *aversive* experiences requires some further remarks.

Negative Definition vs. Focus on the Negative

First, this does not imply that the negative should be the only focus of research on stress and health. We concur with many authors (e.g., Nelson & Simmons, 2003) that positive experiences need much more attention (and, indeed, our discussion of challenge and our advocating situation-specific research on such experiences implies just that). At the same time, we feel that we actually know more about positive processes and outcomes than the "salutogenetic" literature often suggests, and we should carefully examine the results provided by traditional research before suggesting new concepts, lest we run the danger of presenting old wine in new bottles. For instance, we know quite a bit about the characteristics of people who tend to

---

* We realize, of course, that talking of true stress situations is a gross simplification. Many stressful situations are likely to contain positive elements — as, for instance, when not receiving a promotion one had hoped for also implies that certain costs, such as having to move, being responsible for other people, etc., will also not occur. In a similar vein, positive situations can well contain negative or stressful aspects, as when a success is mixed with fears that one cannot sustain that success (cf. Nelson & Simmons, 2003).

† It should be added, however, that this possibility is not without limits: "Many of the hells we are able to finesse into heavens are the minor stressors afflicting the relatively well-off in society.... But when faced with the truly brutal stressors ... it is both bad science and morally unacceptable to preach as an outsider about the techniques for transforming hells into heavens" (Sapolsky, 1999, p. 466).

do well in spite of stressful experiences. They include high self-esteem, internal locus of control, emotional stability, or a tendency to cope in a problem-focused manner (Semmer, 2003; see the section entitled "Individual Belief Systems"). We also know about aspects of the environment that are helpful, most notably control (Steptoe, 2001; Steptoe & Appels, 1989; Bosma et al., 1998, Marmot et al., 1997) and social support (Beehr, 1995; Heinrichs et al., in press; Hemingway & Marmot, 1999; Henderson, 1998; Sarason et al., 1996; Schwarzer & Leppin, 1991, 1992; Steptoe, 2001, Viswesvaran et al., 1999). We should give more weight to positive experiences, but we should not overlook the evidence about positive developments that has accumulated within the negative stress tradition.

Negative Experience vs. Negative Consequences

Second, we want to emphasize that regarding negative *experiences* as the core of stress does not automatically imply negative *consequences* of such experiences. Negative experiences can lead one to acquire self-confidence, effective coping strategies, and the like. This has been shown for stressful situations that have been successfully resolved (Harnish et al., 2000; Schaefer & Moos, 1992; Thoits, 1994; Turner & Avison, 1992). Even quite traumatic experiences can, over time, be reinterpreted as challenges that gave life a new meaning, rearranged priorities, etc. (Tennen & Affleck, 1999). Indeed, many approaches to stress management (and many psychotherapies) can be considered the controlled provocation of stressful situations that one learns to manage (and thus as "inoculations"; Meichenbaum & Fitzpatrick, 1993). The absence of stressful experiences, therefore, is not a meaningful goal. It is important that stressful experiences be modest enough, in number or intensity, to be successfully resolved, thus yielding gains — in coping strategies acquired and in increased self-efficacy — which constitute positive outcomes. We must clearly separate negativity of the ongoing experience (momentary distress) and negativity of the effects of such experiences (development of symptoms and weakening of resilience vs. *increases* in resources and resilience).

CONCEPTUAL ISSUES REGARDING MODELS OF THE STRESS PROCESS

Variables in the stress process include stressors, appraisals, coping responses, and outcomes. These processes operate at different levels of complexity: (1) as single stress episodes; (2) as cycles of stress episodes and recovery, involving multiple events; and (3) as stress involving ongoing conditions that do not necessarily have event character (chronic stress). These different levels of complexity also involve different temporal patterns. Furthermore, they probably are interrelated with one another in ways that are not well understood, because studies typically only examine one of these versions of stress at a time.

Microlevel Stress Episodes

A single stress episode can be viewed as a sequence of stressors, appraisals, coping responses, and outcomes. Each part includes a number of conceptual issues.

Stressors

The classical stress episode, as exemplified, for instance, in many experimental settings, starts with a stimulus configuration that has some probability of eliciting a stress reaction — in other words, a stressor, or a "stress-producing event or condition (SPEC)" (McGrath & Beehr, 1990; Shupe & McGrath, 1998; McGrath & Tschan, 2004; see the section entitled "In the Eye of the Beholder? Social and Individual Meaning" for information on the stressor concept).

Appraisal

With few exceptions, however, a stressor will not elicit a stress reaction automatically; rather, it needs to be evaluated by the individual with regard to the potential damage it contains as well as with regard to the possibilities of coping with that potential damage. The term usually used for these processes is *appraisal* (Lazarus, e.g., 1999), related to threat or harm/loss (primary appraisal) and to coping possibilities (secondary appraisal).* Appraisals do not necessarily require elaborate cognitive processes and often occur very rapidly and without conscious processing (Lazarus, 1999; Zajonc, 1984). Nevertheless, some kind of stimulus check (Leventhal & Scherer, 1987) is necessary to elicit a stress reaction.†

Appraisals are closely connected to the emotional experience. Thus, anger — a very important stress emotion — can be characterized as appraisal of an offense for which the offender is to be blamed (that is, it involves the attribution of responsibility, either through intention or through negligence — Averill, 1983; Schmitt et al., 1991). Fright can be regarded as a response to the appraisal of an "immediate, concrete, and overwhelming physical danger," and shame is experienced when the situation is appraised as "failure to live up to an ego ideal" (Lazarus, 1999, p. 96).

Appraisals of potential SPECs are likely to change rather quickly (reappraisal), as the situation and the behavior of the focal person in dealing with it unfold.

Coping

Coping is the attempt to deal either with the problem itself (problem focused) or with the stressful emotions being elicited by the problem (emotion focused). Although dictionary definitions of coping sometimes imply success, researchers are interested in the question of the relative effectiveness of coping, and so the term cannot be reserved only for successful attempts. Moreover, coping can occur by intrapsychic means as, for example, the redefinition of the situation as challenge rather than threat. In such circumstances, the distinction between appraisal and

---

* The terms *primary* and *secondary* appraisal are somewhat misleading, in that they might suggest a temporal sequence or a priority rather than the focus of attention. However, the terms have been so well established that we will keep using them.

† Of course, one could also argue that stress can be elicited by noxious agents even in unconscious people and in animals that have no nervous system (Selye, 1975). Whether one should call that stress is mainly a semantic question. What is certain (and what Selye, 1975, agreed to as well) is that these phenomena are far from the stress experience typical for human beings (see also Mason, 1975).

coping is blurred, because coping is achieved through reappraisal (see McGrath & Tschan, 2004).

There are many possible distinctions regarding coping, such as intrapsychic vs. behavioral, and approach vs. avoidance. The distinction between problem-focused vs. emotion-focused coping represents the most basic distinction, which is found in practically all classifications of coping. Not only is that distinction quite universal, but so is the empirical evidence that problem-focused coping usually is associated with better well-being (Aldwin & Revenson, 1987; Kohn, 1996; Scheier & Carver, 1992, see Semmer, 2003; Steptoe, 1991). That result is qualified in some studies by an interaction with control, with emotion-focused coping more successful when stressors are not controllable, and problem-focused coping more successful when stressors are controllable (e.g., Forsythe & Compas, 1987). Yet the overall evidence clearly points to adverse effects of emotional coping (Endler, 1998; Kohn, 1996; Semmer, 2003).

Theoretically, one could expect the opposite: there is a logical argument that if stress-related emotions are very strong, one must manage the debilitating emotions before he or she can solve problems rationally (Perrez & Reicherts, 1992). In addition, stress management practices tend to target mainly emotion management — even with regard to work settings, where a focus on work circumstances would seem rather natural (Kahn & Byosiere, 1992; Kompier & Kristensen, 2000; Murphy, 1996) — and the empirical evidence about this type of intervention shows that they can be quite successful (Kaluza, 1997; Murphy, 1996; Semmer & Zapf, in press; van der Klink et al., 2001).

The two bodies of evidence — the apparent inadequacy of emotion-focused coping in many nonexperimental field studies vs. successful interventions aimed at improving emotion-focused coping — tend to live in peaceful (but unacknowledged) coexistence. Like the issue of challenge, we feel that the role of emotion-oriented coping represents somewhat of an unacknowledged enigma in stress research.

The adverse impact of emotion-oriented coping becomes much less surprising, however, if one takes a closer look at how this type of coping is operationalized (see Semmer, 2003). One finds items such as "I get upset and let my emotions out" or "I get upset, and am really aware of it" (Carver et al., 1989), items that tap self-blame (Aldwin & Revenson, 1987; Endler & Parker, 1990; McCrae & Costa, 1986), and items like "I became very tense" (Endler & Parker, 1990) or "I thought about the problem over and over without reaching a decision" (McCrae & Costa, 1986). Nowack (1989) reports a scale named Intrusive Negative Thoughts.

There are many more examples of this, but the point should be clear: Such items measure distress itself more than they measure coping (attempting to deal with a stressful situation). Nothing in these items indicates that one is trying to *regulate* one's emotions. Rather, they seem to be measures of the inability to do so. Some of them, such as rumination, are akin to those involuntary responses to stress that have been shown to aggravate rather than alleviate the course of illness, and to prevent or disrupt coping responses in the strict sense (Compas et al., 1997). It is no wonder that they correlate positively with scales such as anxiety, depression, neuroticism, or psychosomatic complaints (see Semmer, 2003).

If such scales measure the inability to cope rather than an attempt at emotion regulation, they should be negatively related to successful palliative coping. The Semmer research group contrasted a different kind of item (such as "normally, I succeed in calming down" — Perrez & Reicherts, 1992) with a classical emotion-oriented coping measure (Coping Inventory for Stressful Situations [CISS] — Endler & Parker, 1990). As expected, they are correlated negatively with one another, and a scale on Positive Attitude towards Life (Grob et al., 1991) correlates positively with successful palliative coping but negatively with emotion-oriented coping from the CISS (Semmer et al., 2001). Of course, a problem with the successful palliative coping items are that they go too far in the other direction — they tend to include success as part of the item. Given the many indications that high values on scales allegedly measuring emotion-oriented coping are associated with poorer outcomes, however, it is informative to learn that successful regulation of emotions can indeed alleviate stress.

A similar position has been advocated by Stanton and colleagues (Stanton & Franz, 1999; Stanton et al., 2000). They have developed a scale that measures approach-oriented aspects of emotional coping, namely, emotional processing and emotional expression. An emotional approach to coping seems to be beneficial, at least for women, and coping through emotional expression was found to be associated with higher life satisfaction in both sexes.

All these are only first attempts, but they clearly suggest that more work along these lines is necessary and promising. We need instruments that measure emotion-focused coping in a way that matches the definition of coping, which implies doing something about the stress, not simply a measure of negative emotional reactivity to the stress.*

Immediate Outcomes

SPECs of the kind described can have different immediate outcomes. The episode can be resolved (for the moment or permanently), leading to relief and, if the resolution is attributed to one's own effort, pride. If important enough, such an experience can lead to growth and future stress resilience. Alternatively, the episodes can persist or even increase over time, leading to increased distress, diminishing resources, and possibly the triggering of new stress episodes. Even in the positive case, however, there can be costs of coping (Schönpflug & Battmann, 1988). Coping itself, even if successful with regard to the original problem, might carry costs in other domains, as when coping by working overtime enables one to finish an assignment but leads to fatigue and exhaustion or creates problems with one's family (Lepore & Evans, 1996; Schönpflug & Battmann, 1988). Furthermore, coping

* It is also possible that the *attempt* to do something is already predictive of success in the case of problem-oriented coping, as it implies not being overwhelmed by the situation, but that such is not the case for emotion-oriented coping. Measures of emotion-oriented coping in the strict sense (*attempting* to regulate one's emotions) can therefore still not predict outcome, whereas measures of *successful* emotional coping (as in Semmer et al., 2001) will.

requires energy and can lead to energy depletion, implying decreased resources for dealing with new demands (Baumeister et al., 1999).

Cycles of Stress Episodes and Recovery

The single stress episode described so far can be seen as a basic unit in stress experience. Yet a single SPEC is likely to have major long-term consequences only if it is very strong. With regard to more normal daily stressors, such consequences are more likely to the extent that a given stressor tends to reoccur, that several stressors occur near simultaneously, or that some stressful situations tend to trigger others. It is therefore important to consider the processes that follow *after* a stressful episode.

Multiple SPECs

Multiple stressors can be reoccurrences of the same stressor or the more or less simultaneous occurrence of different stressors. Examples of potentially reoccurring stressors would be tight deadlines at work, children who become ill, traffic jams, or antagonistic behavior of other people. Since these recurrences tend to be similar, they imply, at least in principle, a possibility of habituating to them or of developing strategies for more adequate coping, including anticipatory coping by building resources that one can rely on (such as a social network one can rely on for taking care of a child) when the situation occurs again (Beehr & McGrath, 1996). To the extent that this does not happen, the situation is characterized by what McEwen (1998) calls repeated hits: both the SPEC and the distress occur repeatedly.

Reoccurring SPECs imply the same situation (or a variant of it) every time. The situation is somewhat different when several *different* stressors co-occur or follow each other so rapidly that there is no time to recover and build up new resources. Stressors can co-occur for different reasons: (1) the co-occurrence can be incidental, as when one comes home after a bad day at work, only to find the house under water because the pipe has broken; (2) one can be the consequence of the other, as when the broken pipe has caused water to destroy a computer with the only version of an important manuscript; or (3) a SPEC can be the consequence of one's own coping behavior, as when one causes an accident while driving an ill child to the hospital at too high a speed (see McGrath & Tschan, 2004; Repetti & Wood, 1997; Schönpflug & Battmann, 1988). It should be mentioned, however, that seemingly independent co-occurrences can, in fact, be connected in a broader context. For instance, being poor can be connected to many possible causes of stressors that are implied by such aspects as poor housing conditions, few possibilities for preventive coping (insurance, maintenance of the house, etc.), dangers (high crime rates), etc. Thus, to go back to the example cited above, the breaking of the water pipe can be more or less probable due to one's overall living conditions (Taylor & Repetti, 1997).

The crucial element in such sequences is the state of the system when stressor B occurs, due to the effects of stressor A, including the effects of efforts to deal with it. SPECs, even if successfully resolved, are likely to diminish resources, and to rebuild them requires time. It seems useful here to distinguish between energetic and structural resources (Schönpflug & Battmann, 1988). Structural resources represent long-term potential (Hobfoll, 2001, speaks of the resource pool), whereas energetic resources are short-term processes that activate structural ones (Hobfoll, 2001, speaks of investment of resources). Thus, muscle strength is a structural resource, whereas current strength is an energetic one. In some cases, moderate use of energetic resources will build up structural ones in the long run (e.g., exercising will both use energetic resources and diminish them, at the same time building up structural ones). In other cases, structural resources (such as money) are simply used and then can need active efforts to rebuild them.

Applying this to our current discussion, SPECs are likely to diminish energetic resources in the short run (Baumeister et al., 1999). This depletion will be more intense and occur faster, to the extent that structural resources are limited. If there is enough time and structural resources are plenty, energetic resources will be rebuilt, and no negative consequences are likely to occur. To the contrary, as mentioned above, positive developments might take place in that structural resources might be strengthened.

These considerations imply, however, that during the state when energetic resources are depleted and are being rebuilt, vulnerability should be especially high. This is shown in aftereffects of stressful experiences (Cohen, 1980; Glass & Singer, 1972), including carryover from work to private life and vice versa (Frone, 2003; Geurts & Demerouti, 2003; Repetti & Wood, 1997). It is also congruent with findings that one or two life events need not be consequential, but three or more may overtax resources and have an effect on well-being (Grob et al., 1995). By contrast, phases of stress that are followed by phases of recovery and rebuilding of resources are unlikely to have deleterious effects, and can in many cases even have positive effects (Repetti, 1992; Eden, 2001). Again, this applies only to stress episodes that are not in themselves traumatic in character.

Despite the heightened vulnerability in the aftermath of a SPEC, however, there is no automatic increase in distress. During such vulnerable periods, for example, one can well ward off additional stressors by lowering one's standards. On an evening when we come home from work exhausted and frustrated, we can decide not to make a fuss about a child's D in math, not to get upset about the defeat of our favorite football team, or to live with the fact that we did not get promoted although we deserved it. Such a coping strategy is, however, not without limits: if the D in math implies that our child will have to leave a good school, if the failure to get promoted means that we will not be able to pay our debts, and so on, then we can be able to divert our attention away from the stressor for a while, but simply lowering one's expectations cannot be a viable long-term strategy (see Hobfoll, 2001; Sapolsky, 1998; Semmer, 2003). Nevertheless, the possibility has to be considered that the meaning of a stressor changes in light of the occurrence of new stressors, and this effect can imply a reduced impact (Mohr, 2000).

Chronic Conditions

SPECs are conceived as events, with a beginning and an end (although they can last quite long). This can be contrasted with more stable conditions, such as consistently too high demands at work (especially if combined with low rewards — Siegrist, 2002), chronic illness (Gottlieb, 1997), loneliness (Lepore, 1997), or the like.

Of course, the line between events and chronic conditions is difficult to draw, and one can regard chronic conditions as a series of events (Wheaton, 1997). Thus, being in constant threat of becoming unemployed can be reconstructed as episodes where this danger comes to mind, as when considering using much of one's savings for a large investment, when deciding not to protest against the demeaning behavior of a supervisor, or when thinking about the poor working conditions one has to accept. Nevertheless, such episodes are quite distinct from events that have a clear onset and ending. For purposes of illustration, when measured as an event, the demeaning behavior of a supervisor might be categorized as an episode involving conflict with the supervisor, yet it goes well beyond that, because one's reactions to the event are restricted by the implied threat of unemployment (Wheaton, 1997; cf. Grebner et al., in press; Semmer et al., in press).

Thus, even if chronic stress conditions can be translated into recurrent SPECs, their occurrence has another meaning and can induce quite different behavioral, emotional, and physiological responses. These SPECs can be not so much episodes in themselves, but rather expressions of a more or less stable or continuing condition.

Like multiple SPECs, chronic conditions imply no automaticity with regard to consequences. People can endure quite adverse conditions over long periods if they have adequate resources — both external resources such as money, social networks, and social support or power, and internal resources such as health, self-esteem, internal locus of control, etc. (Hobfoll, 2001; Semmer, 2003). Nevertheless, the *risk* of adverse consequences rises when chronic stressors persist, and there is evidence that chronic stressors have more impact than acute SPECs, at least as long as these acute SPECs are not traumatic in themselves (e.g., Beehr et al., 2000; Cohen et al., 1998).

Cumulative Stress Effects as Alterations of System Responsivity

The above discussion implies that SPECs that are not traumatic in themselves and are followed by periods of recovery and rebuilding are not likely to have negative consequences in the long run; quite to the contrary, they are likely to lead to improved resources. Only if one or more is strong enough to be traumatic, or when they accumulate to such a degree that the situation becomes chronic, are negative consequences for health and well-being to be expected. How can this process be conceptualized?

One process that is typically discussed in this context involves chronic alterations of system parameters, as when stressors are associated with (continuously) elevated blood pressure. Normally, blood pressure will return to normal again after a stressing episode. But after prolonged or repeated exposure, it can stay at elevated levels (Grebner et al., 2003; Sterling & Eyer, 1988). Psychologically, such alterations of system parameters can involve chronically heightened anxiety, depression, or hostility. In many cases, psychological and physiological alterations are associated with one another, as in the case of depression, which has been shown to be associated with elevated levels of norepinephrine (Krantz & McCeney, 2002). Often, such changes in basal levels of parameters are signs of physical illness, psychological impairment, or their precursors.

Another important process involves changes in the reactivity of the system, as indicated, for instance, by hyperresponsivity in terms of blood pressure or hormonal reactions to potentially stressful stimuli (Baum & Posluszny, 1999; Kiecolt-Glaser et al., 2002; Krantz & McCeney, 2002; Meijman & Mulder, 1998; Rozanski et al., 1999; Steptoe, 2001; Steptoe & Willemsen, 2002). Besides *hyper*responsivity (which can itself predict more permanent changes in basal levels — Baum & Posluszny, 1999), however, *hypo*responsivity is also increasingly recognized as problematic (Heim et al., 2000; McEwen, 1998; Steptoe, 2001; Sterling & Eyer, 1988). Furthermore, as already mentioned, prolonged responses that are not terminated when a stressful situation is over are indicators of impaired unwinding (Dienstbier, 1992; Frankenhaeuser, 1986; Lundberg & Parr, 2000; McEwen, 1998; Meijman & Mulder, 1998; Sterling & Eyer, 1988). In other words, the capacity of the system to *regulate reactions to stress* is compromised. This indicates reduced resources for dealing with stress.

Relatively constant stressful conditions over a long time can lead to serious outcomes. To the extent that resources are weakened, however, less and less will be needed to lead to symptoms, and eventually rather trivial events can trigger quite serious responses (Krantz & McCeney, 2002). Findings that responses to stress, or to infectious agents, can be different for people who suffer from chronic stress than for people who do not underscore this point (cf. Cohen et al., 1999; Heim et al., 2000; Pike et al., 1997; Roy et al., 1998; Schaubroeck & Ganster, 1993). This also implies that in the interplay between individual and environment, the influence of individual vulnerability becomes stronger as one is in such a downward spiral. If measurement takes place in a later phase only, this can suggest an overemphasis on individual resilience (or lack of it), and the environmental influences that can have played a role in producing this state of affairs can be underestimated. As an example, childhood stressors predict depression in late adolescence, which, in turn, predicts reoccurrence of depressive episodes. Due to this mediating effect, controlling for adolescent depression is likely to render the effect of childhood adversity on adult depression insignificant in statistical models. History of depression will then look like the decisive predictor, and childhood adversity can look less important, although it can be responsible for the vulnerability that is indicated by the initial onset of depression (Kessler & Magee, 1994).

This increased vulnerability has yet another implication. Once resources have been weakened considerably, changes of the environment to the better will no longer suffice for their restoration; rather, some kind of treatment of the stress response (e.g., by stress management training, medication, or psychotherapy) will also be necessary.

All this also has important implications for research. If the constellation of influences changes over time, then findings will be different when they refer to different phases in the development, or weakening, of resistance. If this is not taken into account, effects might not be detected because they apply to subgroups of a population only. Except for the differentiation between studies with healthy participants and studies with patients (cf. Hemingway & Marmot, 1999), such distinctions are not typically made. Prospective studies that run over extended periods *and* include multiple waves of measurement are needed to investigate possible changes in the constellation of predictors.

Outcomes

Outcomes can be discussed at various levels of specificity. For the purpose of the present chapter, it does not seem viable to focus on specific aspects of health and well-being, such as cardiovascular diseases or depression. Rather, we will discuss outcomes in somewhat more general terms, with regard to the psychological, physiological/medical, and social levels, and we will devote a special paragraph to matters of performance.

With regard to the *psychological* level, many specific outcomes have been discussed, including depression (Brown, 2002; Gruen, 1993; Kessler & Magee, 1994), psychosomatic complaints (in the sense of functional problems without identifiable organic substrate — Creed, 1993), burnout (Schaufeli & Enzmann, 1998), and general psychiatric morbidity (Dohrenwend, 2000).

At the *physiological/medical* level, cardiovascular diseases are a rather dominant topic (Hemingway & Marmot, 1999; Krantz & McCeney, 2002; Rozanski et al., 1999; Stansfeld & Marmot, 2002a; Schnall et al., 2000; Siegrist, 2002; Taylor & Repetti, 1997), but illnesses such as cancer and HIV/AIDS (Baum & Posluszny, 1999; Schneiderman et al., 2001), ulcer (Levenstein et al., 1999), and musculoskeletal pain (Bongers et al., 1993; Boos et al., 2000; Elfering et al., 2002; Hurrell, 2001; Linton, 2000; Lundberg & Melin, 2002) have also been investigated, as has general morbidity and mortality (Kiecolt-Glaser et al., 2002; Taylor & Repetti, 1997). Most authors in this literature reach a cautiously positive conclusion about the role of psychosocial variables in predicting disease, with an emphasis on their role as "cofactors in medical conditions, rather than exclusive etiological agents" (Steptoe, 2001, p. 40).

At least as important as outcomes that are direct measures of health and disease, however, are outcomes that can be *precursors* of disease. Many such possibilities have been discussed, involving cardiovascular reactivity, immune regulation, skeletal muscle tension, and hormonal reactions (Baum & Posluszny, 1999; Cacioppo et al., 1998; Cohen & Herbert, 1996; Kiecolt-Glaser et al., 2002; Steptoe, 2001). These processes refer to changes in regulatory processes that indicate reduced resistance to noxious agents. These noxious agents can be biological, as when stress increases the probability of developing a cold after being infected with a virus in a controlled trial (Cohen & Herbert, 1996), or psychological, as when acute stress, especially SPECs triggering anger episodes, trigger cardiac events in people with chronic risk factors (Krantz & McCeney, 2002).

The psychological (or psychiatric) outcomes are important in their own right. At the same time, they have often been found to predict physical illness as well. This is especially well documented for depression (Hemingway & Marmot, 1999; Krantz & McCeney, 2002; Steptoe, 2001; Rozanski et al., 1999; Taylor & Repetti, 1997). Thus, many variables that can be considered outcomes from one point of view can also be considered indicators of vulnerability, while their positive counterparts, such as optimism, emotional stability, and the like, can be considered resources that increase resiliency (Steptoe, 2001; Semmer, 2003). The influence, however, is likely to be bidirectional. Thus, the risk of depression and other symptoms of distress increases with the occurrence of physical health problems, such as back pain (Schade et al., 1999) or diabetes mellitus (Kinder et al., 2002), and diagnosed high blood pressure can increase psychological distress (Steptoe, 2001). Thus, there is a risk of vicious cycles, as exemplified, for instance, in the finding by Schade et al. (1999) that depression both predicts and is predicted by surgical outcome in lower-back-surgery patients.

On the *behavioral* side, health-relevant behaviors such as substance abuse, preventive health care behavior, physical activity, and nutrition have been related to stress, as well as to personal characteristics such as depression that can partly be considered outcomes of stress (Adler & Matthews, 1994; Baum & Posluszny, 1999; Marks et al., 2000). Typically, unhealthy behaviors are seen as mechanisms for coping with stress. Thus, there is evidence for increased consumption of alcohol under stress, provided one believes that alcohol helps to calm one down (Grunberg et al., 1998). In our view, an alternative pattern should receive more attention: many health-related behaviors require self-control. Because self-control can be regarded as a resource that is compromised by stressful experiences and the coping efforts invested in them (Baumeister et al., 1999), stress can simply undermine these self-regulatory mechanisms. This can imply a failure to implement intentions to engage in healthy behavior, such as exercising, which has been shown to be less likely under stressful working conditions (Payne et al., 2002). Conversely, it can imply a lowered ability to refrain from unwanted but habitual behavior, such as smoking or overeating. This is in line with results indicating that stress increases habitual behavior (Barthol & Ku, 1959). This approach emphasizes the undermining of resources as a central element (see Hobfoll, 2001; Hobfoll et al., 1996), with the resource in question being the ability for self-control. The behaviors in question can, but need not, be coping attempts.

Individual behavior is, of course, tightly connected to the *social* level. Social networks and social support are among the most important resources, predicting a wide range of outcomes in terms of both psychological and biological/medical variables (Beehr, 1995; Cohen et al., 2000; Schwarzer & Leppin, 1991, 1992; Steptoe, 2001; Uchino et al., 1996; Viswesvaran et al., 1999). Here, however, we are concerned with social resources as *outcomes*. Diminished social resources are intimately connected with some stressors, as when the death of a loved one implies the loss of support by that person, or when losing a job means losing, or weakening, the social network that went along with it. Beyond this, however, social resources can diminish in times of stress or crisis, simply because they are being (over)used (Lepore, 1997) and because giving social support over an extended period can become a burden to those providing it (Redinbaugh et al., 1995). Whether this occurs depends partly on the individual. Social competences are helpful in building social networks and mobilizing support (Pierce et al., 1996). By way of contrast, people with strong signs of distress, such as those suffering depression, are less attractive to others, so that the very problem they need support for can alienate potential supporters and increase social isolation (Winnubst et al., 1988). Furthermore, supporters often tie their support to certain expectations, for instance, in terms of adequate coping and improvement. If these expectations are not met, supporters can turn away or react with reproach (Silver et al., 1990). People under stress also can provoke more conflict by behaving in an irritated (and irritating) way (O'Brien & DeLongis, 1997), as when the interactions of stressed fathers with their children become more negative (Repetti, 1994), or when chronically ill people vent anger and irritation and, in doing so, provoke anger in significant others who subsequently reduce their support (Lane & Hobfoll, 1992). Finally, distressed people can withdraw socially. This often has positive consequences in the short run, but if used as a strategy too frequently or for too long, it can undermine potentially helpful social networks (Repetti, 1992).

A final category that we want to discuss in terms of outcomes concerns (job) *performance*. This is seldom discussed outside the realm of work psychology. For reasons that we hope will become apparent, however, we believe that it deserves more attention. That is also the reason why we did not simply subsume it under the rubric of behavior.

There are several aspects of job performance that are relevant in the present context. One concerns what is called organizational citizenship behavior (Organ & Paine, 1999) or contextual performance (Borman & Motowidlo, 1997). This essentially refers to the willingness of people to contribute to the well-being of coworkers and the functioning of the organization as a whole by going beyond one's immediate job duties — for instance, by offering help to coworkers, by dealing with problems even when they are outside of one's immediate responsibility, by investing time beyond the formal requirements, and so on. It is for this type of performance that there is the strongest evidence of an empirical relationship with chronic stress (Jex, 1998). A reduced tendency to offer assistance to others has already been found as a correlate of acute stressors by Glass & Singer (1972). The implication for social outcomes is clear: people under stress are less likely to contribute to the well-being of the community as a whole (note the term *citizenship behavior* as used by Organ and Paine). This, in turn, is likely to induce reduced commitment by others to supporting the individual (or group) in question, thus undermining that person's potential resources.

A second type of performance relates to task fulfillment in a narrower sense, that is, the quality of task performance. One might expect this type of performance to deteriorate with stress. Such effects are found in some studies (e.g., Beehr et al., 2000). They tend to be rather weak, however, if one regards global measures of performance. People are quite able to keep up performance under stress for a long time, by increasing effort and by changing work strategies. However, not only is this associated with increased costs for the individual (in terms of fatigue, stress symptoms, etc.), but it also has costs in terms of aspects of task performance that are not so easily seen. When under stress, people set priorities, and they keep up performance by concentrating on the main tasks, at a cost in performance of secondary tasks, such as maintenance operations, seeking feedback about one's actions, keeping up situation awareness, and, as noted earlier, organizational citizenship behaviors. Thus, drivers under stress might look less often into the rearview mirror, workers under stress might omit checking that all screws are tightly secured, etc. (see Hockey, 1997; Matthews et al., 2000; Meijman & Mulder, 1998). Stress, especially if it involves time pressure, is also a major factor that induces people to bend safety rules — for instance, by taking shortcuts, not using safety devices, etc. (Zohar, 2003). So, it is no surprise that stress has been found to be associated with occupational accidents (e.g., Trimpop et al., 2000; Kirkcaldy et al., 1997) and medical malpractice (Jones et al., 1988). Conversely, resources such as autonomy, communication quality, and support by supervisors have been found to be related to safe working practices (Parker et al., 2001).

Such influences on performance, in terms of both citizenship and the changes in secondary task fulfillment, have implications well beyond the workplace: they can not only affect the focal person and his or her colleagues, but also clients, customers, co-members of a community committee, co-users of highways, etc. Through such mechanisms, stress can have an impact not only on one's own health but also on that of others (see Aiken et al., 2002).

A final remark concerns the issue of *specificity vs. generality* of the outcomes and their relationship to stress. Different physiological parameters, such as cardiovascular, endocrine, and immune parameters, correlate with one another (Cacioppo et al., 1998), although their intercorrelation can itself be partly subject to individual differences (Cohen et al., 2000). There is considerable co-morbidity between physical conditions such as cardiovascular disease and psychological problems such as anxiety and depression (Dimsdale, 2001). The latter also are associated with problematic coping strategies and so on (Semmer, 2003). No wonder that researchers tend to find similar predictors and correlates, whichever outcomes they investigate.

Although some specific predictors (e.g., a specific virus) lead to specific outcomes in many fields of medicine, such specificity is less apparent regarding stressors. Instead, there seems to be considerable generality. Many adverse life circumstances tend to cluster — as illustrated by the association between socioeconomic status (SES) and many stress factors, and between SES and general mortality and morbidity and many specific health behaviors (Taylor and Repetti, 1997). So, a picture emerges of both gain and loss spirals with regard to resources of all kinds (Hobfoll, 2001). It is difficult to know *a priori* which predictor is likely to have specific effects. Individual outcomes are also determined by specific individual vulnerabilities or by more or less accidental environmental constellations, such as the presence of a virus that interacts with a general lowering of immunocompetence to produce a certain illness (Steptoe, 2001). Such individual and situational factors are likely to be one reason why associations between a specific SPEC and a given outcome are usually not large and are often inconsistent. Therefore, we should not lose sight of the fact that resourcefulness and vulnerability have considerable generality.

THE MEANING OF STRESSORS, OR STRESS SITUATIONS VIEWED AS PERSON–IN–ENVIRONMENT SETTINGS

IN THE EYE OF THE BEHOLDER? SOCIAL AND INDIVIDUAL MEANING

Since the occurrence of stress depends on individual appraisal, the roles of the individual and, by definition, of individual differences become central. Empirically, this has been corroborated by many findings showing that similar or even identical situations can be perceived and appraised quite differently by different people (Lazarus, 1999). A tradition has therefore developed that focuses on stress as an individual process, and this has led, in turn, to strong reservations about concepts of stressors that refer to events in or characteristics of the environment independent of the individual (Lazarus & Folkman, 1986, p. 75). The meaning of the situation to the individual has therefore become the central focus in many psychological approaches (Perrewé & Zellars, 1999).

Although we agree that the meaning of the situation to the individual is pivotal, we also want to emphasize that *individual* meaning is not totally *idiosyncratic* meaning. After all, shared meaning is one element by which cultures are defined (Erez & Earley, 1993), and it is quite well established that culture also influences appraisal processes and the emotions that go with them (Averill, 1983; Kitayama et al., 1995; Walbott & Scherer, 1995). For instance, when unfair behavior by superiors is found to be less stressful in cultures with high power distance, because such behavior is much more taken for granted (Gudykunst & Ting-Toomey, 1988), or when *collective* self-efficacy acts as a moderator between control at work and stressors in predicting well-being in an Asian culture, but *individual* self-efficacy is the moderator in the more individualistic U.S. culture (Schaubroeck et al., 2000), it becomes clear that individual appraisals have some communalities that are influenced by culture. Meaning is not only individual but also social, and some communalities in situation appraisal can therefore be expected. It is on this basis that one can define stressors as events or circumstances that *increase the probability of stress reactions* for a given population (as we argued in the opening section). Semmer (1992) has argued that there are some stressors that are universal (such as threats to life), some that can be especially important in certain cultures (e.g., losing face in Asian cultures), and some that can be predictive only in certain areas (e.g., the defeat of the local soccer team) or in certain professional groups (e.g., just missing a generally accepted level of statistical significance (e.g., $p = .06$) for psychologists and epidemiologists). In all these groups, there will certainly be individual differences, but the *probability* that a given environmental condition is appraised as stressful and has an effect will be different between identifiable groups.

This leads to a concept of stressors as *risk factors*. Just as a virus does not become harmless simply because it does not kill everybody who is exposed or infected, the idea of stressors does not become a useless concept just because not everybody subjected to them shows stress reactions. Just as some people are more resistant to infection than others, some people are also more resistant to certain stressors than others. Furthermore, identifiable social sets of people will show like resistances. The impact of the virus arises from its biological significance; the impact of stressors arises from their social significance. Thus, it is indeed the meaning of the SPEC that counts, but this meaning is not only individual, but also *social.* Such a probabilistic concept can account for increased risks for a given population without negating individual differences and without being circular (Semmer, 1992; see Hobfoll, 2001; Kahn & Byosiere, 1992, for a similar position).

The fruitfulness of such an approach is convincingly demonstrated by the methodology developed by Brown and associates in studying depression (Brown, 2002; Brown & Andrews, 1986). In this approach, external judges rate the impact of a given life event based on *contextual* (social) information. They consider, for instance, how stressful it is likely to be for an unmarried Catholic medical student to discover that she is pregnant shortly before her final exams but shortly after ending her relationship with her boyfriend. The raters are, of course, blind to the concrete appraisal and affective reaction by that person. This approach has proved extremely valuable in predicting depression (Brown, 2002; see also Dohrenwend, 2000). It illustrates that the *social meaning* of SPECs can reliably be determined by raters who are familiar with the culture in question but who do not know the affective reaction of the individual, and that this information has predictive value.

The Meaning of SPECs

If it is true that the (social) meaning of SPECs is decisive in the stress process, then it should be possible to classify SPECs along these lines. For example, Cutrona & Russell (1990) distinguished between stressors related to social roles, to achievement, and to relationships. In a similar vein, we propose to classify stressors in terms of four facets: role, social interaction (or relationship), goal, and self.

The Role Facet

Many stressful experiences are tied to the fulfillment of social roles. For instance, work is connected to the role of breadwinner (Simon, 1995), and a threat to that role is likely to be one of the reasons why losing one's job is stressful. The interrole conflicts of family interfering with work and especially work interfering with family are frequently encountered problems for working people (Frone, 2003, Geurts & Demerouti, 2003). The latter has been discussed hotly with regard to working women, with many believing that the roles of worker and mother create role overload or conflicts that are stressful. Empirical results, however, yield more support for the role enhancement thesis, that having multiple roles has, on average, positive effects on well-being (Barnett & Hyde, 2001). Stressors from one role, such as spouse, can be put into perspective by having another role, such as worker, and therefore reactivity is decreased (Cleary & Mechanic, 1983; see Semmer, 2003). On the other hand, one role can restrict the possibilities for reacting to demands within another role. If that other role includes caring for dependents who cannot care for themselves, such as children, then demands of a worker role can increase vulnerability to stress associated with the parent role (Cleary & Mechanic, 1983; Frankenhaeuser, 1991).

The role aspect has been prominent in the body of work stemming from one of the oldest and most influential approaches to stress at work, that is, the Michigan model (see Kahn & Byosiere, 1992). That model distinguishes between (1) role conflict, which includes conflicting expectations by different partners in one's role set (intersender conflict), incompatible expectations by the same person (intrasender conflict), conflicts between various roles (role–role or interrole conflict), and conflicts between a role and one's ethical standards (person–role conflict); (2) role ambiguity, that is, unclear expectations and unclear criteria for task fulfillment; and (3) quantitative role overload, which basically amounts to having too much to do within the time given. This model has been historically prominent in studies on stress at work, and the importance of role stress has considerable empirical backing (Beehr & Glazer, forthcoming; Kahn & Byosiere, 1992; Ganster & Schaubroeck, 1991; Sonnentag & Frese, 2003).

Taking on a role makes it part of one's identity, and stress factors affecting a role that is important to one's self-concept, regardless of the specific type of role stress, can have an especially strong impact (Brown, 2002; Simon, 1998).

The Social Interaction Facet

The social interaction of situations includes interactions with people such as family, friends, neighbors, colleagues, or superiors. Stress within interpersonal encounters — conflicts, tensions, insults, humiliations, etc. — are mentioned very prominently throughout the stress literature (O'Brien & DeLongis, 1997). At the same time, benign interactions have great potential to be beneficial, and social support is one of the most important resources available (see below). Social interactions are especially powerful because they invite attributions about a significant other's attitudes toward the focal person, thus touching the self in a very special way (see later discussion of SOS theory in the section entitled "Stress as Offense to Self (SOS)").

The Goal Facet

In a way, all stressors can be construed as interfering with goals such as survival, recognition, status, self-esteem, etc. These types of goals are very general, however. People work toward more specific goals all the time. Of course, workplace activities tend to focus on goal-oriented behavior, and constraints that interfere with reaching specific task goals have been quite well established as stress factors at work (Greiner et al., 1998; Semmer et al., 1996; Spector & Jex, 1998). Personal projects, personal strivings, or related concepts (see Cropanzano et al., 1993; Semmer, 2003) refer to goals at a somewhat intermediate level. These concepts have not played a major role in stress research, although many life events can easily be construed in such terms. Pursuit of such goals and success in reaching them, however, have been linked to well-being in a number of studies (Cantor & Sanderson, 1999; Diener & Lucas, 1999).

The Self Facet

Many stressful experiences are intimately linked to affirming or threatening the self. Having a positive self-image and being positively regarded by others are among the most basic needs we have (Epstein, 1998; Banaji & Prentice, 1994). Not being valued by others can therefore be very stressful, and having to accept negative feedback about oneself can be quite a painful experience as well (Kluger & DeNisi, 1996). People therefore go to pains to maintain favorable images of themselves (Blaine & Crocker, 1993; Sedikides & Strube, 1997; Tesser & Martin, 1996). The important role of self-conscious emotions illustrates this point (Tangney & Fischer, 1995). The first author of this chapter is in the process of elaborating a concept called stress as offense to self, which will be explained in more detail in the "Stress as Offense to Self (SOS)" section.

RESOURCES AND MEANING

Resources have many ways of altering stressful situations or the individual's reaction to them. They can decrease a SPEC's probability, strength, or duration, as when wealth decreases the probability of one's car breaking down (because it is high quality and well maintained) and decreases the probability of additional stressors to follow (because one has enough money to rent a car if necessary). Resources can also change the impact of the SPEC on one's stress response, because one perceives that options are available to deal with it (secondary appraisal in the sense of Lazarus, 1999). Here, we concentrate on the change in meaning of a potentially stressful situation that can come about because of availability of three pivotal kinds of resources: control, social support, and individual belief systems.

Control

The importance of control in dealing with stress has long been recognized (e.g., Averill, 1973; Ganster & Fusilier, 1989; Glass & Singer, 1972). It is especially important that, in many cases, it is not necessary to actually exercise control. It is enough to know one has it (see Glass & Singer, 1972, for an early demonstration of this phenomenon). In other words, the meaning of the situation changes if one knows there is a way out of it.

At the same time — and this aspect has received less attention — exercising control also has implications for one's social relations within the situation, and often these implications pertain to restrictions on the use of such control. Thus, changing one's employer to leave a stressful work situation often helps to improve the situation (Elfering et al., 2000), but changing jobs repeatedly can raise suspicions about one's dependability. Confronting others with demands to change something can induce changes, but if it is done frequently, it can lead to the perception that one is a quarrelsome person. This implies not only that the possibility of exerting control will often have an impact even if it is not used, but also that to some degree use of such power will be constrained by conditions in the situation.

Like many other resources, therefore, control can be eroded by too many attempts to use it (Semmer, 2000).

Social Support

Social support can refer both to concrete changes of a situation accomplished by instrumental support and to changes in the meaning of the situation brought about by emotional support that conveys a message of care and esteem (Burleson et al., 1994a). It is tempting to assume that the most effective type of support depends on the situation — such as instrumental support being most effective if the situation is controllable, and emotional support being most effective if it is not (Cutrona & Russell, 1990). But because we concentrate on the social meaning of support, we want to examine a slightly different view. There is evidence that many forms of instrumental help are perceived as emotional support (Barling et al., 1988). A recent study by Semmer et al. (2003) showed that many instrumental acts were perceived to be helpful precisely because they conveyed a message of care and esteem (which is seen as the essence of social support by many — see Sarason et al., 1996). The value of an emotional support message tied to instrumental forms of support has not received much attention in discussions of social support (see, however, the book by Burleson et al., 1994b). Yet it has been known for a long time that support that does not acknowledge and validate the feelings of the focal person (e.g., by giving unwanted advice, by giving advice too early to be seen as acceptable, or by giving advice with reproaches) cannot be very helpful. It is also clear that even otherwise helpful support can lead to feelings of being inadequate and of having social debts, implying a need to reciprocate, thereby having detrimental side effects (Bowling et al., 2003; Burleson et al., 1994a; Buunk, 1990; Elfering et al., 2002).

It is our contention, therefore, that a given set of statements or actions will be perceived as supportive to the extent that they communicate care and esteem. Whether an action is suited to convey such a message is at least as important as the match between the action and the requirements of the stressful situation. When I am late on my way to the airport and my car will not work, a neighbor offering his or her sympathy, rather than a ride, might be perceived as cynical. If, however, the neighbor is 95 and does not drive any more, offering sympathy can well be appreciated. Conversely, offering a ride and combining it with remarks about the importance of always making sure that one's car is properly maintained, or about the importance of being ready early enough so that one can deal with unexpected problems, are likely to undermine the value of the action, even though it is still instrumentally supportive. Although much of this is known on the basis of research on negative effects of social support, it deserves to be incorporated better within conceptual treatments of social support (Burleson et al., 1994b; Semmer et al., 2003).

Individual Belief Systems

Some personal resources, such as health and fitness, are directly instrumental in dealing with stress. Many others, however, have to do with beliefs that change the meaning of the situation. These include such beliefs as seeing the challenge rather than the threat in the situation (hardiness), perceiving a situation as meaningful and manageable (sense of coherence), expecting things to get better (optimism), assuming as a default option that people are benign (rather than hostile), and assuming that one can overcome difficulties (self-efficacy). Resilient people who have such beliefs also tend to see meaning and purpose in events that happen to them (Semmer, 2003; Taylor et al., 2000). Such a view is likely to be behind many of the positive influences of religious beliefs, because even hardship can be regarded as having a purpose (Pargament, 2002). Moreover, research on talking or writing about traumatic events shows that these are helpful to the extent that they lead to formulation of a coherent and meaningful structure (Smyth & Pennebaker, 1999).

Again, however, it must not be concluded that one can give (benign) meaning to things without limit. Even the strongest proponents of the view that positive beliefs are beneficial for health emphasize that this applies only if the beliefs do not depart drastically from reality (Taylor et al., 2000).

PROMISING THEORETICAL DEVELOPMENTS: EXPLORATIONS INTO THE MEANING OF STRESSORS

Our purpose in this section is not to review all theoretical approaches to stress and health (for a review of current theories see Cooper, 1998 and Adler & Matthews, 1994; Baum & Posluszny, 1999; Cacioppo et al., 1998; Cohen & Herbert, 1996; Kiecolt-Glaser et al., 2002; Krantz & McCeney, 2002; Steptoe, 2001, Taylor et al., 1997; Taylor & Repetti, 1997; Uchino et al., 1996, for relationships between stress and health). Rather, we want to emphasize some promising avenues for theorizing and research, and refer to approaches that exemplify them.

Given the emphasis on both individual and social meaning that we have displayed throughout this chapter, it will come as no surprise that it is in this area where we see some promising developments that we would like to share with our readers. The concept of reciprocity, and thus the exchange perspective, is dominant in two of them. The third one concentrates on offense to self, especially by lack of legitimacy. All three have been developed with a special emphasis on stress at work, but they all seem relevant for other life domains as well, and indeed, they draw on research and theorizing outside of the field of work psychology.

LACK OF RECIPROCITY

Siegrist and colleagues (e.g., Siegrist, 2002; Kuper et al., 2002) have developed the *effort–reward imbalance* model. It is based on the idea that "successful and rewarding exchange through core social roles can reinforce the self and contribute to beneficial effects on health and well-being" (Siegrist, 2002, p. 263). Self-concepts concern self-efficacy, self-esteem, and belonging. Concentrating on the work role as a core role, there are investments in terms of effort, and these are met by rewards in the form of money, esteem, and career opportunities (promotion, security). Effort is determined by the requirements of the job (structural aspect), but also by overcommitment of the person (personal aspect). An imbalance leads to strain both psychologically, in terms of negative emotions, and physiologically, in terms of activation of autonomic nervous system and related neurohormonal reactions. People can expose themselves to situations lacking balanced exchange because they have no choice (e.g., because of the labor market and their lack of skills), because they are overcommitted, or for strategic reasons, that is, to improve their chances for later gains.

The Siegrist model has been investigated in a number of studies (summarized in Siegrist, 2002). Results show that effort–reward imbalance (indicated by the ratio of demands to rewards) is associated with increased coronary heart disease, with prospective studies yielding a relative risk between 2 and 4.5 (with classic behavioral and biomedical risk factors controlled). Other health-related outcomes include subjective health, psychiatric disorders, and alcohol dependence.

We do have some reservations concerning the measurement of overcommitment. Items such as "I get overwhelmed easily by time pressures at work" or "When I get home, I can easily relax and 'switch off' work" (Siegrist, 2002, p. 270) can be regarded as indicators of psychological problems (note the words *overwhelmed* and *relaxed*), rather than as coping style (which is what it is claimed to be). Nevertheless, given the medical and physiological outcomes predicted in longitudinal studies, the status of the model overall is quite impressive.

Although more inspired by sociological theory, the Siegrist model has obvious relations to equity theory, which is more prominent in psychology (Adams, 1965; Buunk & Schaufeli, 1999). Equity considerations are the explicit focus of Schaufeli, Buunk, and their collaborators in the Netherlands, who concentrate on occupational stress and burnout. They show that an imbalance between investments and outcomes predicts burnout, especially its major component of emotional exhaustion (e.g., Bakker et al., 2000; Taris et al., 2001; van Dierendonk et al., 2001). They use somewhat different measures for investment and rewards, but in our view, this strengthens the overall approach, because it demonstrates that effort–reward imbalance, or lack of reciprocity, is a robust predictor that does not depend on a specific operationalization.

The *conceptual* reason why we think this type of approach represents a major breakthrough is the following: Imbalance has been a major concept in stress research for a long time, as the imbalance between what is demanded and the resources needed to meet these demands is at the core of the stress experience. The main question is, "Do demands exceed resources?" which amounts to asking, "Is it bearable?" Effort–reward imbalance, or lack of reciprocity, adds another aspect. Even situations that are stressful and hard to bear can be accepted because bearing them will be rewarded. The question, therefore, is expanded from "Is it bearable?" to "Is it worth bearing?" adding a component of exchange that emphasizes the social embeddedness of the whole process very explicitly. The stress one has to bear is compensated by rewards, and this might influence health outcomes in a positive way. This has interesting implications. For instance, a situation one has gone through can change its meaning in *retrospect.* Having accepted harsh and hectic working conditions for a number of years, only to discover that the promotion envisaged does not occur, can devaluate the effort invested over years.

Reciprocity has, of course, been prominent for a long time in research and theory about social support (Antonucci & Jackson, 1990; Bowling et al., 2003; Buunk,

1990; Elfering et al., 2002). With these theoretical approaches, however, it becomes a construct central not only for dealing with stress by way of support, but also for the very development, maintenance, and impact of stress itself.

Stress as Offense to Self (SOS)

While the approaches dealing with reciprocity start from a perspective of social exchange, Semmer and colleagues in the Bern research group (Semmer & Jacobshagen, in press) starts from the need for high esteem and self-esteem. As noted earlier (see the section entitled "The Self Facet"), having a positive image of oneself and being positively regarded by others are among the most basic needs we have (Epstein, 1998; Banaji & Prentice, 1994; Sedikides & Strube, 1997), and people go to pains to maintain a positive image of themselves as well as a positive social reputation (Blaine & Crocker, 1993; Tesser & Martin, 1996). There is good consensus on this, differences about details notwithstanding. It is therefore surprising that threats to self do not play a very prominent role in research on stress. To be sure, this aspect is often mentioned as important. For instance, in the work by Folkman et al. (1986) threats to self-esteem form a dimension of primary appraisal. But the implications of its central role are usually not considered systematically. Thus, the role of self-esteem (and self-efficacy) in empirical research is mostly confined to regarding it (1) as a resource (e.g., Hobfoll, 2001) and, because self-esteem can be considered part of well-being (Adler & Matthews, 1994; Judge & Bono, 2001), (2) as a dependent variable. Again, the most notable exception is in the area of social support, where feelings of inadequacy as a result of presenting oneself as in need (and possibly, by implication, as unable to cope) have been recognized as a stress factor for a long time (Fisher et al., 1982). Threats to self-esteem are discussed in much more detail there than in the rest of the field (e.g., Goldsmith, 1994).

Stress as offense to self (SOS) can be considered from the perspectives of self-regard and regard by others (or reputation). Stress as threat to *self-regard* refers to experiences of (potential) failure. With Locke et al. (1996), one can distinguish between a competence component of self-esteem and a moral worth component. With regard to moral worth, a violation of accepted norms and rules would be expected to lower self-esteem, and to lead to shame and guilt. With regard to competences, the main threat would be a failure that is attributed internally, leading to lowered self-regard and to shame (Lazarus, 1999; Pekrun & Frese, 1992). Kluger & DeNisi (1996) point out how negative feedback becomes problematic when it leads to turning one's attention to the self. Interestingly, with regard to self-esteem, negative feedback can be the more threatening the more it is seen as valid (Semmer et al., 2002). What all these processes have in common is that they refer to self-respect that is threatened by feelings of being insufficient with regard to standards of achievement or conduct. Stress through insufficiency (SIN) is therefore the part of the SOS concept referring to this kind of self-evaluation.

Stress with regard to *external* evaluations concerns disrespect. Actions by others that carry demeaning, devaluating, (overly) critical, ridiculing, humiliating, careless, or slighting messages are well suited to create stress. Because they violate norms of politeness, respect, and fairness, they are socially *illegitimate*. They are judged to have been avoidable, and so they imply an agent that is responsible for them, either by intention or by neglect. (Il)legitimacy can refer to different kinds of phenomena: legitimacy of social interactions, legitimacy of stressors, and legitimacy of task demands.

Legitimacy of Social Interactions

We have already mentioned social stressors that involve interactions where people feel offended when we discussed the meaning of stressors (see the section entitled "Multiple SPECs"), and considerable evidence supports their prominent role (see O'Brien & DeLongis, 1997). Also, because the message of esteem and care constitutes the essence of social support (Sarason et al., 1996), interactions that do not convey that message, but rather imply a critical or demeaning attitude, will not be helpful and can even be detrimental (Goldsmith, 1994; see the section entitled "Social Support"). Thus, this type of disrespect is well documented.

Nevertheless, some aspects of unsupportive interactions can make more sense from the perspective of disrespect. This refers especially to the aspect of advice, which is both an important part of social support and, as unwelcomed advice, a frequently mentioned problem. Thus, Cutrona and Suhr (1994) report that advice can be welcome if the person giving it has special competence in that area, whereas it will not be welcome when the supported person perceives this competence in himself or herself. The authors discuss this under the rubric of feeling controlled. The SOS perspective suggests an additional mechanism: by giving advice, the supporting person communicates that he or she does not perceive the other to possess the necessary competence to solve the problem — otherwise, it would not be necessary to give the advice. From the perspective of stress as disrespect, therefore, it is the implied attribution of incompetence by the "supporting" person, and therefore a devaluation of the person being "supported," that makes the difference.

Furthermore, advice often is given by saying things such as "You *only* have to…." In doing so, one can inadvertently declare the problem to be a minor one, since otherwise it could not be solved by doing "only…." If the person getting help has been struggling with that problem for a while, he or she will look rather stupid if the problem is so easily resolved. Therefore, people start to defend their problem as being rather complex and not easily resolved. In doing so, they defend themselves as not being so stupid that they could not resolve a minor problem. Finally, the issue of timing is sometimes mentioned in the context of advice, with an emphasis on advice being unwelcome if it comes too early (e.g., Pearlin & McCall, 1990). Why should advice be more welcome when it comes later? The "stress as disrespect" perspective suggests that the difference lies, again, in the acknowledgment of the problem as a real and sincere one, and thus in acknowledging what Pearlin and McCall refer to as legitimizing the distress of the supported person. Getting advice immediately after sketching the problem puts the person down by not acknowledging the complexity of the problem and the legitimacy of the distress involved. It expresses implicitly (that is, by the timing) what the "you only need to …" type of advice does more explicitly: it is a small problem that is easily fixed. By communicating that message, the recipient can feel regarded as not being able to solve a simple problem, or of making a big fuss about a small issue, and thus feel offended. Of course, although there is some evidence on these questions, (e.g., Goldsmith, 1994; Pearlin & McCall, 1990), much of this is speculative at this moment. These considerations can, however, suggest an avenue for analyzing this type of problem.

Legitimacy of Stressors

A second avenue through which legitimacy can play a role concerns the legitimacy of distressing conditions. Consider, for instance, someone who has to work with machines, tools, or materials that do not work properly, such as a computer that keeps breaking down. Such conditions have been established as important stressors (see Semmer et al., 1996; Sonnentag & Frese, 2003; Spector & Jex, 1998). If this situation is attributed to inherent features of the technical device ("After all, computers do break down every once in a while") or to situational necessities ("Our company is struggling to survive, there is simply no money to buy new equipment"), its impact should be less than if it is attributed to intent or neglect ("They take out the profit but don't care about us having acceptable working conditions"). The first type of explanation, of course, legitimizes the situation; the second declares it to be illegitimate.

A number of phenomena that have already been discussed might also be regarded from the perspective of legitimacy. Thus, adequate reward can be seen as legitimizing one's effort (see effort–reward imbalance in the section entitled "Lack of Reciprocity"); finding meaning can be described as a process of finding legitimate reasons for things to happen; and the lower amount of stress induced by supervisors who are not fair in a high-power culture can be seen as stemming from their legitimate right to behave in an arbitrary way (Gudykunst & Ting-Toomey, 1988).

Some evidence for this type of legitimacy comes from studies that find stressors to have less impact if they are a legitimate part of one's core role (Peeters et al., 1995). An example would be nurses that do not find a demanding type of care very stressful ("It's part of the job"), whereas they become very angry when they get the impression that the patient was actually well enough to do, by himself or herself, some of the things he or she demanded from the nurses ("We are a hospital, not a hotel" — Semmer, 2000).

Beyond the mere occurrence of SPECs, therefore, the attributions of (il)legitimacy involved should receive more attention. Again, however, we must caution that such attributions can be very individual, yet at the same time there can be considerable cultural consensus about them. Thus, crimes of passion are commonly judged milder than crimes in cold blood — provided, of course, that the passionate affect is seen as legitimate, because the provocation was violating social rules strongly enough to justify rage.

Legitimacy of Tasks

Situations that are commonly regarded as stressful can be experienced as less stressful when they are legitimate. The other side of this matter has to do with demands that at first sight can look rather normal, or at least not highly stressful, but that are not backed by being a legitimate part of one's role. Strict rules prescribing the clothes to wear are likely to be perfectly acceptable for people who deal with clients, whereas they can be seen as illegitimate by people in the back office, whom clients do not see. Tasks that should be done by others, unreasonable restrictions (the clothes example, bureaucratic rules), or tasks that mainly serve the personal interest of a supervisor (an example from the Berne research program: a secretary having to present all her boss's PowerPoint presentations because he refused to learn how to operate the presentation) would qualify for this. A milder form can be tasks that are unnecessary in the sense that they would not have to be carried out, or could be carried out with less effort, if things were organized better.

This type of phenomenon is currently being investigated in Berne (Semmer & Jacobshagen, 2003). Results so far show (1) that these types of illegitimate demands are, indeed, reported by people; (2) that they occur, as expected, mostly with secondary tasks that are not part of the core role; and (3) that a scale measuring them shows adequate psychometric properties and correlates with measures of well-being as expected.

IMPLICATIONS

The SOS approach can help to organize many different phenomena that are mentioned throughout the stress literature but are seldom connected under a common theme. Focusing on the need for positive regard and self-regard helps to interpret such diverse phenomena as premature advice, the especially strong impact of social stressors, the smaller impact of stressors that are part of one's core role, and the change from an innocuous demand to a stressful demand by lack of legitimacy. Some of these phenomena are well known and organized under a common perspective; others, such as illegitimate demands, are new developments, and instruments are being developed and tested to assess them.

RECIPROCITY AND OFFENSE TO SELF: COMMUNALITIES

Obviously, the approaches depicted here have many features in common. They emphasize fairness — because fairness is a necessary element in the social exchange as depicted by reciprocity approaches, and because fairness is an element of respect in the SOS approach (cf. Miller, 2001). They emphasize esteem — as a possible reward in one case, as an element that determines the stressful character of situations in the other. Both put social exchange and social meaning in the center of their considerations. Of course, reciprocity and equity approaches already have considerable empirical backing, whereas the specific implications of stress as offense to self, such as illegitimate task demands, are just beginning to be explored. But they both illustrate a point that we have emphasized throughout this paper. Cooper et al. (2003) have recently noted that this central point was aptly summarized by Kornhauser in his groundbreaking book *Mental Health of the Industrial Worker* almost 40 years ago: "Mental health is not so much a matter of freedom from specific frustrations as it is an overall balanced relationship to the world which permits a person to maintain realistic, positive belief in himself and his purposeful activities" (Kornhauser, 1965, p. 15). There is now considerable evidence that this "balanced relationship to the world" is related both to mental and to physical health. By giving due attention to these processes, we hope that further developments in the theory of stress and health will be able to get a better understanding of the processes involved.

REFERENCES

Adams, J.S. (1965). Inequity in social exchange. In L. Berkowitz (Ed.), *Advances in Experimental Social Psychology* (Vol. 2, pp. 267–299). New York: Academic Press.

Adler, N. & Matthews, K. (1994). Health psychology: Why do some people get sick and some stay well? *Annual Review of Psychology*, 45, 229–259.

Aiken, L.H., Clarke, S.P., Sloane, D.M., Sochalski, J., & Silber, J.H. (2002). Hospital nurse staffing and patient mortality, nurse burnout, and job dissatisfaction. *Journal of the American Medical Association*, 288, 1987–1993.

Aldwin, C.M. & Revenson, G.A. (1987). Does coping help? A reexamination of the relation between coping and mental health. *Journal of Personality and Social Psychology*, 53, 337–348.

Antonovsky, A. (1991). The structural sources of salutogenic strengths. In C.L. Cooper & R. Payne (Eds.), *Personality and Stress: Individual Differences in the Stress Process* (pp. 67–104). Chichester, U.K.: Wiley.

Antonucci, T.C. & Jackson, J.S. (1990). The role of reciprocity in social support. In B.R. Sarason, I.G. Sarason, & G.R. Pierce (Eds.), *Social Support: An Interactional View* (pp. 173–198). New York: Wiley.

Averill, J.R. (1973). Personal control over aversive stimuli and its relationship to stress. *Psychological Bulletin*, 80, 286–303.

Averill, J.R. (1983). Studies on anger and aggression: Implications for theories of emotion. *American Psychologist*, 38, 1145–1160.

Bakker, A.B., Schaufeli, W.B., Sixma, H.J., Bosveld, W., & van Dierendonck, D. (2000). Patient demands, lack of reciprocity, and burnout: A five-year longitudinal study among general practitioners. *Journal of Organizational Behavior*, 21, 425–441.

Banaji, M.R. & Prentice, D.A. (1994). The self in social contexts. *Annual Review of Psychology*, 45, 297–332.

Barling, J., MacEwen, K.E., & Pratt, L.I. (1988). Manipulating the type and the source of social support: An experimental investigation. *Canadian Journal of Behavioral Science*, 20, 140–153.

Barnett, R.C. & Hyde, J.S. (2001). Women, men, work, and family: an expansionist theory. *American Psychologist*, 56, 781–796.

Barthol, R.P. & Ku, N.D. (1959). Regression under stress to first learned behavior. *Journal of Abnormal and Social Psychology*, 59, 134–136.

Baum, A. & Posluszny, D.M. (1999). Health psychology: Mapping biobehavioral contributions to health and illness. *Annual Review of Psychology*, 50, 137–163.

Baumeister, R.F., Faber, J.E., & Wallace, H.M. (1999). Coping and ego depletion: Recovery after the coping process. In C.R. Snyder (Ed.), *Coping: The Psychology of What Works* (pp. 50–69). New York: Oxford University Press.

Beehr, T.A. (1995). *Psychological Stress in the Workplace*. London: Routledge.

Beehr, T.A. & Glazer, S. (in press). Role stress. In J. Barling, K. Kelloway, & M. Frone (Eds.), *Handbook of Work Stress*. Thousand Oaks, CA: Sage.

Beehr, T.A., Jex, S.M., Stacy, B.A., & Murray, M.A. (2000). Work stressors and coworker support as predictors of individual strain and job performance. *Journal of Organizational Behavior*, 21, 391–405.

Beehr, T.A. & McGrath, J.E. (1996). The methodology of research on coping: Conceptual, strategic, and operational-level issues. In M. Zeidner & N.S. Endler (Eds.), *Handbook of Coping: Theory, Research, Applications* (pp. 65–82). New York: Wiley.

Blaine, B. & Crocker, J. (1993). Self-esteem and self-serving biases in reaction to positive and negative events. An integrative review. In R.F. Baumeister (Ed.), *Self-Esteem: The Puzzle of Low Self-Regard* (pp. 55–85). New York: Plenum Press.

Bolger, N., Davis, A., & Rafaeli, E. (2003). Diary methods: Capturing life as it is lived. *Annual Review of Psychology*, 54, 579–616.

Bongers, P.M., de Winter, C.R., Kompier, M., & Hildebrandt, V.H. (1993). Psychosocial factors at work and musculoskeletal disease. *Scandinavian Journal of Work, Environment and Health*, 19, 297–312.

Boos, N., Semmer, N., Elfering, A., Schade, V., Gall, I., Zanetti, M., Kissling, R. Buchegger, N., Hodler, J., & Main, C. (2000). Natural history of individuals with asymptomatic disc alterations in magnetic resonance imaging. *Spine*, 2, 1484–1492.

Borman, W.C. & Motowidlo, S.J. (1997). Task performance and contextual performance: The meaning for personnel selection research. *Human Performance*, 10, 99–110.

Bosma, H., Stansfeld, S.A., & Marmot, M.G. (1998). Job control, personal characteristics, and heart disease. *Journal of Occupational Health Psychology*, 3, 402–409.

Bowling, N.A., Beehr, T.A., Johnson, A.L., Semmer, N.K., & Hendricks, E.A. (April 2003). Explaining Antecedents of Workplace Social Support: Reciprocity or Attraction? Paper presented at the annual meeting of the Society for Industrial and Organizational Psychology, Orlando FL.

Brown, G.W. (2002). Social roles, context and evolution in the origins of depression. *Journal of Health and Social Behavior*, 43, 255–276.

Brown, G.W. & Andrews, B. (1986). Social support and depression. In M. Appley & R. Trumbull (Eds.), *Dynamics of Stress* (pp. 257–282). New York: Plenum.

Burleson, B.R., Albrecht, T.L., Goldsmith, D.J., & Sarason, I.G. (1994a). Introduction: The communication of social support. In B.R. Burleson, T.L. Albrecht, & I.G. Sarson (Eds.), *Communication of Social Support: Messages, Interactions, Relationships, and Community* (pp. xi–xxx). Thousand Oaks, CA: Sage.

Burleson, B.R., Albrecht, T.L., & Sarason, I.G. (Eds.). (1994b). *Communication of Social Support: Messages, Interactions, Relationships, and Community.* Thousand Oaks, CA: Sage.

Buunk, P.B. (1990). Affiliation and helping interactions within organization: A critical analysis of the role of social support with regard to occupational stress. *European Review of Social Psychology*, 1, 293–322.

Buunk, B.P. & Schaufeli, W.B. (1999). Reciprocity in interpersonal relationships: An evolutionary perspective on its importance for health and well-being. In W. Stroebe & M. Hewstone (Eds.), *European Review of Social Psychology* (Vol. 10, pp. 259–291). Chichester, U.K.: Wiley.

Cacioppo, J.T., Berntson, G.G., Malarkey, W.B., Kiecolt-Glaser, J.K., Sheridan, J.F., Poehlmann, K.M., Burleson, M.H., Ernst, J.M., Hawkley, L.C., & Glaser, R. (1998). Autonomic, neuroendocrine, and immune responses to psychological stress: The reactivity hypothesis. *Annals of the New York Academy of Sciences*, 840, 664–673.

Cantor, N. & Sanderson, C.A. (1999). Life task participation and well-being: The importance of taking part in daily life. In D. Kahneman, E. Diener, & N. Schwarz (Eds.), *Well-Being: The Foundations of Hedonic Psychology* (pp. 230–243). New York: Russell Sage Foundation.

Carver, C.S., Scheier, M.F., & Weintraub, J.K. (1989). Assessing coping strategies: A theoretically based approach. *Journal of Personality and Social Psychology*, 56, 267–283.

Cleary, P.D. & Mechanic, D. (1983). Sex differences in psychological distress among married people. *Journal of Health and Social Behavior*, 24, 111–121.

Cohen, S. (1980). Aftereffects of stress in human performance and social behavior: A review of research and theory. *Psychological Bulletin*, 70, 213–220.

Cohen, S., Doyle, W.J., & Skoner, D.P. (1999). Psychological stress, cytokine production, and severity of upper respiratory illness. *Psychosomatic Medicine*, 61, 175–180.

Cohen, S., Frank, E., Doyle, W.J., Skoner, D.P., Robin, B.S., & Waltney, J.M., Jr. (1998). Types of stressors that increase susceptibility to the common cold in healthy adults. *Health Psychology*, 17, 214–223.

Cohen, S., Gottlieb, B.H., & Underwood, L.G. (2000). Social relationships and health. In S. Cohen, L.G. Underwood, & B.H. Gottlieb (Eds.), *Social Support Measurement and Intervention* (pp. 3–25). New York: Oxford University Press.

Cohen, S., Hamrick, N., Rodriguez, M.S., Feldman, P.J., Rabin, B.S., & Manuck, S.B. (2000). The stability of and intercorrelations among cardiovascular, immune, endocrine, and psychological reactivity. *Annals of Behavioral Medicine*, 22, 171–179.

Cohen, S. & Herbert, T.B. (1996). Health psychology: Psychological factors and physical disease from the perspective of human psychoneuroimmunology. *Annual Review of Psychology*, 47, 113–142.

Cohen, S., Kessler, R.D., & Gordon, L.U. (1997). Strategies for measuring stress in studies of psychiatric and physical disorders. In S. Cohen, R.C. Kessler, & L.U. Gordon (Eds.), *Measuring Stress: A Guide for Health and Social Scientists* (pp. 3–28). New York: Oxford University Press.

Compas, B.E., Connor, J., Osowiecki, D., & Welch, A. (1997). Effortful and involuntary responses to stress: Implications for coping with chronic stress. In B.H. Gottlieb (Ed.), *Coping with Chronic Stress* (pp. 105–130). New York: Plenum.

Cooper, C.L. (Ed.). (1998). *Theories of Organizational Stress*. Oxford, U.K.: Oxford University Press.

Cooper, C.L., Schabracq, M.J. & Winnubst, J.A.M. (2003). Preface. In M.J. Schabracq, J.A. Winnubst, & C.L. Cooper (Eds.), *Handbook of Work and Health Psychology* (2nd ed. pp. xv–xvi). Chichester: Wiley.

Creed, F. (1993). Stress and psychosomatic disorders. In L. Goldberger & S. Breznitz (Eds.), *Handbook of Stress: Theoretical and Clinical Aspects*, 2nd ed. (pp. 496–510). New York: The Free Press.

Cropanzano, R., James, K., & Citera, M. (1993). A goal hierarchy model of personality, motivation, and leadership. *Research in Organizational Behavior*, 15, 267–322.

Cutrona, C.E. & Russell, D.W. (1990). Type of social support and specific stress: Toward a theory of optimal matching. In B.R. Sarason, I.G. Sarason, & G.R. Pierce (Eds.), *Social Support: An Interactional View* (pp. 319–366). New York: Wiley.

Cutrona, C.E. & Suhr, J.A. (1994). Social support communication in the context of marriage: An analysis of couple's supportive interactions. In B.R. Burleson, T.L., Albrecht, & I.G. Sarson (Eds.), *Communication of Social Support: Messages, Interactions, Relationships, and Community* (pp. 113–135). Thousand Oaks, CA: Sage.

Diener, E. & Lucas, R.E. (1999). Personality and subjective well-being. In D. Kahneman, E. Diener, & N. Schwarz (Eds.), *Well-Being: The Foundations of Hedonic Psychology* (pp. 213–229). New York: Russell Sage Foundation.

Dienstbier, R.A. (1992). Mutual impacts of toughening on crises and losses. In L. Montada, S.-H. Filipp, & M.J. Lerner (Eds.), *Life Crises and Experiences of Loss in Adulthood* (pp. 367–384). Hillsdale, NJ: Lawrence Erlbaum.

Dimsdale, J.E. (2001). Comorbidity studies: A core area for psychosomatic research. *Psychosomatic Medicine*, 63, 201–202.

Dohrenwend, B.P. (2000). The role of adversity and stress in psychopathology: Some evidence and its implications for theory and research. *Journal of Health and Social Behavior*, 41, 1–19.

Dohrenwend, B.S. & Dohrenwend, B.P. (1974). *Stressful Life Events: Their Nature and Effects*. New York: Wiley.

Eden, D. (2001). Job stress and respite relief. Overcoming high-tech tethers. In P.L. Perrewé & D.C. Ganster (Eds.), *Exploring Theoretical Mechanisms and Perspectives* (*Research in Occupational Stress and Well-Being*, 1, 143–194). Amsterdam: JAI.

Elfering, A. Grebner, S., Semmer, N.K., & Gerber, H. (2002). Time control, catecholamines and back pain among young nurses. *Scandinavian Journal of Work, Environment and Health*, 28, 386–393.

Elfering, A., Semmer, N.K., & Kälin, W. (2000). Stability and change in job satisfaction at the transition from vocational training into "real work." *Swiss Journal of Psychology*, 59, 256–271.

Elfering, A., Semmer, N.K., Schade, V., Grund, S., & Boos, N. (2002). Supportive colleague, unsupportive supervisor: The role of provider-specific constellations of social support at work in the development of low back pain. *Journal of Occupational Health Psychology*, 7, 130–140.

Endler, N.S. (1998). Stress, anxiety and coping: The multidimensional interaction model. *Canadian Psychology*, 38, 136–153.

Endler, N.S. & Parker, J.D.A. (1990). Multidimensional assessment of coping: A critical evaluation. *Journal of Personality and Social Psychology*, 58, 844–854.

Epstein, S. (1998). Cognitive-experiential self-theory. In D.F. Barone, M. Hersen, & V.B. van Hasselt (Eds.), *Advanced Personality* (pp. 211–238). New York: Plenum.

Erez, M. & Earley, P.C. (1993). *Culture, Self-Identity, and Work*. New York: Oxford University Press.

Fisher, J.D., Nadler, A., & Whitcher-Alagna, S. (1982). Recipient reactions to aid. *Psychological Bulletin*, 91, 27–54.

Folkman, S., Lazarus, R.S., Dunkel-Schetter, C., DeLongis, A., & Gruen, R.J. (1986). Dynamics of a stressful encounter: Cognitive appraisal, coping and encounter outcomes. *Journal of Personality and Social Psychology*, 50, 992–1003.

Forsythe, C.J. & Compas, B.E. (1987). Interaction of cognitive appraisals of stressful events and coping: Testing the goodness of fit hypothesis. *Cognitive Therapy and Research*, 11, 473–485.

Frankenhaeuser, M. (1986). A psychobiological framework for research on human stress and coping. In M.H. Appley & R. Trumbull (Eds.), *Dynamics of Stress: Physiological, Psychological, and Social Perspectives* (pp. 101–116). New York: Plenum Press.

Frankenhaeuser, M. (1991). The psychophysiology of workload, stress, and health: Comparison between the sexes. *Annals of Behavioral Medicine*, 13, 197–204.

Frone, M.R. (2003). Work-family balance. In J.C. Quick & L.E. Tetrick (Eds.), *Handbook of Occupational Health Psychology* (pp. 143–162). Washington, DC: APA.

Ganster, D.C. & Fusilier, M.R. (1989). Control in the workplace. In D.L. Cooper & I.T. Robertson (Eds.), *International Review of Industrial and Organizational Psychology 1989* (pp. 235–280). Chichester, U.K.: Wiley.

Ganster, D.C. & Schaubroeck, J. (1991). Work stress and employee health. *Journal of Management*, 17, 235–271.

Geurts, S.A.E. & Demerouti, E. (2003). Work/non-work interface: A review of theories and findings. In M.J. Schabracq, J.A.M. Winnubst, & C.L. Cooper (Eds.), *Handbook of Work and Health Psychology* (pp. 279–312). Chichester, U.K.: Wiley.

Glass, D.C. & Singer, J.E. (1972). *Urban Stress: Experiments on Noise and Social Stressors.* New York: Academic Press.

Goldsmith, D.J. (1994). The role of facework in supportive communication. In B.R. Burleson, T.L. Albrecht, & I.G. Sarson (Eds.), *Communication of Social Support: Messages, Interactions, Relationships, and Community* (pp. 29–49). Thousand Oaks, CA: Sage.

Gottlieb, B.H. (Ed.). (1997). *Coping with Chronic Stress.* New York: Plenum.

Grebner, S., Elfering, A., & Semmer, N.K. (2003). *Work Experience, Blood Pressure, and Well-Being among Young Workers.* Unpublished manuscript, University of Bern, Switzerland.

Grebner, S., Elfering, A., Semmer, N.K., Kaiser-Probst, C., & Schlapbach, M.-L. (2004). Stressful situations at work and in private life among young workers: An event sampling approach. *Social Indicators Research,* 67, 11–49.

Greiner, B.A., Krause, N., Fisher, J.N. & Ragland, D.R. (1998). Objective stress factors, accidents, and absenteeism in transit operators: A theoretical framework and empirical evidence. *Journal of Occupational Health Psychology,* 3, 130–146.

Grob, A. (1995). Subective well-being nd significant life events across the life span. *Swiss Journal of Psychology,* 54, 3–18.

Grob, A., Lühi, R., Kaiser, F.G., Flammer, A., Mackinnon, A., & Wearing, A. (1991). Berner Gragebogen xm Wohlbefinden Jugendlicher (BFW) [Bern Questionnaire on adolescents' subjective well-being]. *Diagnostica*, 37, 66–76.

Gruen, R.J. (1993). Stress and depression: Toward the development of integrative models. In L. Goldberger & S. Breznitz (Eds.), *Handbook of Stress: Theoretical and Clinical Aspects*, 2nd ed. (pp. 550–569). New York: The Free Press.

Grunberg, L., Moore, S., & Greenberg, E.S. (1998). Work stress and problem alcohol behavior: A test of the spillover model. *Journal of Organizational Behavior,* 19, 487–502.

Gudykunst, W.B. & Ting-Toomey, S. (1988). Culture and affective communication. *American Behavioral Scientist*, 31, 384–400.

Harnish, J.D., Aseltine, R.H., & Gore, S. (2000). Resolution of stressful experiences as an indicator of coping effectiveness in young adults: An event history analysis. *Journal of Health and Social Behavior,* 41, 121–136.

Heim, C., Ehlert, U., & Hellhammer, D.H. (2000). The potential role of hypocortisolism in the pathophysiology of stress-related bodily disorders. *Psychoneuroendocrinology,* 25, 1–35.

Heinrichs, M., Baumgartner, T., Kirschbaum, C., & Ehlert, U. (2003). Social support and oxytocin interact to suppress cortisol and subjective responses to psychosocial stress. *Biological Psychiatry,* 54, 1389–1398.

Hemingway, H. & Marmot, M. (1999). Psychosocial factors in the aetiology and prognosis of coronary heart disease: Systematic review of prospective cohort studies. *British Medical Journal*, 318, 1460–1467.

Henderson, A.S. (1998). Social support: Its present significance for psychiatric epidemiology. In B.P. Dohrendwend (Ed.), *Adversity, Stress, and Psychopathology* (pp. 390–397). New York: Oxford University Press.

Higgins, E.T., Grant, H., & Shah, J. (1999). Self-regulation and quality of life: Emotional and non-emotional life experiences. In D. Kahneman, E. Diener, & N. Schwarz (Eds.), *Well-Being: The Foundations of Hedonic Psychology* (pp. 244–266). New York: Russel Sage Foundation.

Hobfoll, S.E. (2001). The influence of culture, community, and the nested-self in the stress process: Advancing conservation of resources theory. *Applied Psychology: An International Review*, 50, 337–421.

Hobfoll, S.E., Freedy, J.R., Green, B.L., & Solomon, S.D. (1996). Coping in reaction to extreme stress: The roles of resource loss and resource availability. In M. Zeidner & N.S. Endler (Eds.), *Handbook of Coping: Theory, Research, Applications* (pp. 322–349). New York: Wiley.

Hockey, G.R.J. (1997). Compensatory control in the regulation of human performance under stress and high workload: A cognitive-energetical framework. *Biological Psychology*, 45, 73–93.

Holahan, C.J., Moos, R.H., Holahan, C.K., & Cronkite, R.C. (1999). Resource loss, resource gain, and depressive symptoms: A 10-year model. *Journal of Personality and Social Psychology*, 77, 620–629.

Hurrell, J.J. (2001). Psychosocial factors and musculoskeletal disorders. In P.L. Perrewé & D.C. Ganster (Eds.), *Exploring Theoretical Mechanisms and Perspectives. Research in Occupational Stress and Well-Being*, 1, 233–256). Amsterdam: JAI.

Jerusalem, M. & Schwarzer, R. (1992). Self-efficacy as a resource factor in stress appraisal processes. In R. Schwarzer (Ed.), *Self-Efficacy: Thought Control of Action* (pp. 195–213). Washington, DC: Hemisphere.

Jex, S.M. (1998). *Stress and Job Performance*. Thousand Oaks, CA: SAGE.

Jones, J.W., Barge, B.N., Steffy, B.D., Fay, L.M., Kunz, L.K., & Wuebker, L.J. (1988). Stress and medical malpractice: Organizational risk assessment and intervention. *Journal of Applied Psychology*, 73, 727–735.

Judge, T.A. & Bono J.E. (2001). A rose by any other name: Are self-esteem, generalized self-efficacy, neuroticism, and locus of control indicators of a common construct? In B.W. Roberts & R. Hogan (Eds.), *Personality Psychology in the Workplace* (pp. 93–118). Washington, DC, U.S.: American Psychological Association.

Kahn, R.L. & Byosiere, P. (1992). Stress in organizations. In M.D. Dunnette & L.M. Hough (Eds.), *Handbook of Industrial and Organizational Psychology*, Vol. 3 (pp. 571–650). Palo Alto, CA: Consulting Psychologists Press.

Kaluza, G. (1997). Evaluation von Stressbewältigungstrainings in der primären Prävention: eine Metaanalyse (quasi-)experimenteller Feldstudien [Evaluation of stress management trainings in primary prevention: A metaanalysis of (quasi-)experimental field studies]. *Zeitschrift für Gesundheitspsychologie*, 5, 149–169.

Kanfer, R. & Heggestad, E. (1997). Motivational traits and skills. A person-centered approach to work motivation. *Research in Organizational Behavior*, 19, 1–56.

Kessler, R.C. & Magee, W.J. (1994). The disaggregation of vulnerability to depression as a function of the determinants of onset and recurrence. In W.R. Avison & I.H. Gotlib (Eds.), *Stress and Mental Health* (pp. 239–258). New York: Plenum.

Kiecolt-Glaser, J.K., McGuire, L., Tobles, T.F., & Glaser, R. (2002). Emotions, morbidity, and mortality: New perspectives from psychoneuroimmunology. *Annual Review of Psychology*, 53, 83–107.

Kinder, L.S., Kamarck, T.W., Baum, A., & Orchard, T.J. (2002). Depressive symptomatology and coronary heart disease in type I diabetes mellitus: A study of possible mechanisms. *Health Psychology*, 21, 542–552.

Kirkcaldy, B.D., Trimpop, R., & Cooper, C.L. (1997). Working hours, job stress, work satisfaction and accident rates among medical practitioners, consultants and allied personnel. *International Journal of Stress Management*, 4, 79–98.

Kirschbaum, C., Pirke, K.M., & Hellhammer, D.H. (1993). The "Trier Social Stress Test": a tool for investigating psychobiological stress responses in a laboratory setting. *Neuropsychobiology*, 28, 76–81.

Kitayama, S., Markus, H.R., & Matsumoto, H. (1995). Culture, self, and emotion: A cultural perspective on "self-conscious" emotions. In J.P. Tangney & K.W. Fischer (Eds.), *Self-Conscious Emotions* (pp. 439–464). New York: Guilford Press.

Kluger A.N. & DeNisi, A. (1996). The effects of feedback interventions on performance: A historical review, a meta-analysis, and a preliminary feedback intervention theory. *Psychological Bulletin*, 119, 254–284.

Klumb, P.L. & Perrez, M. (2004). Why time-sampling studies can enrich work-leisure research. Introduction to the special issue on intensive time sampling of work and leisure activities. *Social Indicators Research*, 67, 1–10.

Kohn, P. (1996). On coping adaptively with daily hassles. In M. Zeidner & N.S. Endler (Eds.), *Handbook of Coping: Theory, Research, Applications* (pp. 181–201). New York: Wiley.

Kompier, M.A.J. & Kristensen, T.S. (2000). Organizational work stress interventions in a theoretical, methodological and practical context. In J. Dunham (Ed.), *Stress in the Workplace: Past, Present and Future* (pp. 164–190). London: Whurr Publishers.

Kornhauser, A. (1965). *Mental Health of the Industrial Worker.* New York: Wiley.

Krantz, D.S. & McCeney, M.K. (2002). Effects of psychological and social factors on organic disease: A critical assessment of research on coronary heart disease. *Annual Review of Psychology*, 53, 341–369.

Kuper, H., Singh-Manoux, A., Siegrist, J., & Marmot, M. (2002). When reciprocity fails: Effort-reward imbalance in relation to coronary heart disease and health functioning within the Whitehall II study. *Occupational and Environmental Medicine*, 59, 777–784.

Lane, C. & Hobfoll, S.E. (1992). How loss affects anger and alienates potential supporters. *Journal of Consulting and Clinical Psychology*, 60, 935–942.

Lazarus, R.S. (1999). *Stress and Emotions: A New Synthesis*. London: Free Association Books.

Lazarus, R.S. & Folkman, S. (1984). *Stress, Appraisal, and Coping*. New York: Springer.

Lazarus, R.S. & Folkman, S. (1986). Cognitive theories of stress and the issue of circularity. In M. Appley & R. Trumbull (Eds.), *Dynamics of Stress* (pp. 63–80). New York: Plenum.

Lepore, S.J. (1997). Social-environmental influences on the chronic stress process. In B.H. Gottlieb (Ed.), *Coping with Chronic Stress* (pp. 133–160). New York: Plenum.

Lepore, S.J. & Evans, G.W. (1996). Coping with multiple stressors in the environment. In M. Zeidner & N.S. Endler (Eds.), *Handbook of Coping: Theory, Research, Applications* (pp. 350–377). New York: Wiley.

Levenstein, S., Ackerman S., Kiecolt-Glaser, J.K., & Dubois, A. (1999). Stress and peptic ulcer disease. *Journal of the American Medical Association*, 181, 10–11.

Leventhal, H. & Scherer, K. (1987). The relationship of emotion to cognition: A functional approach to a semantic controversy. *Cognition and Emotion*, 1, 3–28.

Linton, S.J. (2000). Psychological risk factors for neck and back pain. In A. Nachemson & E. Jonsson (Eds.), *Neck and Back Pain: The Scientific Evidence of Causes, Diagnosis, and Treatment* (pp. 57–78). Philadelphia: Lippincott Williams & Wilkins.

Locke, E.A., McClear, K., & Knight, D. (1996). Self-esteem and work. In C.L. Cooper & I.T. Robertson (Eds.), *International Review of Industrial and Organizational Psychology 1996*, Vol. 11 (pp. 1–328). Chichester, U.K.: Wiley.

Lundberg, U. & Melin, B. (2002). Stress in the development of musculoskeletal pain. In S.J. Linton (Ed.), *New Avenues for the Prevention of Chronic Musculoskeletal Pain and Disability* (pp. 165–179). Amsterdam: Elsevier.

Lundberg, U. & Parr, D. (2000). Neurohormonal factors, stress, health, and gender. In R.M. Eisler & M. Hersen (Eds.), *Handbook of Gender, Culture, and Health* (pp. 21–41). Mahwah, NJ: Erlbaum.

Marks, D.F., Murray, M., Evans, B., & Willig, C. (2000). *Health Psychology: Theory, Research and Practice*. London: Sage.

Marmot, M.G., Bosma, H., Hemingway, H., Brunner, E., & Stansfeld, S. (1997). Contribution of job control and other risk factors to social variations in coronary heart disease incidence. *The Lancet*, 350, 235–239.

Mason, J.W. (1975). A historical view of the stress field. *Journal of Human Stress*, 1, 6–12 (Part I); 1, 22–36 (Part II).

Matthews, G., Davies, D.R., Westerman, S.J., & Stammers, R.B. (2000). *Human Performance: Cognition, Stress and Individual Differences*. Hove, U.K.: Psychology Press.

McClelland, D.C. (1987). *Human Motivation*. Cambridge, U.K.: Cambridge University Press.

McCrae, R.R. & Costa, P.T. (1986). Personality, coping, and coping effectiveness in an adult sample. *Journal of Personality*, 54, 385–405.

McEwen, B. (1998). Protective and damaging effects of stress mediators. *New England Journal of Medicine*, 338, 171–179.

McGrath, J.E. & Beehr, T.A. (1990). Time and the stress process: Some temporal issues in the conceptualization and measurement of stress. *Stress Medicine*, 6, 93–104.

McGrath, J.E. & Tschan, F. (2004). *Temporal Matters in Social Psychology*. Washington, DC: American Psychological Association.

McLean, D.E. & Link, B.G. (1994). Unraveling complexity: Strategies to refine concepts, measures, and research designs in the study of live events and mental health. In W.R. Avison & I.H. Gotlib (Eds.), *Stress and Mental Health: Contemporary Issues and Prospects for the Future* (pp. 14–42). New York: Plenum.

Meichenbaum, D. & Fitzpatrick, D. (1993). A constructivist narrative perspective on stress and coping: Stress inoculation applications. In L. Goldberger & S. Breznitz (Eds.), *Handbook of Stress: Theoretical and Clinical Aspects*, 2nd ed. (pp. 706–723). New York: The Free Press.

Meijman, T.F. & Mulder, G. (1998). Psychological aspects of workload. In P.J.D. Drenth, H. Thierry, & C.J. de Wolff (Eds.), *Work Psychology*, Vol. 2, *Handbook of Work and Organizational Psychology*, 2nd ed. (pp. 5–33). Hove, U.K.: Psychology Press.

Miller, D.T. (2001). Disrespect and the experience of injustice. *Annual Review of Psychology*, 52, 527–553.

Murphy, L.R. (1996). Stress management in work settings: A critical review of the health effects. *American Journal of Health Promotion*, 11, 112–135.

Nelson, D.L. & Simmons, B.L. (2003). Health psychology and work stress: A more positive approach. In J.C. Quick & L.E. Tetrick (Eds.), *Handbook of Occupational Health Psychology* (pp. 97–119). Washington, DC: American Psychological Association.

Nowack, K.M. (1989). Coping style, cognitive hardiness, and health status. *Journal of Behavioral Medicine*, 12, 145–158.

O'Brien, T.B. & DeLongis, A. (1997). Coping with chronic stress: An interpersonal perspective. In B.H. Gottlieb (Ed.), *Coping with Chronic Stress* (pp. 161–190). New York: Plenum.

Organ, D.W. & Paine, J.B. (1999). A new kind of performance for industrial and organizational psychology: Recent contributions to the study of organizational citizenship behavior. In C.L. Cooper & I.T. Robertson (Eds.), *International Review of Industrial and Organizational Psychology 1999*, Vol. 14 (pp. 337–368). Chichester, U.K.: Wiley.

Ouelette, S.C. (1993). Inquiries into hardiness. In L. Goldberger & S. Breznitz (Eds.), *Handbook of Stress: Theoretical and Clinical Aspects*, 2nd ed. (pp. 77–100). New York: The Free Press.

Pargament, K.I. (2002). The bitter and the sweet: An evaluation of the costs and benefits of religiousness. *Psychological Inquiry*, 13, 168–181.

Parker, S.K., Axtell, C.M., & Turner, N. (2001). Designing a safer workplace: Importance of job autonomy, communication quality, and supportive supervisors. *Journal of Occupational Health Psychology*, 6, 211–228.

Paykel, E.S. (1974). Life stress and psychiatric disorder: Application of the clinical approach. In B.S. Dohrenwend & B.P. Dohrenwend (Eds.), *Stressful Life Events: Their Nature and Effects* (pp. 135–149). New York: Wiley.

Payne, N., Jones, F., & Harris, P. (2002). The impact of working life on health behavior: The effect of job strain on the cognitive predictors of exercise. *Journal of Occupational Health Psychology*, 7, 342–353.

Pearlin, L.I. & McCall, M.E. (1990). Occupational stress and marital support: A description of microprocesses. In J. Eckenrode & S. Gore (Eds.), *Stress between Work and Family* (pp. 39–60). New York: Plenum.

Peeters, M.C.W., Schaufeli, W.B., & Buunk, B.P. (1995). The role of attributions in the cognitive appraisal of work-related stressful events: an event-recording approach. *Work and Stress*, 9, 463–474.

Pekrun, R. & Frese, M. (1992). Emotions in work and achievement. In C.L. Cooper & I.T. Robertson (Eds.), *International Review of Industrial and Organizational Psychology 1992*, Vol. 7 (pp. 153–200). Chichester, U.K.: Wiley.

Perrewé, P.L. & Zellars, K.L. (1999). An examination of attributions and emotions in the transactional approach to the organizational stress process. *Journal of Organizational Behavior*, 20, 739–752.

Perrez, M. & Reicherts, M. (1992). *Stress, Coping, and Health*. Seattle: Hogrefe & Huber.

Pierce, G.R., Sarason, I.G., & Sarason, B.R. (1996). Coping and social support. In M. Zeidner & N.S. Endler (Eds.), *Handbook of Coping: Theory, Research, Applications* (pp. 434–451). New York: Wiley.

Pike, J.L., Smith, T.L., Hauger, R.L., Nicassio, P.M., Patterson, T.L., McClintick, J., Costlow, C., & Irwin, M.R. (1997). Chronic life stress alters sympathetic, neuroendocrine, and immune responsivity to an acute psychological stressor in humans. *Psychosomatic Medicine*, 59, 447–457.

Rahe, R.H. (1974). The pathway between subjects' recent life changes and their near-future illness reports: Representative results and methodological issues. In B.S. Dohrenwend & B.P. Dohrenwend (Eds.), *Stressful Life Events: Their Nature and Effects* (pp. 73–86). New York: Wiley.

Redinbaugh, E.M., MacCallum, R.C., & Kiecolt-Glaser, J.K. (1995). Recurrent syndromal depression in caregivers. *Psychology and Aging*, 10, 358–368.

Repetti, R.L. (1992). Social withdrawal as a short-term coping response to daily stressors. In H.W. Friedman (Ed.), *Hostility, Coping, and Health* (pp. 15–165). Washington, DC: American Psychological Association.

Repetti, R.L. (1994). Short-term and long-term processes linking job stressors to father-child interactions. *Social Development*, 3, 1–15.

Repetti, R.L. & Wood, J. (1997). Families accommodation to chronic stress: Unintended and unnoticed processes. In B.H. Gottlieb (Ed.), *Coping with Chronic Stress* (pp. 191–220). New York: Plenum.

Roy, M.P., Steptoe, A., & Kirschbaum, C. (1998). Life events and social support as moderators of individual differences in cardiovascular and cortisol reactivity. *Journal of Personality and Social Psychology*, 75, 1273–1281.

Rozanski, A., Blumenthal, J.A., & Kaplan, J. (1999). Impact of psychological factors on the pathogenesis of cardiovascular disease and implications for therapy. *Circulation*, 99, 2192–2217.

Sapolsky, R.M. (1998). *Why Zebras Don't Get Ulcers: An Updated Guide to Stress, Stress-Related Diseases, and Coping*. New York: Freeman.

Sapolsky, R.M. (1999). The psychophysiology and pathophysiology of unhappiness. In D. Kahneman, E. Diener, & N. Schwarz (Eds.), *Well-Being: The Foundations of Hedonic Psychology* (pp. 453–469). New York: Russel Sage Foundation.

Sarason, I.G., Johnson, J.H., & Siegel, J.M. (1979). Assessing the impact of life changes: Development of the Life Experiences Survey. In I.G. Sarason & C.D. Spielberger (Eds.), *Stress and Anxiety*, Vol. 6 (pp. 131–149). New York: Hemisphere.

Sarason, I.G., Sarason, B.R., Brock, D.M., & Pierce, G.R. (1996). Social support: Current status, current issues. In C.D. Spielberger, I.G. Sarason, J.M.T. Brebner, E. Greenglass, P. Laungani, & A.M. O'Roark (Eds.), *Stress and Emotion: Anxiety, Anger, and Curiosity*, Vol. 16 (pp. 3–27). Washington, DC: Taylor & Francis.

Schade, V., Semmer, N., Main, Ch., Hora, J., & Boos, N. (1999). The impact of clinical, morphological, psychosocial and work-related factors on the outcome of lumbar discectomy. *Pain*, 80, 239–249.

Schaefer, J.A. & Moos, R.H. (1992). Life crises and personal growth. In B.N. Carpenter (Ed.), *Personal Coping: Theory, Research, and Application* (pp. 149–170). Westport, CT: Praeger.

Schaubroeck, J. & Ganster, D.C. (1993). Chronic demands and responsivity to challenge. *Journal of Applied Psychology*, 78, 73–85.

Schaubroeck, J., Lam, S.S.K., & Xie, J.L. (2000). Collective efficacy versus self-efficacy in coping responses to stressors and control: A cross-cultural study. *Journal of Applied Psychology*, 85, 512–525.

Schaufeli, W.B. & Enzmann, D. (1998). *The Burnout Companion to Study and Practice: A Critical Analysis*. London: Taylor & Francis.

Scheier, M.F. & Carver, C.S. (1992). Effects of optimism on psychological and physical well-being: Theoretical overview and empirical update. *Cognitive Therapy and Research*, 16, 201–228.

Schmitt, M., Hoser, K., & Schwenkmezger, P. (1991). Schadensverantwortlichkeit und Ärger [Responsibility for damage and anger]. *Zeitschrift für Experimentelle und Angewandte Psychologie*, 38, 634–647.

Schnall, P.L., Belkic, K., Landsbergis, P., & Baker, D. (Eds.). (2000). The workplace and cardiovascular disease. *Occupational Medicine: State of the Art Review*, 15.

Schneiderman, N., Antoni, M.H., Saab, P.G., & Ironson, G. (2001). Health psychology: Psychosocial and biobehavioral aspects of chronic disease management. *Annual Review of Psychology*, 52, 555–580.

Schönpflug, W. & Battmann, W. (1988). The costs and benefits of coping. In S. Fisher & J. Reason (Eds.), *Handbook of Life Stress, Cognition and Health* (pp. 699–713). Chichester, U.K.: Wiley.

Schwarzer, R. & Leppin, A. (1991). Social support and health: A theoretical and empirical overview. *Journal of Social and Personal Relationships*, 8, 99–127.

Schwarzer, R. & Leppin, A. (1992). Social support and mental health: A conceptual and empirical overview. In L. Montada, S.-H. Filipp, & M.J. Lerner (Eds.), *Life Crises and Experiences of Loss in Adulthood* (pp. 435–458). Hillsdale, NJ: Lawrence Erlbaum.

Sedikides, C. & Strube, M.J. (1997). Self-evaluation: To thine own self be good, to thine own self be sure, to thine own self be true, and to thine own self be better. In M.P. Zanna (Ed.), *Advances in Experimental Social Psychology*, Vol. 29 (pp. 209–269). New York: Academic Press.

Seligman, M.E.P. & Csikszentmihalyi, M. (2000). Positive psychology. *American Psychologist*, 55, 5–14.

Selye, H. (1975). Confusion and controversy in the stress field. *Journal of Human Stress*, 1, 37–44.

Selye, H. (1993). History of the stress concept. In L. Goldberger & S. Breznitz (Eds.), *Handbook of Stress: Theoretical and Clinical Aspects*, 2nd ed. (pp. 7–17). New York: The Free Press.

Semmer, N. (1992). One man's meat, another man's poison? Stressors and their cultural background. In M. v. Cranach, W. Doise, & G. Mugny (Eds.), *Social Representations and the Social Bases of Knowledge* (pp. 153–158). Berne: Huber.

Semmer, N.K. (2000). Control at work: Issues of specificity, generality, and legitimacy. In W.J. Perrig & A. Grob (Eds.), *Control of Human Behavior, Mental Processes, and Consciousness: Essays in Honour of the 60th Birthday of August Flammer* (pp. 714–741). Mahwah, NJ: Erlbaum.

Semmer, N.K. (2003). Individual differences, work stress and health. In M.J. Schabracq, J.A. Winnubst, & C.L. Cooper (Eds.), *Handbook of Work and Health Psychology*, 2nd ed. (pp. 83–120). Chichester, U.K.: Wiley.

Semmer, N.K., Elfering, A., Jacobshagen, N., Perrot, T., & Boos, N. (2003). *The Emotional Significance of Instrumental Support.* Unpublished manuscript, University of Berne, Switzerland.

Semmer, N.K., Grebner, S., & Elfering, A. (2004). Beyond self-report: Using observational, physiological, and situation-based measures in research on occupational stress. In P. Perrewé & D.C. Ganster, (Eds.), *Research in Occupational Stress and Well-Being,* Vol. 3, pp. 205–263. Amsterdam: Elsevier.

Semmer, N.K. & Jacobshagen, N. (2003). Ego Threat as a Core Element of Occupational Stress: The Concept of "Stress as Disrespect." Paper presented at the 50th Anniversary Conference of the Department of Psychology of the University of Stockholm, June 14, 2003.

Semmer, N.K. & Jacobshagen, N. (2003). Selbstwert und Wertschätzung als Themen der arbeitspsychologischen Stressforschung [Self-esteem and respect as topics of research on occupational stress]. In K.-C. Hamborg & H. Holling (Eds.), *Innovative Personal- und Organisationsentwicklung*.(S. 131–155), Göttingen, Germany: Hogrefe.

Semmer, N.K., Kaelin, W., Elfering, A., & Dauwalder, J.P. (2001). *Work Experience and Quality of Life in Switzerland: Work, Stress, and Personality Development*, Report to the Swiss National Science Foundation. University of Berne, Department of Psychology.

Semmer, N.K., Tschan, F., Keller-Schuhmacher, K., Minelli, M., Walliser, F., Dunckel, H., & Jerusel, S. (2002). The dark side of accurate feedback: Some side effects of a tailor-made system for measuring work performance. In R.D. Pritchard, H. Holling, F. Lammers, & B.D. Clark (Eds.), *Improving Organizational Performance with the Productivity Measurement and Enhancement System: An International Collaboration* (pp. 147–163). New York: Nova Science.

Semmer, N.K. & Zapf, D. (In press). Gesundheits- und verhaltensbezogene Interventionen in Organisationen [Health- and behavior-related interventions at the work site]. In H. Schuler (Hrsg.), *Organisationspsychologie (Enzyklopädie der Psychologie)*. Göttingen, Germany: Hogrefe.

Semmer, N., Zapf, D., & Greif, S. (1996). "Shared job strain." A new approach for assessing the validity of job stress measurements. *Journal of Occupational and Organizational Psychology*, 69, 293–310.

Shupe, E.I. & McGrath, J. (1998). Stress and the sojourner. In C.L. Cooper (Ed.), *Theories of Organizational Stress* (pp. 86–100). Oxford: Oxford University Press.

Siegrist, J. (2002). Effort-reward imbalance at work and health. In P.L. Perrewé & D.C. Ganster (Eds.), *Historical and Current Perspectives on Stress and Health*, Vol. 2, *Research in Occupational Stress and Well-Being* (pp. 261–291). Amsterdam: JAI.

Silver, R.C., Wortman, C.B., & Crofton, C. (1990). The role of coping in support provision: The self-presentational dilemma of victims of life crises. In B.R. Sarason, I.G. Sarason, & G.R. Pierce (Eds.), *Social Support: An Interactional View* (pp. 397–426). New York: Wiley.

Simon, R.W. (1995). Gender, multiple roles, role meaning, and mental health. *Journal of Health and Social Behavior*, 36, 182–194.

Simon, R.W. (1998). Assessing sex differences in vulnerability among employed parents: The importance of marital status. *Journal of Health and Social Behavior*, 39, 38–54.

Smyth, J.M. & Pennebaker, J.W. (1999). Sharing one's story: Translating emotional experiences into words as a coping tool. In C.R. Snyder (Ed.), *Coping: The Psychology of What Works* (pp. 70–89). New York: Oxford University Press.

Sonnentag, S. & Frese, M. (2003). Stress in organizations. In W.C. Borman, D.R. Ilgen, & R.J. Klimoski (Eds.), *Handbook of Psychology*, Vol. 12, *Industrial and Organizational Psychology* (pp. 453–491). Hoboken, NJ: Wiley.

Spector, P. & Jex, S. (1998). Development of four self-report measures of job stressors and strain: Interpersonal Conflict at Work Scale, Organizational Constraints Scale, Quantitative Workload Inventory, and Physical Symptoms Inventory. *Journal of Occupational Health Psychology*, 3, 356–367.

Stansfeld, S. & Marmot, M. (Eds.). (2002a). *Stress and the Heart: Psychosocial Pathways to Coronary Heart Disease*. London: BMJ Books.

Stanton, A.L. & Franz, R. (1999). Focusing on emotion: An adaptive coping strategy? In C.R. Snyder (Ed.), *Coping: The Psychology of What Works* (pp. 90–118). New York: Oxford University Press.

Stanton, A.L., Kirk, S.B., Cameron, C.L., & Danoff-Burg, S. (2000). Coping through emotional approach: Scale construction and validation. *Journal of Personality and Social Psychology*, 78, 1150–1169.

Steptoe, A. (1991). Psychological coping, individual differences and physiological stress responses. In C.L. Cooper & R. Payne, (Eds.), *Personality and Stress: Individual Differences in the Stress Process* (pp. 205–233). Chichester, U.K.: Wiley.

Steptoe, A. (2001). Psychophysiological bases of disease. In D.W. Johnston & M. Johnston (Eds.), *Health Psychology*, Vol. 8, *Comprehensive Clinical Psychology* (pp. 39–78). Amsterdam: Elsevier.

Steptoe, A. & Appels, A. (Eds.). (1989). *Stress, Personal Control and Health*. Chichester, U.K.: John Wiley.

Steptoe, A. & Willemsen, G. (2002). Psychophysiological responsivity in coronary heart disease. In S. Stansfeld & M. Marmot (Eds.), *Stress and the Heart: Psychosocial Pathways to Coronary Heart Disease* (pp. 168–180). London: BMJ Books.

Sterling, P. & Eyer, J. (1988). Allostasis: A new paradigm to explain arousal pathology. In S. Fisher & J. Reason (Eds.), *Handbook of Life Stress, Cognition and Health* (pp. 629–649). Chichester, U.K.: Wiley.

Tangney, J.P. & Fischer, K.W. (Eds.). (1995). *Self-Conscious Emotions.* New York: Guilford Press.

Taris, T.W., Peeters, M.C.W., Le Blanc, P.M., Schreurs, P.J.G., & Schaufeli, W.B. (2001). From inequity to burnout: The role of job stress. *Journal of Occupational Health Psychology*, 6, 303–323.

Taylor, S.E., Kemeny, M.E., Reed, G.M., Bower, J.E., & Gruenewald, T.L. (2000). Psychological resource, positive illusions, and health. *American Psychologist*, 55, 99–109.

Taylor, S.E. & Repetti, R.L. (1997). Health psychology: What is an unhealthy environment and how does it get under the skin? *Annual Review of Psychology*, 48, 411–447.

Tennen, H. & Affleck, G. (1999). Finding benefits in adversity. In C.R. Snyder (Ed.), *Coping: The Psychology of What Works* (pp. 279–304). New York: Oxford University Press.

Tesser, A. & Martin, L. (1996). The psychology of evaluation. In E.T. Higgins & A.W. Kruglanski (Eds.), *Social Psychology: Handbook of Basic Principles* (pp. 400–432). New York: Guilford.

Thoits, P.A. (1994). Stressors and problem-solving: The individual as psychological activist. *Journal of Health and Social Behavior*, 35, 143–159.

Tice, D.M. (1993). The social motivations of people with low self-esteem. In R. Baumeister (Ed.), *Self-Esteem: The Puzzle of Low Self-Regard* (pp. 37–53). New York: Plenum.

Trimpop, R., Kirkcaldy, B., Athanasou, J., & Cooper, C. (2000). Individual differences in working hours, work perceptions and accident rates in veterinary surgeries. *Work and Stress*, 14, 181–188.

Turner, R.J. & Avison, W.R. (1992). Innovations in the measurement of life stress: Crisis theory and the significance of event resolution. *Journal of Health and Social Behavior*, 33, 36–50.

Uchino, B.N., Cacioppo, J.T., & Kiecolt-Glaser, J.K. (1996). The relationship between social support and physiological processes: A review with emphasis on underlying mechanisms and implications for health. *Psychological Bulletin*, 119, 488–531.

Van der Klink, J.J.L., Blonk, R.W.B., Schene, A.H., & van Dijk, F.J.H. (2001). The benefits of interventions for work-related stress. *American Journal of Public Health*, 91, 270–276.

Van Dierendonk, D., Schaufeli, W.B., & Buunk B.P. (2001). Burnout and inequity among human service professionals: A longitudinal study. *Journal of Occupational Health Psychology*, 6, 43–52.

Vinokur, A. & Selzer, M.L. (1975). Desirable versus undesirable life events: their relationship to stress and mental distress. *Journal of Personality and Social Psychology*, 32, 329–337.

Viswesvaran, C., Sanchez, J., & Fisher, J. (1999). The role of social support in the process of work stress: A meta-analysis. *Journal of Vocational Behavior*, 54, 314–334.

Walbott, H.G. & Scherer, K.R. (1995). Cultural determinants in experiencing shame and guilt. In J.P. Tangney & K.W. Fischer (Eds.), *Self-Conscious Emotions* (pp. 465–487). New York: Guilford Press.

Wheaton, B. (1997). The nature of chronic stress. In B.H. Gottlieb (Ed.), *Coping with Chronic Stress* (pp. 43–73). New York: Plenum.

Winnubst, J.A.M., Buunk B.P., & Marcelissen, F.H.g. (1988). Social support and stress. In S. Fisher & J. Reason (Eds.), *Handbook of Life Stress, Cognition and Health* (pp. 511–528). Chichester, U.K: Wiley.

Zajonc, R.B. (1984). On the primacy of affect. *American Psychologist*, 39, 117–123.

Zohar, D. (2003). Safety climate: Conceptual and measurement issues. In J.C. Quick & L.E. Tetrick (Eds.), *Handbook of Occupational Health Psychology* (pp. 123–142). Washington, DC: American Psychological Association.

2 Stress and Cancer: The Critical Research

Susanne Oksbjerg Dalton
and Christoffer Johansen

CONTENTS

INTRODUCTION

Belief in the existence of a relationship between psychological factors, such as stress and depression, and physical disease can be traced a long time back. Galen first noted that "melancholic women were more prone to cancer than those of sanguine temperament,"[1] and the emotional state as a causative factor in cancer has attracted attention continuously since then. It was not until the past few decades that the relationship between psychological factors and cancer began to be systematically investigated with the necessary research tools. With the findings that the biochemical effects of emotional states can have a suppressive effect on the immune system, the scientific field of psycho-oncology emerged, focusing on psychological states associated with cancer. Despite a lack of evidence substantiating stress as a cause of cancer, 42% of long-term breast cancer survivors in a Canadian study felt stress had

0-8493-1820-3/05/$0.00+$1.50

caused or precipitated their breast cancer.[2] The popular literature directed at cancer patients and survivors highlights the role of stress. There is no necessary connection between believing a claim and requiring evidence for such a belief. Cancer patients in common with many people develop their own attributions for symptoms and illness, which can be highly personalized, externalized, and associated with specific health behaviors used to combat the illness.[3,4] The yearning to find psychological explanations for physical diseases runs deep.

Definition of Psychological Stress

There is no definitive consensus existing on the concept of psychological stress today. Cannon, back in 1914, introduced the fight-or-flight response, describing the discharge of the noradrenergic nervous system induced by an upsetting life situation.[5] Selye defined stress as the "non-specific response of the body to any demand made upon it,"[6] and more recently, Lazarus stated that "stress occurs where there are demands on the person which tax or exceed his adjustive resources."[7] These definitions have served as a broad framework for the linking of stress with cancer, and in addition to this, the critical role of one's self-perception of stress due to different life demands and stressors is now generally recognized. Most of the epidemiological evidence on stress and cancer has been using life events as a marker for stress — due in part to the fact that obtaining reliable data is relatively easy. Other psychological factors linked to cancer also fall under the broader stress reaction model, and some of the more rigorously investigated factors include depression and personality traits.[8]

Stress and Immune Dysregulation

The prevailing hypothesis linking stress with cancer is that stress impairs immune function, which in turn predisposes the person to initiation or progression of neoplastic disease.[9,10] It is through the impact that these behavioral and psychological factors have on the cellular immune response, including natural killer (NK) cell function, that they can ultimately affect the occurrence and progression of certain tumors.

One recurrent concern regarding stress-related immunological changes has been the question of the significance of the immune system for cancer. Cancer comprises a heterogeneous group of diseases with multiple etiologies, and immunological involvement varies across different cancers. A series of studies have shown that suppression of cellular immunity, as in patients with congenital immunoinsufficiencies,[11] AIDS,[12] or organ transplants,[13] increases the risk for certain types of tumors.

Additionally, it has been questioned whether stress-related immune changes are of either the type or magnitude to influence tumor growth and metastases,[14] although there is some evidence that NK cells play a role in resisting the progression and metastatic spread of tumors once they have developed.[10]

The evidence that stress can dysregulate NK cell function, including depressing the stimulatory response of NK cells to cytokines, stems from diverse studies, including students undergoing exams[15] or caregivers for demented spouses,[16] or from evaluating the reaction to the loss of spouse[17] or to marital problems in newlyweds.[18,19]

Stress and Cellular DNA Repair and Apoptosis

A more direct action of stress on the initiation or production of abnormal cells independent of the immune system has also been suggested. A linkage between emotional distress and DNA repair was demonstrated by greater impairment in ability to repair damaged cellular DNA in newly diagnosed nonmedicated psychiatric patients, compared with controls.[20] Those who were depressed had the poorest repair of the psychiatric patients. It is possible that stress might have direct effects on carcinogenesis through alteration in DNA repair, as well as affecting the ability of the specific and innate immune responses to eliminate growth transformed and also fully malignant cells. Stress has also been found to have an impact on apoptosis, a process of genetically programmed alterations in cell structure that leads to failure of proliferation and differentiation, and eventual cell suicide.[21] Control of the expression of apoptosis is critical to the function of several cell types, including target cells of cytotoxic effector cells, and hence inhibition of apoptosis could result in suppression of the immune function. This was, for instance, demonstrated in a lower rate of apoptosis in students undergoing examination stress.[22]

All these physiological changes could operate independently or in conjunction with the stress-induced immune dysregulation described earlier. If these interpretations are correct, then psychosocial stressors could ultimately lead to progressive accumulation of errors within cell genomes as well as to the reduction of tumor-specific and innate immune responses.[10]

Stress and Cancer through Behavioral Pathways

Other plausible hypotheses include the idea that any effect of depression on cancer risk is indirect, mediated by the intervening effects of cancer-related health behaviors,[23,24] such as smoking, alcohol intake, low intake of fruit and vegetables, and lack of physical activity. This is based on the assumption that individuals who are under stress are more likely to engage in these kinds of unhealthy behavior patterns, which aim to reduce the threat or to cope with the emotions aroused by the stressful experience.

Research suggests a link between stress and smoking behavior in terms of smoking initiation,[25,26] relapse,[27–29] and the amount smoked.[30] An explanation for these behaviors has been suggested to be that stress causes an increased urge for smoking, which can be modified by smoking.[31–33] This is an explanation quite similar to that of the tension reduction theory suggested in alcohol research,[34] where tension refers to states such as fear, anxiety, depression, and distress. According to this model, an individual who feels tense or anxious as a result of an external stressor and believes that alcohol will reduce this tension (the expected outcome) might drink alcohol to improve his mood. The association between negative mood and drinking behavior is supported in the literature[35,36] and thus is parallel with the findings on smoking, indicating an indirect link between stress and cancer risk, as both smoking and alcohol use are well-established risk factors for some forms of cancer.[37,38]

In regard to diet, most research has focused on the individual change model, which predicts that stress only causes changes in eating in vulnerable groups of individuals.[39] For example, the effect of stress on eating habits has been found to be related to both weight[40] and levels of dieting.[41] However, these findings are not consistent and other studies have described no differences according to either gender or dieting, and this has led to an introduction of the stress-eating paradox, describing how at some times stress causes overeating and at others it causes undereating, without any clear pattern emerging.[42]

In summary, stress can result in increases in the consumption of alcohol and smoking and in a reduction in the amount of exercise, and can have detrimental effects on diet. These indirect mechanisms for stress to influence cancer risk are probably very complex and present great challenges to the design and analytical approaches for studies evaluating this hypothetical pathway.

ASSOCIATION AND CAUSAL RELATIONSHIP

Causation criteria have been developed that are generally and internationally accepted for the assessment of the accumulated evidence derived from the results of a number of studies, but also for an individual study. There are three factors that could explain an apparent association between stress and cancer apart from a true causal association: bias, confounding, and chance.[43]

First, bias in the observations that are made includes recall of the exposure under study, in this case the various operationalizations of stress. The case-control study has been the study design most often used to evaluate the relationship between stress and cancer. One of the inherent problems in this design is that people who have been diagnosed with cancer might be more likely to recall and report previous exposure than people who have not had cancer. The aforementioned tendency to attribute cancer, at least in part, to psychological stress makes it likely that recall bias can lead to more reports of cases of, for example, severe emotional disturbances resulting from major life events. In an attempt to reduce the potential for recall bias, many investigators have conducted case-control studies with a so-called limited prospective design. That is, reports on stress are obtained from patients who have symptoms but have not yet been given a definitive diagnosis. An assessment of psychological factors just before the confirmation of diagnosis cannot be considered independent of the outcome. In the case of women investigated for possible breast cancer, they were found to often correctly predict their definitive diagnosis, possibly based on their own bodily symptoms or interpretation of communication with their doctors.[44]

Apart from recall bias, other forms of bias can skew the results, in both limited case-control studies and proper case-control studies; however, as there is no such thing as a perfect scientific study, the methodological limitations have to be taken into account when evaluating the contribution of a study to the sum of knowledge in the area.

Second, confounding could lead to a situation in which the relationship with cancer appears stronger or weaker than it truly is due to a relation between the apparent causal factor and another factor that is also in itself associated with either increase or decrease in the risk for cancer. Earlier studies of the association between cancer and psychological variables did not have the possibility to include information of possible competing risk factors in the study design, and consequently, the results appear separated from the evidence of carcinogenic risk of these other factors. There is substantial evidence emerging on how psychological stress influences lifestyle, especially smoking, which is a strong risk factor for some forms of cancer — so strong, perhaps, that not accounting for it in the analysis of these cancer forms will render the interpretation of results difficult, and even when accounting for it, often raises the question of whether there can be some residual confounding not accounted for. Also, other lifestyle factors, such as alcohol consumption, exercise, diet, etc., fit the definition of a confounder when discussing stress and cancer, although their role is generally not so well established, or at least not as prominent, as in the case of smoking.

Third, an apparent association can also be due to chance variation, and although this is partly accounted for by the statistical methods used in the analyses of data, often a series of psychological factors or a number of cancer sites are analyzed and the question of a chance finding must always be considered.

The bulk of literature on stress and cancer is huge and the standard diverse. To bring our understanding further, it is necessary to set high standards when interpreting the empirical evidence. This research area is dealing with often somewhat "softer" data, which some can dismiss as out of hand data and others will support with almost religious fervor. But the stringent design and methodological standards must apply to this field of research as to any other scientific research, to challenge and bridge the gap between psyche and soma, and also to bring different research strategies — the "soft" and the "hard" — together as complementary instead of opposites. The following literature discussion will concentrate on those studies concerning life events as possible risk factors for cancer, only touching on some of the many other psychosocial factors used to operationalize stress in other studies. Further, although we acknowledge the major contributions to the field and substantial efforts to elucidate this relationship using case-control studies and limited prospective studies, we have restricted our discussion to only those studies of prospective cohorts or based on register linkage using incident cancer cases as endpoints, to avoid at least some of the methodological issues outlined above, inherent in those retrospective designs.

MAJOR LIFE EVENTS AND RISK FOR CANCER: EVIDENCE FROM THE LITERATURE

RECORD LINKAGE STUDIES

Several record linkage studies have investigated the relationship between single major life events and risk for cancer.[45–53] These studies are all relatively large, with the number of cancer cases spanning from 461 to 19,020, and with the follow-up time ranging from 5 to 27 years. The investigated life events include loss of a spouse or a child and the experience of severe illness in offspring.

Loss of Spouse

Several record linkage studies have investigated the risk for cancer after the loss of one's partner, either by death or by divorce. An English study comprising 1% of the population of England and Wales in the 1971 census[45] found no increase for cancer at any site after the death of a spouse after 5 years of follow-up in women, although the risk was nonsignificantly increased in men. Two studies from Norway and Denmark, respectively, found no increase after widowhood or divorce for cancer of all sites[46] or for breast cancer[47] in large population-based cohorts of women, using registry-based data. However, a recent large Swedish population-based study found a pattern of some cancers with increased risks and some with decreased risks in widows/widowers or divorced persons, compared to married persons.[48] Although not all statistically significant findings, a consistent pattern was that the effects in the divorced were always stronger than on those in widows/widowers, irrespective of the direction of the effect.[48] There seemed to be a balance between increased risks at tobacco-, alcohol-, and human papilloma virus-associated cancer sites and decreased risks at most other sites,[48] indicating that the effect of the change in life status could be mediated by specific lifestyle changes.

Loss of Child or Experience of Severe Illness in Child

Other linkage studies have evaluated the loss of a child using registry-based data. Using the same Norwegian cohort as mentioned above, no risk for cancer overall, or for any specific cancer site, was observed in bereaved mothers.[49] The effect of bereavement was studied in Israelis who had lost an adult son in war or in an accident.[50] No effect on total cancer risk was observed; however, an increased risk for lymphatic and hematopoietic cancers and for malignant melanoma was observed in parents who had lost their son at war or in accidents, as well as for respiratory tract cancers in those parents who lost a son in an accident.[50] Also, in a Danish population-based study of parents who lost a child,[51] a slightly increased risk for overall cancer was observed in bereaved mothers after 7 to 18 years of follow-up. This seemed to be mainly due to an increase in risk for smoking-related malignancies, whereas there was no observed risk for breast cancer, alcohol-related cancers, virus- or immune-related cancers, or hormone-related cancers, supporting an indirect effect of stress via increased smoking.

The experience of serious illness in offspring has also been evaluated using registry-based data. In a Danish nationwide follow-up of parents whose children had developed cancer,[52] no increase in risk for overall cancer or for any particular cancer site was observed, and there was no increase in risk during any period of follow-up after the stressful event. Further, the only increased risk in parents with a child who had been diagnosed with schizophrenia was for lung cancer in mothers,[53] offering indirect support of the pathway through behavioral changes.

Each of these studies was population based and obtained unbiased data on life events using administrative registries and ascertained endpoints as incident cancer cases through cancer registries. Although all studies adjusted for age, most of them were stratified by follow-up time, and some adjusted for factors such as education, residence, number of children, etc.; none of these studies were able to take into account lifestyle factors. This of course limits conclusions, but the consistency in the few positive findings does indicate that any effect of stress on cancer risk seems to be limited to cancer forms associated with adverse lifestyle factors.

Another point often put forward in regard to these record linkage studies is that the individual mastering of the stressful event is not taken into account, as these studies are evaluating group means. Although no one will question that the loss of a loved one or experience of serious illness in one's child is stressful to all people, regardless of personality, coping style, and social support or network, still the context in which the event occurs, for instance, whether death of the partner or child is sudden or following an extended illness, cannot be taken into account. However, if there is a threshold effect for stress on cancer risk, it is very likely that the exposure is a strain of such level and duration that most of the exposed cohort members in the above-mentioned studies would be considered above this threshold.

Prospective Cohort Studies

Two prospective studies have evaluated the association between major life events and risk for breast cancer. In an American cohort of 1,213 women, a 2.5-fold risk for breast cancer was observed after 15 years of follow-up in women whose mother had died during their childhood, based on only six cases. More recent life events were not associated with an increased risk.[54] The study obtained unbiased data on life events in childhood; however, some of the more recent life events were ascertained at follow-up, leading to a possibility of recall bias. Further, the follow-up endpoint was self-reported, clearly casting doubt on the validity of the case ascertainment, and there was no adjustment for reproductive factors, which are known to be associated with breast cancer.

In a recent cohort study from Finland, both the number and nature of stressful life events were ascertained in 10,808 women from the Finnish twin cohort.[55] Exposure data were obtained by self-report at baseline in combination with additional information on other risk factors for breast cancer, as well as on stress of daily activities, life satisfaction, and neuroticism. Incident breast cancer cases were identified through linkage with the Finnish Cancer Registry. After 17 years of follow-up, an increase in breast cancer risk was reported to be 7% per one event.[55] Three life events were in themselves associated with increase in breast cancer risk: divorce/separation, death of a husband, and death of a close friend or relative. The power of this recent and well-conducted study lies particularly in that many of the previous drawbacks from other studies have been addressed. There is information on well-established risk factors for breast cancer, and thus confounding is better accounted for than in most other studies, and also, the authors attempt to take into account whether an individual's personality, experience of daily stress, and mood could play a role. This adjustment was performed, although these factors in themselves in other analyses from the same cohort were found to be of no influence on breast cancer risk independently.[56,57] However, the rationale is that it is an individual's reaction to life events stress rather than the events per se that might be important. One limitation is the self-report of the life events, although the factors with the largest impact were generally not underreported.[58] This study suggests that breast cancer risk is influenced by life events stress independently of behavioral changes brought about by the psychological stress (adjustment for body mass index, weight change, alcohol use, smoking, and physical activity), and curiously, that the effect is not mediated or modified by self-perceptions of daily stress, adverse personality, or suboptimal mood.

In summary, in regard to breast cancer, the evidence from prospective cohorts does in fact suggest an effect of specific life events on risk. On the other hand, this was not supported by the large population-based studies based on information from administrative registers. The findings of increased risk for smoking-associated cancers in particular from the record linkage studies differ from the results from the prospective Finnish cohort, suggesting that the effects of life events are not mediated by obesity, weight gain, alcohol use, smoking, or physical inactivity. However, this is the first study attempting to evaluate whether it is the life event per se or some behavioral correlate of this that is behind an altered risk. This finding clearly cannot stand alone and calls for confirmation in future well-designed prospective studies of both breast cancer and other cancer sites.

DEPRESSION AND THE RISK FOR CANCER

Other varieties of psychological stress have been evaluated in regard to cancer, among them depression. Studies including both record linkage studies and prospective cohorts have investigated the association between depression and cancer risk.

Record Linkage Studies

In an American study of 923 depressed inpatients who were followed for up to 19 years, the risk for cancers at all sites was increased in comparison with the background population when the first 2 years were excluded from the analysis.[59] The excess risk appeared to be due to cancers of the breast, endometrium, or skin. In a nationwide Danish cohort study of 66,648 women hospitalized with affective disorders, no increase in risk for breast cancer was found after up to 25 years of follow-up.[60] In another Danish study, the cohort was extended to include all adults hospitalized for depressive disorder, and an increased risk for smoking-related cancers in both men and women hospitalized with reactive depression or dysthymia was reported.[61]

Prospective Cohort Studies

In a cohort of 2,018 middle-aged men who were followed for 20 years, depressed mood at baseline was associated with an increased risk for cancer at all sites during the first 10 years of follow-up.[62] Six subsequent cohort studies of population-based samples comprising 1,529 to 6,913 subjects followed for 10 to 17 years failed to confirm an increased risk for total cancer.[63–68] Only some of these studies provided risk estimates for cancers at specific cancer sites, including increased risk for lung cancer,[63,67] smoking-related cancers,[65] and breast cancer.[68] One study of 4,825 elderly patients assessed in depressed mood three times over a 6-year period before start of follow-up showed an increased risk for all cancers after an average follow-up of 3.8 years.[69] In that study the analyses of site-specific cancers revealed no predominant association with smoking-related cancers. Two prospective cohorts of 8,932 and 1,213 women, who were followed up for breast cancer for 13 and 15 years, respectively, were evaluated for depression.[54,70] One study showed no significant increase,[70] whereas the other showed a 14-fold increase in women with both major depression and dysthymia.[54]

Several explanations for the apparently disparate results can be put forward. In the relatively small samples available, the follow-up periods of 10 to 20 years in most studies might not have been adequate for examining cancer as an endpoint. Thus, the role of chance cannot be ruled out in interpretation of the findings.

Depression was defined psychometrically (as a continuous variable) in some of the prospective studies[62–65,69,70] and psychiatrically in others.[54,66–68] Therefore, the incidence of cancer was either expressed as a function of the degree of depression or compared with that of the general population, so the resulting information might not be comparable. Also, problems of lack of specificity arise, as no fewer than ten different instruments — eight standardized scales and two personal structured interviews — were used to assess depression or depressed mood.

SOME CONSIDERATIONS

The study of life events alone can be a somewhat incomplete approach. It might be that life events stressors, when examined in conjunction with vulnerability factors such as personality, coping style, emotional and behavioral patterns, and social support, will enable the relative impact of components of psychosocial stress to be teased apart. The cancer-prone personality described by Greer and Watson[71] and Temoshok[72] is believed to predispose an individual to developing cancer. This personality is purported to be maladaptive under conditions of prolonged or severe stress, increasing rather than reducing the impact of stressors. Hilakivi-Clarke[73] has made another attempt to outline a comprehensive model that includes life events stress, personality, and social support influencing the ability to cope and mediating, in this case, breast cancer risk. The crucial factor in this particular model is not the stressor per se, but the complex interaction between stressors, personality, and social support that affect an individual's ability to cope. This is a model compatible with more general models of stress and illness where life events are conceptualized as provoking agents for illness, are influenced by specific vulnerability factors such as social support, and are proposed to increase the impact of life events and consequently the resulting stress and strain.[74] In the available research published in the stress and cancer area, only a few methodologically sound studies consider life events stress together with other psychosocial aspects that might predict the effect of the stress on the individual. This is a difficult and complex task; however, an example of this approach is the prospective study from Finland evaluating the effect of life events on risk for breast cancer taking into account some aspects of personality and experience of daily stress and mood.[55]

Psychological stress, perhaps alternatively to major life events stress, should be assessed by a less specific measure more likely to reveal stable, intraindividual aspects of stress, although prospective evidence evaluating daily job strain[75] and perceived stress of daily activities[56] showed no association with breast cancer. Further, consideration of the role of social support as a buffer to the psychological impact of stressful life events has to the best of our knowledge not been evaluated prospectively. However, social support as an independent factor was evaluated in a prospective study using an unspecified self-report measure of social support, finding no association with breast cancer.[76] But most of the research on of the role of social support in cancer has generally focused on the ability to mitigate the impact of diagnosis, adjustment to illness, and prognosis.[77,78]

All in all, to what degree stress has a causal role in cancer is not completely clarified; however, based on the scientific evidence, it seems that the etiological fraction, i.e., the number of cases of cancer that stress can explain, is limited. Although some studies have observed a relationship between major life events stress and risk for some cancers, these findings must be interpreted with caution until repeated in other well-conducted prospective studies. The majority of the scientific evidence fails to support the direct association between stress and cancer, and this is reassuring information to those who believe the opposite, but also from a public health point of view. Some findings, however, point to the unfortunate effects that life events stress might have on lifestyle factors, such as smoking. This underlines the need for careful consideration of whether health behaviors should be treated as mediating factors rather than confounding factors in future studies of prospective character. This might have great implications for our understanding of a possible association between psychological stress and cancer risk.

REFERENCES

1. LeShan, L., Psychological states as factors in the development of malignant disease: A critical review. *J. Natl. Cancer Inst.*, 22, 1, 1959.
2. Stewart, D.E. et al. Attributions of cause and recurrence in long-term breast cancer survivors. *Psycho-oncology*, 10, 179, 2001.
3. Cassileth, B.R. et al. Psychosocial correlates of survival in advanced malignant disease. *N. Engl. J. Med.*, 312, 1551, 1985.
4. Stewart, D.E. et al. What makes women tired? *J. Wom. Health*, 7, 69, 1998.
5. Cannon, W.B. The emergency function of the adrenal medulla in pain and the major emotions. *Am. J. Physiol.*, 33, 356, 1914.
6. Selye, H. *The Stress of Life*. McGraw-Hill, New York, 1956.
7. Lazarus, RS. *Patterns of Adjustment*. McGraw-Hill, New York, 1976.
8. Fox, B.H. The role of psychological factors in cancer incidence and prognosis. *Oncology*, 9, 245, 1995.
9. Ader, R., Cohen, N., and Felten, D. Psychoneuroimmunology: Interaction between the nervous system and the immune system. *Lancet*, 345, 99, 1995.
10. Kiecolt-Glaser, J.K. et al. Psycho-oncology and cancer: Psychoneuroimmunology and cancer. *Ann. Oncol.*, 13, 165, 2002.
11. Kinlen, L.J. Immunosuppressive therapy and acquired immunological disorders. *Cancer Res.*, 52, 5474, 1992.

12. Johnson, C.C. et al. Cancer incidence among an HIV-infected cohort. *Am. J. Epidemiol.*, 146, 470, 1997.
13. Birkeland, S.A. et al. Cancer risk after renal transplantation in the Nordic countries, 1964–1986. *Int. J. Cancer*, 60, 183, 1995.
14. Herbert, T.B. and Cohen, S. Stress and immunity in humans: A meta-analytic review. *Psychosom. Med.*, 55, 364, 1993.
15. Dobbin, J.P. et al. Cytokine production and lymphocyte transformation during stress. *Brain Behav. Immun.*, 5, 339, 1991.
16. Irwin, M. et al. Impaired natural killer cell activity during bereavement. *Brain Behav. Immun.*, 1, 98, 1987.
17. Esterling, B.A. et al. Chronic stress, social support, and persistent alterations in the natural killer cell response to cytokines in older adults. *Health Psychol.*, 13, 291, 1994.
18. Irwin, M. et al. Plasma cortisol and natural killer cell activity during bereavement. *Biol. Psychiatry*, 24, 173, 1988.
19. Kiecolt-Glaser, J.K. et al. Negative behaviour during marital conflict is associated with immunological downregulation. *Psychosom. Med.*, 55, 395, 1993.
20. Kiecolt-Glaser, J.K. et al. Distress and DNA repair in human lymphocytes. *J. Behav. Med.*, 8, 311, 1985.
21. Kerr, J.F.R., Wyllie, A.H., and Currie, A.R. Apoptosis: A basic biological phenomenon with wide-ranging implications in tissue kinetics. *Br. J. Cancer*, 26, 239, 1972.
22. Tomei, L.E. et al. Psychological stress and phorbol ester inhibition of radiation-induced apoptosis in human PBLs. *Psychiatry Res.*, 33, 59, 1990.
23. Smith, T.W. and Gallo, L.C. Personality traits as risk factors for physical illness. In *Handbook of Health Psychology*, Baum, A., Revenson, T., and Singer, J. Eds. Lawrence Erlbaum, Hillsdale, NJ, 2000, pp. 139–172.
24. Ogden, J. *Health Psychology. A Textbook*. Open University Press, Buckingham, 2000.
25. Wills, T.A. and Shiffman, S. Coping and substance use: A conceptual framework. In *Coping and Substance Abuse*, Shiffman, S. and Wills, T.A., Eds. Academic Press, New York, 1985, pp. 3–24.
26. Koval, J.J. and Pederson, L.L. Stress-coping and other psychosocial risk factors: A model for smoking in grade 6 students. *Addict. Behav.*, 24, 207, 1999.
27. Lichtenstein, E. et al. Patterns of smoking relapse. *Health Psychol.*, 5, 29, 1986.
28. Carey, M.P. et al. Stress and unaided smoking cessation: A prospective investigation. *J. Consult. Clin. Psychol.*, 61, 831, 1993.
29. McKee, S.A. et al. Sex differences in the effects of stressful life events on change in smoking status. *Addiction*, 98, 847, 2003.
30. Anda, R.F. et al. Depression and the dynamics of smoking. A national perspective. *J.A.M.A.*, 264, 1541, 1990.
31. Gilbert, D.G. and Spielberger, C.D. Effects of smoking on heart rate, anxiety, and feelings of success during social interaction. *J. Behav. Med.*, 10, 629, 1987.
32. Perkins, K.A. and Grobe, J.E. Increased desire to smoke during acute stress. *Br. J. Addict.*, 87, 1037, 1992.
33. Niaura, R. et al. Response to social stress, urge to smoke and smoking cessation. *Addict. Behav.*, 27, 241, 2002.
34. Cappell, H. and Greeley, J. Alcohol and tension reduction: An update on research and theory. In *Psychological Theories of Drinking and Alcoholism*, Blane, H.T. and Leonard, K.E., Eds. Guilford Press, New York, 1987.
35. Violanti, J., Marshall, J., and Howe, B. Police occupational demands, psychological distress and the coping function of alcohol. *J. Occup. Med.*, 25, 455, 1983.

36. Schuckitt, M.A. Alcohol and depression: A clinical perspective. *Acta Psychiatr. Scand.*, 377, 28, 1994.
37. Dreyer, L. et al. Avoidable cancers in the Nordic countries. Tobacco smoking. *A.P.M.I.S.*, 105, 9, 1997.
38. Dreyer, L. et al. Avoidable cancers in the Nordic countries. Alcohol consumption. *A.P.M.I.S.*, 105, 48, 1997.
39. Greeno, C.G. and Wing, R.R. Stress-induced eating. *Psychol. Bull.*, 115, 444, 1994.
40. Baucom, D.H. and Aiken, P.A. Effect of depressed mood in eating among obese and nonobese dieting and nondieting persons. *J. Pers. Soc. Psychol.*, 41, 577, 1981.
41. Cools, J., Schotte, D.E., and McNally, R.J. Emotional arousal and overeating in restrained eaters. *J. Abnorm. Psychol.*, 101, 348, 1992.
42. Stone, A.A. and Brownell, K.D. The stress-eating paradox: Multiple daily measurements in adult males and females. *Psychol. Health*, 9, 425, 1994.
43. Hennekens, C.H. and Buring, J.E. *Epidemiology in Medicine*. Little Brown, Boston, 1987.
44. Schwarz, R. and Geyer, S. Social and psychological differences between cancer and non-cancer patients: Cause or consequence of the disease. *Psychother. Psychosom.*, 41, 195, 1984.
45. Jones, D.R., Goldblatt, P.O., and Leon, D.A. Bereavement and cancer: Some data on deaths of spouses from the longitudinal study of Office of Population Censuses and Surveys. *B.M.J.*, 289, 461, 1984.
46. Kvikstad, A. et al. Death of a husband or marital divorce related to risk of breast cancer in middle-aged women. A nested case-control study among Norwegian women born 1935–1954. *Eur. J. Cancer*, 30A, 473, 1994.
47. Ewertz, M. Bereavement and breast cancer. *Cancer*, 53, 701, 1986.
48. Hemminki, K. and Li, X. Lifestyle and cancer: Effect of widowhood and divorce. *Cancer Epidemiol. Biomarkers Prev.*, 12, 899, 2003.
49. Kvikstad, A. and Vatten, L.J. Risk and prognosis of cancer in middle-aged women who have experienced the death of a child. *Int. J. Cancer*, 67, 165, 1996.
50. Levav, I. et al. Cancer incidence and survival following bereavement. *Am. J. Public Health*, 90, 1601, 2000.
51. Li, J. et al. Cancer incidence in parents who lost a child. A nationwide study in Denmark. *Cancer*, 95, 2237, 2002.
52. Johansen, C. and Olsen, J.H. Psychological stress, cancer incidence and mortality from non-malignant diseases. *Br. J. Cancer*, 75, 144, 1997.
53. Dalton, S.O. et al. Major life event: A diagnosis of schizophrenia in offspring and risk for cancer. *Br. J. Cancer,* 30, 1364, 2004.
54. Jacobs, J.R. and Bovasso, G. Early and chronic stress and their relation to breast cancer. *Psychol. Med.*, 30, 669, 2000.
55. Lillberg, K. et al. Stressful life events and risk of breast cancer in 10,808 women: A cohort study. *Am. J. Epidemiol.*, 157, 415, 2003.
56. Lillberg, K. et al. Stress of daily activities and risk of breast cancer: A prospective cohort study in Finland. *Int. J. Cancer*, 91, 888, 2001.
57. Lillberg, K. et al. A prospective study of life satisfaction, neuroticism and breast cancer risk (Finland). *Cancer Causes Control*, 13, 191, 2002.
58. Funch, D.P. and Marshall, J.R. Measuring life stress: Factors affecting fall-off in the reporting of life events. *J. Health Soc. Behav.*, 25, 453, 1984.
59. Friedman, G.D. Psychiatrically-diagnosed depression and subsequent cancer. *Cancer Epidemiol. Biomarkers Prev.*, 3, 11, 1994.

60. Hjerl, K. et al. Breast cancer risk among women with psychiatric admission with affective or neurotic disorders: A nationwide cohort study in Denmark. *Br. J. Cancer*, 81, 907, 1999.
61. Dalton, S.O. et al. Depression and cancer risk: A register-based study of patients hospitalized with affective disorders, Denmark, 1969–1993. *Am. J. Epidemiol.*, 155, 1088, 2002.
62. Persky, V.W. et al. Personality and risk of cancer: 20-year follow-up of the Western Electric Study. *Psychosom. Med.*, 49, 435, 1987.
63. Kaplan, G.A. and Reynolds, P. Depression and cancer mortality and morbidity: Prospective evidence from the Alameda County Study. *J. Behav. Med.*, 11, 1, 1988.
64. Zonderman, A.B., Costa, P.T., and McCrae, R.R. Depression as a risk for cancer morbidity and mortality in a nationally representative sample. *J.A.M.A.*, 262, 1191, 1989.
65. Linkins, R.W. and Comstock, G.W. Depressed mood and development of cancer. *Am. J. Epidemiol.*, 132, 962, 1990.
66. Vogt, T. et al. Mental health status as a predictor of morbidity and mortality: A 15-year follow-up of members of a health maintenance organization. *Am. J. Public Health*, 84, 227, 1994.
67. Knekt, P. et al. Elevated lung cancer risk among persons with depressed mood. *Am. J. Epidemiol.*, 144, 1096, 1996.
68. Gallo, J.J. et al. Major depression and cancer: The 13-year follow-up of the Baltimore Epidemiologic Catchment Area sample (United States). *Cancer Causes Control*, 11, 751, 2000.
69. Penninx, B.W.J.H. et al. Chronically depressed mood and cancer risk in older persons. *J. Natl. Cancer Inst.*, 90, 1888, 1998.
70. Hahn, R.C. and Petitti, D.B. Minnesota Multiphasic Personality Inventory-rated depression and the incidence of breast cancer. *Cancer*, 61, 845, 1988.
71. Greer, S. and Watson, M. Towards a psychobiological model of cancer: Psychological considerations. *Soc. Sci. Med.*, 20, 773, 1985.
72. Temoshok, L. Personality, coping style, emotion and cancer: Towards an integrative model. *Cancer Surv.*, 6, 545, 1987.
73. Hilakivi-Clarke, L. et al. Psychosocial factors in the development and progression of breast cancer. *Breast Cancer Res. Treat.*, 29, 141, 1993.
74. Brown, G.W. and Harris, T.O. *Life Events and Illness*. Guilford Press, New York, 1989.
75. Achat, H., Kawachi, I., Byrne, C., Hankinson, S.E., and Colditz, G.A.A. Prospective study of job strain and risk of breast cancer. *Int. J. Epidemiol.*, 29, 622–628, 2000.
76. Bleiker, E.M. et al. Personality factors and breast cancer development: A prospective longitudinal study. *J. Natl. Cancer Inst.*, 88, 1478, 1996.
77. Kornblith, A.B. et al. Social support as a buffer to the psychological impact of stressful life events in women with breast cancer. *Cancer*, 91, 443, 2001.
78. De Boer, M.F. et al. Psychosocial correlates of cancer relapse and survival: A literature review. *Patient Educ. Couns.*, 37, 215, 1999.

3 Stress and Cancer: The Practice

Lone Ross, Ellen Boesen, and Christoffer Johansen

CONTENTS

How do cancer patients cope with the stress related to the diagnosis, treatment, and changed perspective of life? What is the impact of psychology on survival? What does it mean to think positive? These and other questions all reflect the popular idea that psychological factors can influence survival from cancer. This idea became prevalent in the population partly based on a small study published in 1979 by Greer and co-workers.[1] In this study it was observed that women who used "fighting spirit" as their coping style lived longer than women who used other coping styles. In support of this finding, other studies have reported that helplessness/hopelessness predicted a poorer outcome. It is very important to investigate to what degree coping style influences the outcome following a cancer disease, as it can be possible for patients to improve their chance of survival by becoming more focused on their ways of coping with the disease. The results of two randomized studies of psychosocial intervention, by Spiegel et al.[2] and Fawzy et al.,[3] which showed remarkable increases in the length of survival of breast cancer patients and of patients with malignant melanoma, respectively, led the public to believe that psychosocial support for cancer patients can affect their prognosis. In addition, psychological interventions aimed at changing and enhancing the use of certain ways of coping with cancer are believed to be beneficial in terms of emotional well-being by the patients themselves, their families, and many health care professionals. Over the past 30 to 40 years, several intervention strategies have been used in an attempt to improve emotional adjustment and survival.

Even if reliable, valid associations can be established between psychosocial intervention and subsequent improvement in length of survival, the mechanisms underlying this effect have yet to be determined. Several explanations have been proposed. Kiecolt-Glaser and Glaser[4] suggested that psychological stress is directly

0-8493-1820-3/05/$0.00+$1.50

linked to immune downregulation, and that distress or depression is associated with poorer repair of damaged DNA and alterations in apoptosis. These adverse effects are hypothesized to be amenable to psychosocial intervention. An indirect biological effect could be mediated by healthier behavior after psychosocial intervention, i.e., reductions in smoking habits and alcohol consumption, improved nutrition and physical activity, and compliance with medical regimens.[5]

DOES COPING AFFECT THE PROGNOSIS OF CANCER DISEASES?

In a recent review of studies focused on the association between coping and prognosis, the authors identified 26 prospective studies that investigated the survival question and 11 studies that investigated time to recurrence.[6] The authors identified 10 studies that investigated the association between a coping style named fighting spirit (information seeking and high degree of activities associated with behavioral changes) and survival; however, only two studies reported a positive effect of this way to cope with a cancer disease. In three of four studies, fighting spirit was associated with a reduced risk for recurrence, but the largest and most well conducted study did not confirm this association.[7] In eight studies a coping style labeled "active or problem focused" was the focus, and one study did report an effect during 7 years of follow-up.[8] None of these studies reported an effect of this coping style on time to recurrence. In 12 studies, a coping style defined as helplessness/hopelessness (giving up all hope that cure is possible) was investigated, but only two small studies reported that this particular coping style was associated with a poorer survival. When looking at this coping style as a predictor of recurrence, the findings were mixed, and methodological problems in the five studies that investigated this particular hypothesis made it impossible to draw any firm conclusion. The authors noted that the most recently published study on this association[7] did report an association when comparing those with high and low scores on the Helplessness/Hopelessness Scale but not when it was the predominant coping style.[6] In 15 studies that investigated the association between denial and avoidance (not wanting to talk about the cancer diagnosis, avoiding all situations associated with the status as a cancer patient), there was little evidence that these coping styles influenced survival, and only one of eight studies reported a positive effect on time to recurrence. Four studies of an acceptable quality explored the effect of stoic acceptance and fatalism (accepting the diagnosis, not believing in the effect of one's own activities, believing that the disease is one's destiny), and none of these studies reported an effect on survival. Likewise, the evidence for an effect associated with recurrence was weak. Anxious coping, anxious preoccupation, or depressive coping was investigated in ten studies, and in three small studies an effect was observed. None of these studies reported that these ways of coping would influence time to recurrence of the cancer disease. Suppression of emotions and emotion-focused coping was the focus in six studies, but only in one study did this coping style influence survival.[6]

How people feel, think, and behave is of the greatest importance for how they live after a cancer diagnosis. By live, we mean how they adapt to the challenges in life facing a serious and often chronic condition. The term *coping* has been observed as a psychological issue isolated from the physical part of human beings, reflecting the intention to demonstrate that psychological components had an independent effect on health. However, as demonstrated above, there is only weak evidence from clinical and epidemiological studies that coping styles influence survival or time to recurrence. Concurrently with the development of more refined research methods for investigating this hypothesis, the evidence weakens, illustrated by the differences between the design and outcome of the original study by Greer and co-workers published in 1979[1] and the replication published by the same group 20 years later.[7] Studies comparing groups of patients that use different coping styles are threatened by confounding by other characteristics of these patients that might be associated with their prognosis. Thus, the groups of cancer patients cannot be compared. Confounding by other characteristics might be overcome in randomized intervention studies where it is attempted to change the coping styles of a group of patients and to compare the prognosis of this group of patients with a control group that has not received this intervention. Such intervention studies could reveal to what extent it is possible to help cancer patients to cope with the disease in a way that improves well-being and perhaps also the prognosis.

HOW CAN THE WELL-BEING OF CANCER PATIENTS BE IMPROVED?

Research has shown that patients with poor problem-solving abilities and feelings of lack of control also report higher levels of depressive symptoms and anxiety that require interventions aimed at improving coping skills and thereby reducing depression and anxiety.[9–11] Interventions that aim to increase self-efficacy seem to promote better adjustment to cancer.[12] In a meta-analysis of psychosocial intervention components, interventions with a greater number of components related to social cognitive theory gave better quality of life outcomes than interventions with fewer or no such components.[13]

In a recent review published in 2002,[14] we identified 35 randomized studies that have addressed the effect of psychosocial intervention on well-being, most of them applying components related to cognitive theory, without assessing survival.[15–50] In studies in which different intervention strategies were compared, no clear pattern emerged. A randomized study from 1986 by Cain et al.[39] involved a comparison of individual and group counseling and support. At the end of the 8-week intervention, the patients given individual counseling reported significantly less anxiety than those receiving group counseling or the control group, and at the 6-month follow-up, the patients in both intervention groups reported significantly less anxiety and depression than patients in the control group.[39] The intervention used in two studies of Fawzy et al.[51] and Fawzy,[33] respectively, was similar but was used in a group setting in the former study and in an individual setting in the latter. Patients in the intervention group in the group setting improved their coping skills, whereas no significant effect on coping was observed in the individual setting.[52]

A study by Telch & Telch[41] showed that training in coping techniques was more effective than supportive therapy, whereas another study by Evans & Connis[43] found the opposite to be true. With regard to the effectiveness of various intervention strategies in reducing anxiety and depression, 12 studies focused on psychological education. Of these studies, eight showed a positive effect[15,25,27,31,39,41,43,53] and four showed no effect.[28,37,40,51] In four studies of long-term (>6 months) psychotherapeutic intervention, a positive effect on well-being was observed in two studies[46,54] and no effect was observed in two other studies.[38,55] Likewise, a short-term psychotherapeutic intervention had a positive effect on well-being in two studies[41,43] and no effect in two others.[21,24] Short-term provision of information alone had a beneficial effect in three studies[20,35,42] and no effect in one other study.[30] As information is part of psychological education, these two strategies appear to be more effective than supportive psychotherapy, regardless of duration, showing the importance of including education and information in psychosocial interventions.

The optimal timing of an intervention has not been fully elucidated. In many reports, the time between diagnosis and intervention was not given, probably because the patient population was heterogeneous in this regard. In a study by Edgar et al.,[56] the same intervention was provided immediately after the initial diagnosis of cancer and 4 months later. The group that received the intervention later was significantly less depressed, anxious, and worried 8 months after inclusion and continued to be less worried about their illness compared with the group given early intervention was 4 months later. In another study by Cunningham et al.,[57] a 6-week intervention consisting of supportive therapy and training in coping strategies was compared with the same intervention provided during an intensive weekend program. At 6 and 19 weeks' follow-up, no difference in well-being was found between the two groups.

The hypothesis that only patients with severe psychological distress benefit from psychosocial intervention was supported by the results of five studies that included only patients who were found on screening to be suffering from psychological distress:[25,27,41,43,46] all these studies found a significant effect on anxiety or depression.[31,37,38,45]

In summing up results from these 35 studies, we encountered several problems, as the comparability of the results of the studies on well-being was reduced by differences in the time between diagnosis of cancer and inclusion in the study, in patient populations, in intervention strategies, and in outcomes. Furthermore, most of the studies suffered from methodological flaws. The randomization procedure and the characteristics of nonresponders were often not adequately described, and long-term follow-up was rare. The intention-to-treat principle might not have been followed in some of the analyses, which would violate the principle of randomization and possibly result in an overestimate of the benefit, if only highly motivated patients experiencing a beneficial effect were included in the analyses.

The results of the studies were not consistent, as 15 of 25 studies in which anxiety and depression were assessed immediately after the end of the intervention showed a significant positive effect.[15,20,23,25,27,31,35,36,39,41–43,46,53,54] Most of the findings were, however, in the predicted direction, and the lack of significance in some studies might have been due to lack of power, as the study populations were generally small. Of the five studies in which more than 100 patients were included and anxiety and depression were measured,[25,29,30,35,38] two showed a positive effect at the end of the intervention.[25,35] In general, methods have improved over the past decade; however, consideration only of studies conducted during that period revealed the same degree of inconsistency as in the total group of studies, precluding a clear conclusion.[23–38,42–50]

A meta-analysis conducted in 1995 of published randomized studies of psychosocial intervention included 15 of the studies described above.[58] The analysis showed a significant, small to moderate effect on emotional adjustment, which covered a number of scales of mood state, fear and anxiety, depression, denial or repression, self-esteem, locus of control, satisfaction with medical care, other attitudes, personality traits, and other types of emotional adjustment or distress. It is not clear whether anxiety and depression had an independent effect. A meta-analysis conducted in 1999 of studies published before 1993 of psychological interventions among cancer patients included nine of the studies described above and several nonrandomized studies.[59] A moderate positive effect was found on anxiety, although the size of the effect was reduced when only randomized studies of high quality and with a sample size of more than 40 patients were included. A moderate positive effect for depression was found, but inclusion only of randomized studies of high quality and with a sample size of more than 40 patients reduced the size of the effect to a clinically negligible value. Group therapy tended to be more effective than individual therapy, and psychoeducational interventions appeared to be particularly effective. Furthermore, short-term interventions seemed to be more effective than long-term ones, and the most experienced therapists tended to be the most effective. The effect on anxiety and depression tended to be greater in patient groups who were found on screening to suffer from psychological distress, when compared with unscreened populations.[59] Although it is difficult to conduct a meta-analysis of heterogeneous studies, the results of this meta-analysis are convincing and support our conclusion that psychosocial intervention can have a weak effect on well-being and can be most relevant in populations screened for psychological distress. In addition, results suggest that interventions including an educational element can be most effective in reducing distress.

IS IT POSSIBLE TO IMPROVE THE PROGNOSIS OF CANCER PATIENTS?

We have identified nine randomized psychosocial intervention studies in which the length of survival of cancer patients has been assessed. In these studies, various intervention strategies were employed.

In a study from 1982 by Linn et al.,[55] 120 men with advanced cancer were included. The intervention group received individual counseling when needed for 1 year or until the patient died. No difference in survival was observed after 1 year of follow-up between the intervention group and the control group. The intervention group reported significantly better quality of life than the control group, and in addition, the intervention group reported significantly less depression after 3 months of intervention.

In a study by Spiegel et al.,[2,54,60] including 86 women with metastasizing breast cancer, the intervention consisted of group therapy for 1 year and instruction in self-hypnosis to control physical pain. No significant difference in the degree of depression was observed at the end of the intervention, but the intervention group reported significantly less anxiety[54] and pain intensity[60] than the control group.[60] In an analysis 10 years later,[2] the women in the intervention group were found to have lived on average 18 months longer than the women in the control group; however, the survival curve for the intervention group was found to be similar to that of the background population, whereas the curve for the control group showed appreciably worse survival.[61] The explanations could be that the women in this study differed somehow from the background population at baseline, that randomization to the control group had a negative effect on survival, or that more women with a poor prognosis were randomized to the control group by chance.[61] Although this study was well conducted, it needed to be replicated, and this is currently under way in the U.S. and has been done in Canada.[62]

In a study from 1993 by Fawzy et al.,[3,51] 80 patients with malignant melanoma were randomized to psychoeducational group therapy once a week for 6 weeks or to a control group. At the 6-year follow-up, a significant reduction in mortality was seen in the intervention group, when compared with the control group, when the 68 patients with stage I disease (no metastases) were considered.[3] Results from a 10-year follow-up showed that participation in the intervention group remained predictive of survival, however weakened since the 6-year follow-up.[63] The patients in the intervention group reported significantly less depression and mood disturbance than the control group at the 6-month follow-up.[51] After randomization, 25% of the patients in the control group dropped out of the study, which could possibly have biased the results.

In a study by Ilnyckyj et al.,[64] composed of 127 patients with various cancers, the intervention consisted of weekly group sessions for 6 months, professionally led for either the first 3 months (n = 30) or the full 6 months (n = 31). These two intervention groups were compared with a group of cancer patients who met weekly for 6 months with no professional leadership (n = 35) and with a control group of patients who did not participate in group meetings (n = 31). Owing to the withdrawal of a considerable number of patients from the group with no professional leadership, 21 patients who had not been randomized were added after 3 months. Survival at 11 years of follow-up was analyzed both including and excluding these 21 patients. In both cases, no significant difference in survival was observed.[64] The time between diagnosis of the cancer and inclusion in the study was not reported.

A study by Cunningham et al.[65,66] was composed of 66 women with metastatic breast cancer. The intervention consisted of 35 weekly 2-h sessions of supportive and cognitive behavioral therapy and an intensive weekend course of training in coping skills. The control group received a home study cognitive behavior package. Patients in the intervention group experienced significantly more anxious preoccupation and less helplessness than the controls, but no improvements in mood or quality of life were recorded.[66] At the 5-year follow-up, no significant difference in survival was found between the two groups.[65] The survival curves of the two groups in this study closely resembled that of the intervention group in the study of Spiegel et al.[2] The study of Cunningham et al. was well conducted, but offering the control group a home study cognitive behavioral package might have weakened the study, as the two groups might have tended to become more similar. In addition, this study, like most of these studies, had a relatively small sample size. The Kaplan–Meier plot of survival after a first metastasis does not, however, indicate lack of strength as an explanation for the negative finding, as the survival curves of the intervention and control groups were identical.[65]

In a study by Edelman et al.,[53,67] 121 women with metastatic breast cancer were randomized and the intervention group received eight weekly sessions of cognitive behavioral therapy, a family night, and three further monthly sessions. The intervention group showed reduced total mood disturbance and depression at the assessment immediately after therapy, but these improvements were not seen at the 3- and 6-month follow-ups.[53] No significant difference in survival was observed between the intervention group and the control group at the 5-year follow-up.[67] A major drawback of this well-conducted study is that 19 of the 62 patients who were randomized to the intervention group subsequently dropped out. This might have weakened the study, as the survival analysis was done on an intention-to-treat basis. However, an analysis of survival after exclusion of the dropouts did not alter the result.

In a study by Kuchler et al.,[68] 271 patients with a primary diagnosis of gastrointestinal cancer were randomized to individual psychotherapy during the hospital stay or to a control group. Quality of life was measured but not reported. A significant difference in survival was observed between the intervention group and the control group after 2 years of follow-up. After randomization, 34 patients in the control group requested transfer to the intervention group and 10 patients in the intervention group requested transfer to the control group. Because an intention-to-treat analysis was used, the patients remained in their originally assigned groups for the analysis. Owing to the crossover, the true prognostic effect of the intervention was probably underestimated.

A study by McCorkle et al.[69] was composed of 375 postsurgical cancer patients aged 60 or more who were randomized to an intervention or a control group. The intervention consisted of three home visits and five telephone calls from specialized nurses over 4 weeks. The patients in the intervention group and their family caregivers received comprehensive clinical assessments, monitoring, and teaching, and the nurses functioned as a liaison with health care settings and providers in the provision of technical and psychological support. No significant differences in the degree of depression were observed between the two groups at the 3- and 6-month follow-ups. A significant positive effect on survival was reported after 44 months of follow-up.

In a study by Goodwin et al.,[62] a replication of Spiegel's results was attempted. The 235 women with metastatic breast cancer who entered the study were randomized to weekly supportive-expressive group therapy for 1 year or to a control group. A multivariate Cox model including different biological prognostic variables showed no significant effect of the intervention on survival. Analyses of mood revealed a significant effect of the intervention, particularly for the women who were initially more distressed. Likewise, the effect of the intervention on the experience of pain and suffering or hurt was only significant for the women with high baseline scores of pain and suffering.

In summary, four studies reported a significant effect on survival, whereas five studies failed to demonstrate such an effect. Two of the four studies that found a positive effect on survival found a beneficial effect on well-being during follow-up,[2,3] and one study had no information on well-being.[68] In contrast to this, three of the five studies that failed to find an effect on survival reported a positive effect on well-being that either did not persist or only existed for a subgroup of patients with high baseline scores of mood disturbance or pain. [55,62,67]

The nine studies of the effect of interventions on survival were generally well conducted, but three had a sample size of fewer than 90 persons,[2,3,65] which would have increased the possibility that a positive or detrimental effect would be observed on the basis of a few atypical patients. The two studies with a sample size greater than 250 both showed improved survival,[68,69] but the follow-up in these two studies was less than 4 years, which reduces the conclusiveness of the results. Two other studies that showed a benefit with regard to survival had follow-up periods of 10 years.[2,63]

No consistent pattern of an effect on survival emerged with different intervention strategies. In the study of McCorkle et al.,[69] the intervention not only was psychosocial but also included clinical assessment. The results can therefore indicate an effect on prognosis of optimized medical treatment.

It has been proposed that psychosocial intervention affects the prognosis only of patients with early-stage cancer, as the natural course of more advanced stages might obviate a possible effect of psychosocial factors. Indeed, except for one study of patients with diseases in various stages,[64] all studies failing to find an effect on survival included late-stage patients.[55,62,65,67] The four studies that found an effect on survival of psychosocial intervention[2,3,68,69] included patients with late-stage cancer,[2] patients with cancers known to have a poor prognosis,[68] a study population that was heterogeneous in terms of stage,[69] and patients with early-stage cancer,[3] thus precluding any clear conclusion.

If psychosocial intervention is capable of prolonging survival by improving the well-being, which in turn improves the immune functioning, it seems unlikely that an intervention that does not affect psychological well-being could affect survival. This perception is supported by the finding that studies that showed no persistent effect on well-being also did not show a beneficial effect on survival.[55,67] It had also been proposed that intervention does not enhance survival, but rather, that randomization to a control group decreases the length of survival. Patients who are randomized to the control group in psychosocial intervention studies might be disappointed that they are not receiving an intervention that they consider might have been helpful. However, in a study in Sweden by Berglund et al.,[70] in which 73 nonparticipants were compared with 199 cancer patients participating in a randomized study of the effect of psychosocial intervention and physical training, no negative effect of randomization to the control group was observed on psychosocial variables over time when controls were compared with nonparticipants.

None of the studies included in this review showed that any effect on prognosis was mediated by alteration of the immune system. However, a positive effect on survival was observed in the study of patients with malignant melanoma,[3] an immune-related cancer form.[71] This was the only study in which immune parameters were assessed.[3,72] Although changes in these parameters were indeed observed, these were unrelated to survival.[3] As changes in health behavior were not measured in any of the studies, the possible mechanism is unknown.

CONCLUSION

The results of a large number of studies fail to demonstrate a conclusive effect of coping style and psychosocial intervention on survival or psychological well-being. Several explanations are possible. First, different intervention strategies were used in different studies, and perhaps only some of them affect prognosis or well-being, and in only certain patient groups. Second, the effect can be weak, accounting for the inconsistent results found for the generally small study populations. Third, the effect of the interventions might have been diluted by the inclusion of unselected patient groups rather than being restricted to selected groups of patients in need of psychosocial support.

To make progress in this field of research, large-scale studies are needed that allow evaluation of a possibly small effect. Identifying patients in need of psychosocial intervention by screening for psychological distress or available social support could enhance an effect on well-being. Sound methods regarding the randomization procedure and assessment of outcomes should be used, and international collaboration might be considered to increase the study size and comparability of the findings. Future studies on survival should address the possible mechanisms underlying an improved prognosis.

It has been suggested that the identification of a patient's coping styles might be of importance because treatment of unhealthy coping styles might be helpful for the patient. We want to emphasize that such intervention cannot be justified at this point if conducted with the aim of improving survival or prolonging time to recurrence. However, even if the effect of psychosocial intervention on endpoints such as survival, anxiety, and depression is found to be weak, it might have other, more subtle benefits, which are difficult to measure but which might justify implementation of psychosocial programs in the clinical treatment of cancer patients. The emerging field of rehabilitation among cancer patients points to new aspects in psychosocial cancer treatment.

REFERENCES

1. Greer, S., Morris, T., and Pettingale, K. Psychological response to breast cancer: Effect on outcome, *Lancet*, 2, 785, 1979.
2. Spiegel, D. et al. Effect of psychosocial treatment on survival of patients with metastatic breast cancer, *Lancet*, II, 888, 1989.
3. Fawzy, F.I. et al. Malignant melanoma. Effects of an early structured psychiatric intervention, coping, and affective state on recurrence and survival 6 years later, *Arch Gen Psychiatry*, 50, 681, 1993.
4. Kiecolt-Glaser, J. and Glaser, R. Psychoneuroimmunology and cancer: Fact or fiction? *Eur J Cancer*, 35, 1603, 1999.
5. Cohen, S. and Rabin, B. Psychologic stress, immunity, and cancer, *J Natl Cancer Inst*, 90, 3, 1998.

6. Petticrew, M., Bell, R., and Hunter, D. Influence of psychological coping on survival and recurrence in people with cancer: Systematic review, *BMJ*, 325, 1066, 2002.
7. Watson, M. et al. Influence of psychological response on survival in breast cancer: A population-based cohort study, *Lancet*, 354, 1331, 1999.
8. Faller, H. et al. Coping, distress, and survival among patients with lung cancer, *Arch Gen Psychiatry*, 56, 756, 1999.
9. Nezu, A.M. et al. Relevance of problem-solving therapy to psychosocial oncology, *J Psychosoc Oncol*, 16, 5, 1999.
10. Brennan, J. Adjustment to cancer: Coping or personal transition, *Psycho-oncology*, 10, 1, 2001.
11. Taylor, S.E. et al. Self-generated feelings of control and adjustment to physical illness, *J Soc Issues*, 47, 91, 1991.
12. Lev, E.L. Bandura's theory of self-efficacy: Applications to oncology, *Sch Inq Nurs Pract*, 11, 21, 1997.
13. Graves, K.D. Social cognitive theory and cancer patients' quality of life: A meta-analysis of psychosocial intervention components, *Health Psychol*, 22, 210, 2003.
14. Ross, L. et al. Mind and cancer. Does psychosocial intervention improve survival and psychological well-being? *Eur J Cancer*, 38, 1447, 2002.
15. Johnson, J. The effects of a patient education course on persons with a chronic illness, *Cancer Nurs*, 5, 117, 1982.
16. Jacobs, C. et al. Behavior of cancer patients: A randomized study of the effects of education and peer support groups, *Am J Clin Oncol*, 6, 347, 1983.
17. Watson, P.G. The effects of short-term postoperative counseling on cancer/ostomy patients, *Cancer Nurs*, 6, 21, 1983.
18. Forester, B., Kornfeld, D.S., and Fleiss, J.L. Psychotherapy during radiotherapy: Effects on emotional and physical distress, *Am J Psychiatry*, 142, 22, 1985.
19. Rimer, B. et al. Enhancing cancer pain control regimens through patient education, *Patient Educ Couns*, 10, 267, 1987.
20. Ali, N.S. and Khalil, H.Z. Effect of psychoeducational intervention on anxiety among Egyptian bladder cancer patients, *Cancer Nurs*, 12, 236, 1989.
21. Hagopian, G. and Rubenstein, J. Effects of telephone call interventions on patients' well-being in a radiation therapy department, *Cancer Nurs*, 13, 339, 1990.
22. Lerman, C. et al. Effects of coping style and relaxation on cancer chemotherapy side effects and emotional responses, *Cancer Nurs*, 13, 308, 1990.
23. Bindemann, S., Soukop, M., and Kaye, S. Randomised controlled study of relaxation training, *Eur J Cancer*, 27, 170, 1991.
24. Connor, SR. Denial in terminal illness: To intervene or not to intervene, *Hosp J*, 8, 1, 1992.
25. Greer, S. et al. Adjuvant psychological therapy for patients with cancer: A prospective randomised trial, *BMJ*, 304, 675, 1992.
26. Moorey, S. et al. Adjuvant psychological therapy for patients with cancer: Outcome at one year, *Psycho-oncology*, 3, 39, 1994.
27. Pruitt, B.T. et al. An educational intervention for newly-diagnosed cancer patients undergoing radiotherapy, *Psycho-oncology*, 2, 55, 1993.
28. Berglund, G. et al. A randomized study of a rehabilitation program for cancer patients: The 'Starting Again' group, *Psycho-oncology*, 3, 109, 1994.
29. Berglund, G. et al. One-year follow-up of the "Starting Again" group rehabilitation programme for cancer patients, *Eur J Cancer*, 30A, 1744, 1994.
30. Brandberg, Y. et al. Information to patients with malignant melanoma: A randomized group study, *Patient Educ Couns*, 23, 97, 1994.

31. Marchioro, G. et al. The impact of a psychological intervention on quality of life in non-metastatic breast cancer, *Eur J Cancer*, 32A, 1612, 1996.
32. de Wit, R. et al. A pain education program for chronic cancer pain patients: Follow-up results from a randomized controlled trial, *Pain*, 73, 55, 1997.
33. Fawzy, N.W. A psychoeducational nursing intervention to enhance coping and affective state in newly diagnosed malignant melanoma patients, *Cancer Nurs*, 18, 427, 1995.
34. Davison, B. and Degner, L. Empowerment of men newly diagnosed with prostate cancer, *Cancer Nurs*, 20, 187, 1997.
35. McQuellon, R. et al. Reducing distress in cancer patients with an orientation program, *Psycho-oncology*, 7, 207, 1997.
36. Speca, M. et al. A randomized, wait-list controlled clinical trial: The effect of a mindfulness meditation-based stress reduction program on mood and symptoms of stress in cancer outpatients, *Psychosom Med*, 62, 613, 2000.
37. Fukui, S. et al. A psychosocial group intervention for Japanese women with primary breast carcinoma. A randomized controlled trial, *Cancer*, 89, 1026, 2000.
38. Classen, C. et al. Supportive-expressive group therapy and distress in patients with metastatic breast cancer, *Arch Gen Psychiatry*, 58, 494, 2001.
39. Cain, E.N. et al. Psychosocial benefits of a cancer support group, *Cancer*, 57, 183, 1986.
40. Davis, H. Effects of biofeedback and cognitive therapy on stress in patients with breast cancer, *Psychol Rep*, 59, 967, 1986.
41. Telch, C.F. and Telch, M.J. Group coping skills instruction and supportive group therapy for cancer patients: A comparison of strategies, *J Consult Clin Psychol*, 54, 802, 1986.
42. Burish, T., Snyder, S., and Jenkins, R. Preparing patients for cancer chemotherapy: Effect of coping preparation and relaxation interventions, *J Consult Clin Psychol*, 59, 518, 1991.
43. Evans, R.L. and Connis, R.T. Comparison of brief group therapies for depressed cancer patients receiving radiation treatment, *Public Health Rep*, 110, 306, 1995.
44. Johnson, J. Coping with radiation therapy: Optimism and the effect of preparatory interventions, *Res Nurs Health*, 19, 3, 1996.
45. Burton, M. et al. A randomized controlled trial of preoperative psychological preparation for mastectomy, *Psycho-oncology*, 4, 1, 1995.
46. Mantovani, G. et al. Impact of psychosocial intervention on the quality of life of elderly cancer patients, *Psycho-oncology*, 5, 127, 1996.
47. Braden, C., Mishel, M., and Longman, A. Self-help intervention project. Women receiving breast cancer treatment, *Cancer Pract*, 6, 87, 1998.
48. Walker, B., Nail, L., and Croyle, R. Does emotional expression make a difference in reactions to breast cancer? *Oncol Nurs Forum*, 26, 1025, 1999.
49. Helgeson, V. et al. Education and peer discussion group interventions and adjustment to breast cancer, *Arch Gen Psychiatry*, 56, 340, 1999.
50. Herth, K. Enhancing hope in people with a first recurrence of cancer, *J Adv Nurs*, 32, 1431, 2000.
51. Fawzy, F.I. et al. A structured psychiatric intervention for cancer patients. I. Changes over time in methods of coping and affective disturbance, *Arch Gen Psychiatry*, 47, 720, 1990.
52. Fawzy, F.I. and Fawzy, N.W. Group therapy in the cancer setting, *J Psychosom Res*, 45, 191, 1998.
53. Edelman, S., Bell, D., and Kidman, A. A group cognitive behaviour therapy programme with metastatic breast cancer patients, *Psycho-oncology*, 8, 295, 1999.

54. Spiegel, D., Bloom, J.R., and Yalom, I. Group support for patients with metastatic cancer, *Arch Gen Psychiatry*, 38, 527, 1981.
55. Linn, M.W., Linn, B.S., and Harris, R. Effects of counseling for late stage cancer patients, *Cancer*, 49, 1048, 1982.
56. Edgar, L., Rosberger, Z., and Nowlis, D. Coping with cancer during the first year after diagnosis. Assessment and intervention, *Cancer*, 69, 817, 1992.
57. Cunningham, A.J. et al. A randomised comparison of two forms of a brief, group, psychoeducational program for cancer patients: Weekly sessions versus a "weekend intensive," *Int J Psychiatry Med*, 25, 173, 1995.
58. Meyer, T.J. and Mark, M.M. Effects of psychosocial interventions with adult cancer patients: A meta-analysis of randomized experiments, *Health Psychol*, 14, 101, 1995.
59. Sheard, T. and Maguire, P. The effect of psychological interventions on anxiety and depression in cancer patients: Results of two meta-analyses, *Br J Cancer*, 80, 1770, 1999.
60. Spiegel, D. and Bloom, J.R. Group therapy and hypnosis reduce metastatic breast carcinoma pain, *Psychosom Med*, 45, 333, 1983.
61. Fox, B.H. Some problems and some solutions in research on psychotherapeutic intervention in cancer, *Support Care Cancer*, 3, 257, 1995.
62. Goodwin, P. et al. The effect of group psychosocial support on survival in metastatic breast cancer, *N Engl J Med*, 345, 1719, 2001.
63. Fawzy, F.I., Canada, A.L., and Fawzy, N.W. Malignant melanoma: Effects of a brief, structured psychiatric intervention on survival and recurrence at 10-year follow-up, *Arch Gen Psychiatry*, 60, 100, 2003.
64. Ilnyckyj, A. et al. A randomized controlled trial of psychotherapeutic intervention in cancer patients, *Ann R Coll Phys Surg Can*, 27, 93, 1994.
65. Cunningham, A. et al. A randomized controlled trial of the effects of group psychological therapy on survival in women with metastatic breast cancer, *Psycho-oncology*, 7, 508, 1998.
66. Edmonds, C., Lockwood, G., and Cunningham, A. Psychological response to long term group therapy: A randomized trial with metastatic breast cancer patients, *Psycho-oncology*, 8, 74, 1999.
67. Edelman, S. et al. Effects of group CBT on the survival time of patients with metastatic breast cancer, *Psycho-oncology*, 8, 474, 1999.
68. Kuchler, T. et al. Impact of psychotherapeutic support on gastrointestinal cancer patients undergoing surgery: Survival results of a trial, *Hepato-gastroenterology*, 46, 322, 1999.
69. McCorkle, R. et al. A specialized home care intervention improves survival among older post-surgical cancer patients, *J Am Geriatr Soc*, 48, 1707, 2000.
70. Berglund, G. et al. Is the wish to participate in a cancer rehabilitation program an indicator of the need? Comparisons of participants and non-participants in a randomized study, *Psycho-oncology*, 6, 35, 1997.
71. Maeurer, M. and Lotze, M. Immune responses to melanoma antigens, in *Cutaneous Melanoma*, 3rd ed., Balch, C., Houghton, A., Sober, A., and Soong, S.-J., Eds., Quality Medical Publishing, St. Louis, 1998, p. 517.
72. Fawzy, F.I. et al. A structured psychiatric intervention for cancer patients. II. Changes over time in immunological measures, *Arch Gen Psychiatry*, 47, 729, 1990.

4 Stress and Prevention of Cardiovascular Disease

Töres Theorell

CONTENTS

The present chapter deals with life conditions that could be of significance to the risk of cardiovascular disease. The understanding of these conditions could be of importance to programs aiming at the prevention of cardiovascular disease. Such strategies will be discussed. The clinical context and the mechanisms that might be of importance to individual counseling to the patient with cardiovascular disease will be discussed in more detail in another chapter.

When the relationship between stress and heart disease is being discussed, it is important to distinguish between different levels in a hypothetical chain of causes, since this can have a very important relationship with targeted actions aiming at reduced stress. In my own terminology, stress equals energy mobilization in all situations that require energy (see Figure 4.1).[1,2] This is close to Selye's stress concept.[3] Life conditions that can evoke stress are labeled stressors. Stressors are handled by the individual according to a psychobiological program (coping). Coping patterns[4] arise in interplay between genes and environment. The individual's way of reacting psychologically and biologically is thus determined by the individual's

0-8493-1820-3/05/$0.00+$1.50

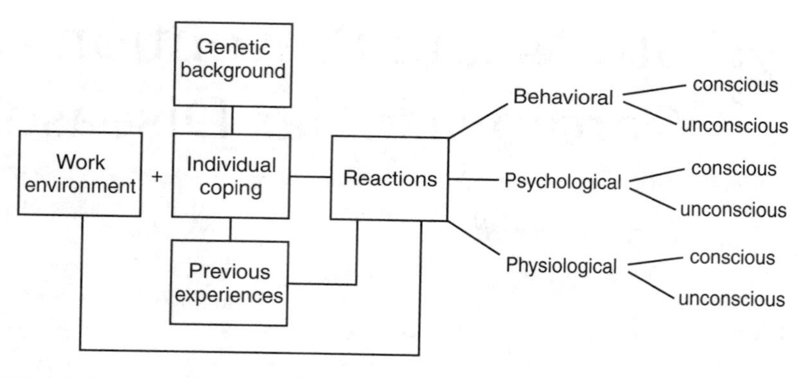

FIGURE 4.1 Theoretical model of the interaction between the environment, the individual, and his or her reactions. (Adapted from Kagan and Levi, in *Society, Stress and Disease. The Psychosocial Environment and Psychosomatic Diseases,* Levi, L. (Ed.), Oxford University Press, London, 1971.)

genetic makeup in interplay with total life experiences from childhood all the way to his or her present years. A continuous remodeling of the psychobiological program takes place. According to this reasoning, stress prevention of potential importance to cardiovascular disease could deal with both the environment and the individual. Both kinds of stress prevention could be labeled primary prevention. When the environment is the target, the number of stressors should be lowered or the conditions that protect against adverse stress reactions strengthened. When the individual is the target, the aim is to strengthen the individual's coping pattern. The stress reactions themselves could also be the target for action pharmacologically or psychologically, but that is mostly a clinical problem.

The presentation will be organized in relation to the general model. First we shall discuss stressors, and then individual programs.

STRESSORS AT WORK AND OUTSIDE WORK

Several of the concepts and theoretical models that are used in work stress prevention could be applied to life outside work as well. Of course, the interplay between conditions at work and conditions outside work is also important. It is necessary, however, to start with a general overview of stressors at work and outside work that have been discussed in the literature.

STRESSORS AT WORK

Cooper and Marshall[5] as well as Landsbergis et al.[6] have described a wide spectrum of possible work stressors. Stressors could be divided into physical and psychosocial, but also into long-lasting and more acute stressors. Such categorizations, however, suffer from several difficulties. First of all, it is not always possible to differentiate between psychosocial and physical stressors. For instance, a noisy work environment does induce a physical problem since the noise itself can cause hearing loss and hypertension.[7] However, it can also change the psychosocial work environment. In a recent study in a coronary care unit, we observed that for the staff several aspects of the psychosocial environment, such as perceived psychological demands and staff ratings of quality of care, improved after the acoustic conditions had improved. The roof was equipped with sound-absorbing tiles.[8] When the intelligibility of the spoken word improves and there is less need for repetition and raised voices, there can very well be a reduced feeling of frustration. The patients also felt that they received better care during the period with improved acoustics, and they also showed a decreased pulse amplitude (difference between systolic and diastolic blood pressure) during the night hours in the ward, possibly a consequence of fewer awakenings at night.[9] In the real world, it might not be meaningful to differentiate between physical and psychosocial stressors.

The stressors are easily identifiable for workers in different occupations. Each occupation has its own mix of physical and psychosocial stressors. It is always necessary to explore in detail the kinds of stressors that characterize a given work site. In such an effort, the detailed list of stressors is very useful. In work site interventions and in work design, however, it is also necessary to summarize stressors in such a way that a more general plan of action is possible. That is why the broader theoretical models are useful since they can provide a map for action. The most commonly used models of this broader type are the demand–control–support (DCS) and effort–reward imbalance (ERI) models. These two models seem to supplement each another in the sense that if they are used simultaneously, predictions of cardiovascular disease risk improve (see below).

The demand–control model was introduced by Karasek.[10] It was subsequently expanded to include support — the demand–control–support model.[11,12] It was empirically tested in relation to cardiovascular disease in several studies during the 1980s.[12] It has always been an environmental model. While it is certainly true that different individuals can perceive one and the same situation differently, it is still possible to describe the organizational context of a work site from a collective point of view. All three main dimensions could be affected by work design. *Psychological demands* include quantitative (amount per time unit) as well as qualitative (difficulty) demands. *Decision latitude* includes authority over decisions (possibility for employees to influence decisions regarding daily work) and *intellectual discretion* (possibility for employees to develop skills and knowledge so that they can make decisions regarding their work). *Social support* includes support from workmates as well as from superiors. Each one of the subdimensions of the three main dimensions could of course be explored separately, and this can be very important in certain situations. Kristensen et al.[13] have argued that a differentiation between cognitive (for instance, demands on the memory function) and emotional (to be emotionally engaged, for instance, in patients) demands can be very important since excessive cognitive demands in general relate to good health and emotional demands in general to adverse health effects. While in most of the epidemiological cardiovascular literature decision latitude includes both intellectual discretion and authority over decisions, many recent reports in this area have been focused on decision authority only, since this relates most directly to work organization. It could sometimes be important to differentiate between support from workmates and support from superiors.[14] Figure 4.2 shows the interaction between the three basic elements of the DCS model. The

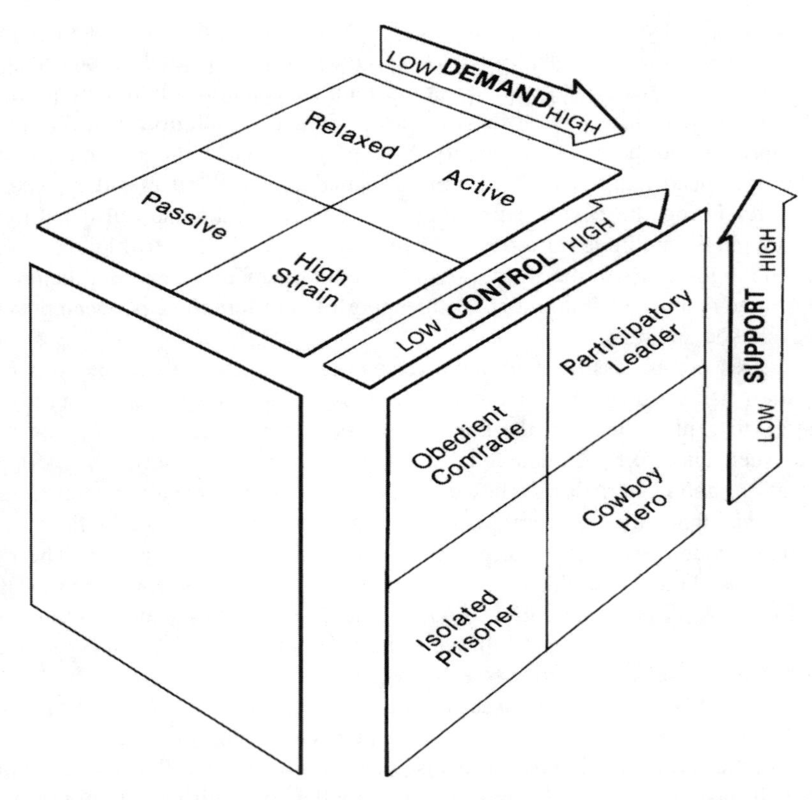

FIGURE 4.2 A three-dimensional model of the psychosocial work environment.

theory states that the ideal combination is to have reasonable demands, good decision latitude, and good support, while the worst combination is to have excessive demands in combination with low decision latitude (job strain) and poor support (iso-strain).

The effort–reward imbalance model has been introduced by Siegrist.[15] This theory states that there must be balance between efforts and rewards. The effort dimension has two components, one intrinsic (commitment) and one extrinsic, the latter being similar to the psychological demand dimension in the demand–control–support model. The reward dimension has three components: material (salary and related material rewards), social (promotion prospects and social prestige associated with the job), and psychological (self-esteem). In the early studies, intrinsic and extrinsic efforts were added together, while in most recent studies, they have been separated.

What relationship is there between the job stress models and risk of cardiovascular disease? Numerous studies have explored the relationship between job strain (the combination of high psychological demands and low decision latitude) and cardiovascular disease. Most of these studies have been cross-sectional, but also, several prospective ones have been published. The cross-sectional examination includes an assessment of psychosocial situation/stress and a health examination at the same time. The prospective examination includes assessment of psychosocial situation/stress at one point in time and an examination of cardiovascular health on a later occasion. The prospective study has a higher regard scientifically because it is possible to disentangle the possible temporal relationships. All studies published before 2000 have been summarized by Schnall et al.[16] Several conclusions could be drawn from that review. The majority of the published cross-sectional and prospective studies showed a relationship in the expected dimension — low decision latitude and job strain predict higher risk of cardiovascular disease. The relationships mostly held after adjustment for age, serum lipids, body mass index, smoking habits, and social class. In two of the prospective studies, the effects of personality characteristics (type A behavior in the Framingham study and negative affectivity in the Whitehall II study) were also studied as possible confounders. The total impression is that the relationships held also after adjustment for these individual characteristics. In the Schnall et al. review from 2000, decision latitude was more important in the predictions than psychological demands. Totally negative findings (no relationship with either job strain or decision latitude) were associated with:

- *Indirect assessments* (imputed assessments based upon job title and known characteristics of psychosocial environments for men and women in different ages in different occupations) rather than self-ratings.
- *Higher age* rather than ages below 55. In some of the studies including older subjects, retirement has taken place in a large proportion of the participants during follow-up.
- *Lack of dispersion* of psychosocial working conditions. For instance, subjects in one occupation might have too homogenous working conditions. This limits the possibility to establish relationships.
- *Nonrepresentative samples*. One study[17] was based upon consecutive subjects going through coronary angiography in a large university clinic. Neither cross-sectional nor prospective results confirmed any relationship between demands and decision latitude on the one hand and clinical outcomes (including progression of coronary atherosclerosis) on the other hand. The difficulty of interpreting the results in this study arises due to the fact that the participants had been subjected to angiography for very different reasons. Subjects without objectively verifiable coronary atherosclerosis with a high degree of anxiety and pronounced tendency to complain about life conditions, including those at work, might be more likely to be subjected to coronary angiography than nonanxious subjects without coronary atherosclerosis. This can give rise to serious bias against the hypothesis.

In two of the most recent large-scale studies, high demand and low decision latitude (job strain) have provided more precise predictions of cardiovascular disease than low decision latitude alone. This is the case with the most recent follow-up of the Whitehall II study[18] and the Finnish follow-up study.[19] On the other hand, there is conflicting evidence regarding a possible true interaction between the effects of high psychological demands and low decision latitude on risk.[20] A study by

Hallqvist[21] has shown that this discrepancy in findings can be due to differences in the operational definitions of demands and decision latitude. It has also been pointed out that the assessment of psychological demand is methodologically more difficult than the assessment of decision latitude.[22]

Men and Women, Blue-Collar and White-Collar Workers, Younger and Older Workers

More studies of the demand–control model and cardiovascular disease have been performed in men than in women. So far, the studies that have been performed on women show that women as well as men in high-demand and low-decision-latitude jobs have increased risk of developing cardiovascular disease.

Low decision latitude is more common in lower social classes, whereas high psychological demands are more often reported by subjects in higher social classes. There is evidence supporting the assumption that job strain has a more pronounced effect on cardiovascular risk in blue-collar workers than in white-collar workers.

Findings of associations between the demand–control model and cardiovascular disease have been stronger below age 55 than above. This can be due to the fact that aging is such a strong explanatory factor in itself that other risk factors lose importance in the higher working ages.

The Relationship between the Demand–Control–Support Model and Biological Risk Factors

With regard to the demand–control model and risk factors for cardiovascular disease, findings are less clear than for heart disease. It is, of course, important to know to what extent the association between job strain and myocardial infarction risk is due mainly to physiological mechanisms — and if so which ones — or what effects it has on lifestyle. *Serum lipids* have not shown unequivocal relationships with the demand–control model. *Plasma fibrinogen*, which is related to both coagulation and inflammatory processes, seems to be associated with job strain.[23] A growing literature is indicating that there can be relationships between stress and the *activity in the immune system*, for instance, endothelial activity, interleukin-6 (IL-6), and C-reactive protein.[24] A recent study by our group showed that a small difference between morning and midday serum cortisol levels (a possible indicator of exhaustion) was related to a high IL-6 activity, and in men a low decision latitude was related to a high IL-6 activity.[25]

With regard to *systolic and diastolic blood pressure*, most of the research has supported the assumption that high demands in combination with low decision latitude are associated with high blood pressure, and that continuously high or rising levels of job strain are associated with rising systolic and/or diastolic blood pressure. Reviews of published research have supported this conclusion for blood pressure monitoring during activities at work.[26] However, the results from studies of conventional blood pressure recordings (in the medical examination, after resting) have been diverging.

One longitudinal study has also shown that increasing job strain is associated with increased energy mobilization (mirrored in rising blood pressure levels during work hours) and decreased regeneration (mirrored in decreasing serum testosterone levels in men).[27,28]

An epidemiological study of industrial workers in Israel showed that smoking was more common in workers with adverse job conditions than in others.[29] However, most of the research exploring the relationship between the demand–control model and risk factors has shown that the relationship cannot be explained by effects on lifestyle such as diet, smoking, and physical exercise. Hence, it is likely that there is an independent effect of job strain on physiological stress mechanisms, which could be through stress effects in the direction of reduced regeneration and disturbances in energy regulation, blood pressure regulation, coagulation, and inflammation. Social support at work has been less extensively examined. However, lack of social support in general has been shown to be associated with acceleration of coronary atherosclerosis in women.[30]

In summary, there is considerable evidence supporting the demand–control hypothesis in relation to cardiovascular disease. Particularly strong evidence has been found for men below age 55 in blue-collar jobs. There is evidence indicating that some of this relationship can be mediated by blood pressure regulation and effects on coagulation mechanisms.

Effort–Reward Imbalance

There is a growing number of published studies of the ERI model in relation to heart disease. The most extensive test was done in the Whitehall Study, which showed high coronary heart disease incidence in high-effort and low-reward jobs. When the decision authority component of the demand–control model was combined with the ERI model (intrinsic and extrinsic efforts combined), particularly strong relationships were found.[31,32] A Swedish case-control study based upon SHEEP (Stockholm Heart Epidemiology Program) showed similar results, although in this case self-reported job strain was combined with extrinsic effort–reward imbalance (for terminology, see above). This combination was particularly predictive of being in the myocardial infarction case group for men. In women, the combination of intrinsic effort (commitment) and self-reported job strain was particularly important in relation to being a case. This difference can be of significance to the establishment of prevention programs for men and women. Since women and men have different labor markets,[33] the differences that were observed in this study could be related to differences in the conditions in "male" (with a majority of men) and "female" (with a majority of women) jobs.

Several studies have shown relationships between ERI and biological mechanisms, the most established ones being blood pressure[34] and serum lipids, and in particular, the relationship between adverse (LDL or low density lipoprotein) and protective (HDL or high density lipoprotein) cholesterol.[35]

Shift Work (with Some of the Work Shift at Night Hours)

The effects of shift work (changing between night and day work) on myocardial infarction risk have been studied for many years. There is growing consensus among researchers that exposure to such shift work can increase myocardial infarction risk and that there can be accumulated risk over time (increasing risk up to 20 years of exposure, after which even decreased risk has been observed — which can be due to a late "healthy worker effect") (for reviews, see Knutsson et al.[36] and Steenland[37]). The mechanism behind this association has been discussed. There can be a direct physiological effect mediated by catecholamines[38] or effects via life habits. It has been found, for instance, that shift workers tend to have a more unhealthy diet than others, and that such a diet can have particularly damaging effects at "odd" meal hours.[39]

Stressors Outside Work

The most widely studied stressor outside work is lack of social support. This can exert its effect *directly* (lack of support, which is a basic need in humans, being a stressor in itself) or *indirectly* (lack of constructive support in stressful situations, inducing a deterioration in expectations and coping). Reviews[40,41] have shown that social network (which is the objective framework for support) and social support (which could be regarded as the functional aspect of network) are strong independent risk factors for myocardial infarction, perhaps more so in men than in women. That social support/network can interact with stressors has been shown in an epidemiological study of myocardial infarction risk in men. This showed that men with pronounced type A behavior had a much higher risk of developing myocardial infarction if there was at the same time a poor social network.[42] Similarly, in a longitudinal study, one immunological parameter, serum immunoglobulin G, showed an increase when job strain (increasing job demands in relation to decision latitude) increased. However, most of this rise took place in subjects with poor social support in the general life situation.[43]

A possible difference between men and women with regard to the effect of social support has been discussed in the literature. In women more often than in men, a large social network can mean more social obligations and therefore constitute a stressor. However, social support does have a protective role for both women and men, although the mechanisms can be different.[44]

Critical Life Events

Two different theories have been tested in relation to the relationship between critical life events and risk of myocardial infarction. The first one deals with *change per se*, the theory being that when a large number of changes that require adaptation occur within a short period, there will be increasing illness susceptibility in general. This theory has been tested by means of two methods, questionnaire and interview (for a review, see Theorell et al.[45]). From retrospective studies, there is support for this theory. Thus, there seems to be a buildup of life events requiring adaptation during the months preceding myocardial infarction. However, the few studies that have been prospective or have used more sophisticated methodology do not give substantial support to this general theory. This can be due to methodological flaws, such as inadequate grouping of events or insufficient attention to the time factor. The second theory deals with effects of *specific changes*, such as retirement, unemployment, migration, and bereavement. For some such events, there is evidence for a relationship. The clearest evidence has been shown for unemployment. Accordingly, long-lasting unemployment is associated with increased myocardial infarction risk.[46] For the other events mentioned in the examples, the evidence seems to be nonconclusive. Loss of a close relative has been associated with increased risk in several studies, but the evidence is conflicting. A recent large prospective Danish study showed that parents who had lost a child had increased risk (approximately 20%) of developing a myocardial infarction during several years of follow-up.[47]

For certain areas, particularly changes at work inducing overload, family conflicts, and negative life events in general,[48–50] there is additional evidence pointing at a relationship. With regard to job changes triggering a myocardial infarction, some events (such as "being praised by the boss" or an event where "pressure of competition was felt") were more important in a 7-day perspective (week before myocardial infarction). Others (such as "high-pressure deadline") had a more immediate effect (day before).

It should be pointed out that a low habitual level of life events can be associated with increased risk of developing hypertension (see Theorell et al.[51]). Positive and negative life events can have very different effects, and hence there is an argument regarding the rationale of adding up positive and negative life events to sum scores. The proponents of this argue that an accumulation of important adaptation-requiring life events within a short period will increase illness risks regardless of whether they are positive or negative.[52] The antagonists claim that positive and negative life events indeed have opposite effects. This depends very much on outcomes. For instance, positive and negative life events, regardless of sign, can increase the incidence of angina pectoris attacks in subjects with known coronary heart disease.[53] On the other hand, a longitudinal study showed that positive and negative life events had opposite effects on blood pressure and serum triglycerides — improvement after positive and deterioration after negative life events.[53,54]

In summary, there is evidence pointing in the direction of a relationship between certain kinds of life events and subsequent elevation of myocardial infarction risk.

Coping Mechanisms

The importance of coping in relation to coronary heart disease and its risk factors has been shown in several studies. In men, type A behavior was discussed extensively in relation to coronary heart disease. During recent years, hostility has been replacing type A behavior as a more precise aspect of coping. Cynical attitudes to family members and workmates are probably the crucial element. There might be a systematic difference between men and women. Accordingly, hostility as a risk factor can be of greater importance to men than to women.[55] On the other hand, a passive-submissive coping behavior can be a more important predictor of myocardial infarction risk in women.[56]

Open and covert coping patterns can be of importance for subjects who are exposed to situations at work when they have been treated in an unfair way. Covert ways of coping were shown to be associated with high blood pressure, especially in men.[57]

Areas for Possible Preventive Strategies — a Summary

Accordingly, there is evidence of a relationship between the following psychosocial factors and myocardial infarction risk:

- Job stressors
  - Low level of decision latitude and job strain (high demand in combination with low decision latitude)
  - Effort–reward imbalance
  - Shift work
- Stressors outside work
  - Lack of social support/network
  - Family conflicts
  - Specific life events such as unemployment and loss of a child
- Coping strategies
  - Hostility (mainly men)
  - Passive submissiveness (mainly women)

SPECIFIC STRATEGIES FOR DIFFERENT STRESSORS

Only a few studies have been published that present data on the evaluation of programs designed to improve the relationship between demands, decision latitude, and social support at work, and how such programs influence cardiovascular health. Of course, it is important to keep the level of psychological demands on a reasonable level. The employer has to take responsibility for the monitoring of demands. However, as long as demands are kept on a reasonable level, most of the organizational improvement has to be focused on the improvement of decision latitude and social support. An excellent review of the theoretical basis for interventions aiming at improved decision latitude and social support has been published by Wahlstedt,[58] who emphasizes that the preparatory work is crucial. The initiative should ideally come from employees. If the employer or some other party takes the initiative, there has to be a preparatory phase during which all other parties become prepared for the change.

There are special programs for improving decision latitude, and controlled evaluation studies of such programs show improved health or psychological conditions after they have been instituted,[59,60] but there are very few studies that show specific effects on cardiovascular risk factors or illness. The psychosocial working conditions are systematically examined using questionnaires, interviews, or observations. The information is fed back to the organization. Conditions that can be deleterious are identified, and after this a dialogue follows. Groups of employees are assigned to prepare written background material for improvement of the identified problems. They should do this within a given time period, and a discussion should follow regarding possible actions to be taken. A small-scale study[61] was based upon a psychosocial intervention process including a questionnaire examination of psychosocial environment and individual factors, feedback (to individuals as well as to the organization), and group discussions. This program was associated with improved decision latitude as well as with improved social support and a subsequent improvement of serum lipid patterns. This was found despite the fact that there were no effects on dietary habits or physical activity. No similar effects were observed in a control population. In the female participants in this study, serum lipids improved more in the experimental part of the organization than in the control part.

The evaluation of another approach has been described by Theorell.[62] The managers in an insurance company were taught psychosocial factors (communication; individual, group, and organization stress and improvement processes) during a program that lasted for a year (2 hours every second week). Their subordinates were followed before and after the program, and these subjects were compared with employees in another part of the same company. Serum cortisol decreased in the employees in the experimental part of the organization, whereas no such change was observed in the control group of employees. The questionnaire data showed that authority over decisions improved in the employees in the experimental group and deteriorated in the control group.

In summary, the available theoretical job stress models could be used as a basis for interventions that can decrease cardiovascular risk. In most programs that have been evaluated, such a psychosocial job site intervention has been part of a general program aiming at improved health, and it has been difficult to disentangle the independent effect of the psychosocial intervention itself. Practical experience has shown that the combination of individual counseling and group interventions is more likely to succeed than interventions that only include one of these two components.

Similarly, there is evidence indicating that improved coping by means of programs for stress management or improved coping in general has the potential to reduce the risk of cardiovascular disease.

Individual Teaching of Stress Management (Improved Coping)

In secondary prevention of cardiovascular disease, several individual stress management principles have been applied, the most extensively studied one being type A behavior modification. This has been shown to be effective in preventing new events by two different groups of researchers, Friedman et al.[63] and Burell and Granlund,[64] although the latter group has pointed out that women and men need different approaches, and as pointed out above, female and male coping patterns associated with increased risk are different. This means that it is possible to reduce the incidence of new events of coronary heart disease in subjects (particularly men) who have had a first myocardial infarction by introducing a behavior modification program aimed at reduced type A behavior. This behavior has three main components: speed and impatience, excessive work involvement, and hostility. Group discussions and video recordings for self-reflection are important components. Reduced type A behavior has been shown to be associated with a reduced number of coronary risk factors as well. A related concept that constitutes the basis for another type of intervention is cynical hostility.[55] The focus is on reduction of cynical hostility, which has been considered to be the core concept of type A behavior and the component that has the strongest relationship with myocardial infarction risk. Cynical hostility is a life attitude, and the program aims at reducing a hostile attitude to other people by means of group work, video recordings (used for self-reflection), and seminars. So far, no publication based upon a controlled intervention study has shown that this program has reduced the number of heart disease cases during follow-up, although it seems to have the potential to do so.

There is an extensive literature indicating that teaching of relaxation techniques can reduce coronary risk. One example is transcendental meditation.[65] Another example is yoga, which has been combined with psychophysiological feedback in an individualized program that was based upon group interventions in work sites. The participants were employees who had been screened for coronary heart disease risk factors. Those with high risk were offered the opportunity to participate in this program. The evaluation was based upon the follow-up after 5 years of subjects who had been randomly allocated to either the intervention (yoga and biofeedback) or control group.[66] The results showed not only that there was a lasting effect on blood pressure recorded at rest, but also that the number of coronary disease events were reduced in the intervention group in the 5-year follow-up. This is one of the few studies that have shown a primary prevention effect.

REFERENCES

1. Kagan, A. and Levi, L. Adaptation of the psychosocial environment to man's abilities and needs. In *Society, Stress and Disease. The Psychosocial Environment and Psychosomatic Diseases*, Levi, L. (Ed.). Oxford University Press, London, 1971.
2. Theorell, T. Health promotion research. In *Health Promotion in the Work Place*, Badura, B. and Kickbusch, I. (Eds.). Oxford University Press, London, 251–266,1991.
3. Selye, H. *The Stress of Life*. McGraw-Hill, New York, 1956.
4. Lazarus, R.S. and Folkman, S. *Stress, Appraisal and Coping*. Springer, New York, 1984.
5. Cooper, C.L. and Marshall, J. Occupational sources of stress: A review of the literature relating to coronary heart disease and mental ill health. *J Occup Psychol*, 49, 11–28, 1976.
6. Landsbergis, P.A. et al. Work stressors and cardiovascular disease. *Work*, 17, 191–208, 2001.
7. Belkic, K. et al. Evidence for mediating econeurocardiologic mechanisms. *Occup Med*, 15, 117–162, 2000.
8. Blomkvist, V. et al. Acoustics and psychosocial environment in intensive coronary care. Accepted for publication in *Occup Environ Med*, 2003.
9. Hagerman, I. et al. Influence of intensive coronary care acoustics on the quality of care and physiological state of patients. *Int J Cardiol*, in press, 2003.
10. Karasek, R.A. Job demands, job decision latitude and mental strain: Implications for job redesign. *Admin Sci Q*, 24, 285–307, 1979.
11. Johnson, J.V. and Hall, E.M. Job strain, workplace support and cardiovascular disease: A cross-sectional study of a random sample of the Swedish working population. *Am J Public Health*, 78, 1336–1342, 1988.
12. Karasek, R. and Theorell, T. *Healthy Work*. Basic Books, New York, 1990.

13. Kristensen, T.S. et al. How to measure quantitative demands at work? Results from a national Danish study. Submitted.
14. Oxenstierna, G. et al. The Double Source Support Model and Its Relationship to Poor Health. *Scand J Pub Health*, in review, 2003.
15. Siegrist, J. Adverse effects of high-effort/low-reward conditions. *J Occup Health Psychol*, 1, 27–41, 1996.
16. Belkic, K. et al. Psychosocial factors: Review of the empirical data among men. In: *Occupational Medicine. The Workplace and Cardiovascular Disease*. Schnall, P. et al. (Eds.), Hanley & Belfus, Inc., Philadelphia, 34–46. 2000.
17. Hlatky, M.A. et al. Job strain and the prevalence and outcome of coronary artery disease. *Circulation*, 92, 327–333, 1995.
18. Kuper, H. and Marmot, M. Intimations of mortality: Perceived age of leaving middle age as a predictor of future health outcomes within the Whitehall II study. *Age Ageing*, 32, 178–184, 2003.
19. Kivimäki, M. et al. Sickness absence as a global measure of health: Evidence from mortality in the Whitehall II prospective cohort study. *BMJ*, 16, 327–364, 2003.
20. Kristensen, T.S. Job stress and cardiovascular disease: A theoretic critical review. *J Occup Health Psychol*, 1, 246–260, 1996.
21. Hallqvist, J. Is the effect of job strain on myocardial infarction risk due to interaction between high psychological demands and low decision latitude? Results from Stockholm Heart Epidemiology Program (SHEEP). *Soc Sci Med*, 46, 1405–1415, 1998.
22. Theorell, T. and Karasek, R.A. Current issues relating to psychosocial job strain and cardiovascular disease research. *J Occup Health Psychol*, 1, 9–26, 1996.
23. Theorell, T. Job stress and fibrinogen. Editorials. *Eur Heart J*, 23, 1799–1801, 2002.
24. Ghiadoni, L. et al. Mental stress induces transient endothelial dysfunction in humans. *Circulation*, 14, 2473–2478, 2000.
25. Theorell, T., Hasselhorn, H.-M., and the MUSIC Norrtälje Study Group. Endocrinological and immunological variables sensitive to psychosocial factors of possible relevance to work-related musculoskeletal disorders. *Work Stress*, 16, 154–165, 2002.
26. Belkic, K. et al. Psychosocial factors: Review of the empirical data among men. In: *Occupational Medicine. The Workplace and Cardiovascular Disease*. Schnall, P. et al. (Eds.), Hanley & Belfus, Inc., Philadelphia, Table 4, 2000.
27. Theorell, T. et al. Changes in job strain in relation to changes in physiological state: A longitudinal study. *Scand J Work Environ Health*, 14, 189–196, 1988.
28. Theorell, T., Karasek, R.A., and Eneroth, P. Job strain variations in relation to plasma testosterone fluctuations in working men: A longitudinal study. *J Intern. Med*, 227, 31–36, 1990.
29. Melamed, S. et al. Repetitive work, work underload and coronary heart disease risk factors among blue collar workers: The CORDIS study. *J Psychosom Res*, 39, 19–29, 1995.
30. Orth-Gomer, K. et al. Social relations and extent and severity of coronary artery disease. The Stockholm Female Coronary Risk Study. *Eur Heart J*, 19, 1648–1656, 1998.
31. Bosma, H., Peter, R., Siegrist, J., and Marmot, M. Two alternative job stress models and the risk of coronary heart disease. *Am J Public Health*, 88, 68–74, 1998.
32. Peter, R. et al. Theory and methods. Psychosocial work environment and myocardial infarction: Improving risk estimation by combining two complementary job stress models in the SHEEP study. *J Epidemiol Commun Health*, 56, 294–300, 2002.

33. Hall, E.M. Women's Work: An Inquiry into the Health Effects of Invisible and Visible Labor. Doctoral thesis, Karolinska Institutet, Stockholm, 1990.
34. Peter, R. et al. High effort, low reward and cardiovascular risk factors in employed Swedish men and women: Baseline results from the WOLF-study. *J Epidemiol Commun Health*, 52, 540–547, 1998.
35. Siegrist, J. Adverse health effects of high effort/low reward condition. *J Occup Health Psychol*, 1, 27–41, 1996.
36. Knutsson, A. et al. Increased risk of ischemic heart disease in shift work. *Lancet*, 8498, 89–92, 1986.
37. Steenland, K. Shift work, long hours and cardiovascular disease: A review. *Occup Med State Art Rev*, 15, 7–10, 2000.
38. Theorell, T. and Åkerstedt, T. Day and night work: Changes in cholesterol, uric acid, glucose and potassium in serum and in circadian patterns of urinary catecholamine excretion. A longitudinal cross-over study of railway workers. *Acta Med Scand*, 200, 47–53, 1976.
39. Lennernäs, M. Nutrition and Shift Work. Doctoral thesis, Uppsala University, Sweden, 1993.
40. Berkman, L.F. The role of social relations in health promotion. *Psychosom Med*, 57, 245–254, 1995.
41. Blom, M. et al. Social relations in women with coronary heart disease: The effects of work and marital stress. *J Cardiovasc Risk*, 10, 201–206, 2003.
42. Orth-Gomer, K. and Unden, A.L. Type A behavior, social support, and coronary risk: Interaction and significance for mortality in cardiac patients. *Psychosom Med*, 52, 59–72, 1990.
43. Theorell, T., Orth-Gomer, K., and Eneroth, P. Slow-reacting immunoglobulin in relation to social support and changes in job strain: A preliminary note. *Psychosom Med*, 52, 511–516, 1990.
44. Berkman, L.F. and Orth-Gomér, K. Prevention of cardiovascular morbidity and mortality: Role of social relations. In *Behavioral Medicine Approaches to Cardiovascular Disease Prevention*, Orth-Goméer, K. and Schneiderman, N. (Eds.). Lawrence Erlbaum Associates, Publishers, Hahwah, NJ, 1996, pp. 51–67.
45. Theorell, T. et al. Critical life events, infections, and symptoms during the year preceding chronic fatigue syndrome (CFS): An examination of CFS patients and subjects with a nonspecific life crisis. *Psychosom Med*, 61, 304–310, 1999.
46. Janlert, U. Unemployment as a disease and diseases of the unemployed. *Scand J Work Environ Health*, 23 (Suppl 3), 79–83, 1997.
47. Li, J., Hansen, D., Mortensen, P.B., and Olsen, J. Myocardial infarction in parents who lost a child. A nationwide prospective cohort study in Denmark. *Circulation*, 106, 1634–1639, 2002.
48. Theorell, T. and Flodérus-Myrhed, B. "Workload" and risk of myocardial infarction: A prospective psychosocial analysis. *Int J Epidemiol*, 6, 17–21, 1977.
49. Möller, J. Case-Crossover Studies of the Triggering of Disease. Myocardial Infarction and Ménière's Disease. Thesis, Karolinska Institutet, Stockholm, 2003.
50. Welin, C. Psychosocial Factors in Myocardial Infarction Patients: A Case-Control Study. Doctoral dissertation, Göteborg University, Sweden, 1995.
51. Theorell, T. et al. Young men with high blood pressure report few recent life events. *J Psychosom Res*, 30, 243–249, 1986.
52. Rahe, R.H. Life change, stress responsivity, and captivity research. *Psychosom Med*, 52, 373–396, 1990.

53. Theorell, T. and Emlund, N. On physiological effects of positive and negative life changes: A longitudinal study. *J Psychosom Res*, 37, 653–659, 1993.
54. Edwards, J.R. and Cooper, C.I. The impact of positive psychological stress and physical health: A review and theoretical framework. *Soc Sci Med*, 27, 1447–1459, 1988.
55. Williams, R.W. and Virginia, P. Managing hostile thoughts, feelings, and actions: The LifeSkills approach. In *Coping with Stress: Effective People and Processes*, Snyder, C.R. (Ed.). 2001, pp. 137–153.
56. Orth-Gomer, K. Psychosocial risk factor profile in women with coronary heart disease. In *Women, Stress, and Heart Disease*, Orth-Gomer, K. and Chesney, M. (Eds.), Mahwah, NJ: Lawrence Erlbaum Associates, 1998, pp. 25–38.
57. Theorell, T. Coping with unfair treatment at work: What is the relationship between coping and hypertension in middle-aged men and women? *Psychother Psychosom*, 69, 86–94, 2000.
58. Wahlstedt, K. Postal work: Work organizational changes as tools to improve health. *Acta Univ Uppsaliensis*, Doctoral thesis, Uppsala, Sweden, 2001.
59. Jackson, S. Participation in decision making as a strategy for reducing job related strain. *J Appl Psychol*, 68, 3–19, 1983.
60. Bond, F.W. and Bunce, D. Job control mediates change in work organization intervention for stress reduction. *J Occup Health Psychol*, 6, 290–302, 2001.
61. Orth-Gomér, K. Lipid lowering through work stress reduction. *Int J Behav Med*, 1, 204–214, 1994.
62. Theorell, T. Employee effects of an educational program for managers at an insurance company. *Psychosom Med*, 63, 724–733, 2001.
63. Friedman, M. et al. Alteration of type A behavior and its effect on cardiac recurrences in post myocardial infarction patients: Summary results of the recurrent coronary prevention project. *Am Heart J*, 112, 653–665, 1986.
64. Burell, G. and Granlund, B. Women's hearts need special treatment. *Int J Behav Med*, 9, 228–242, 2002.
65. King, M.S. and D'Cruz, C. Transcendental meditation, hypertension and heart disease. *Aust Fam Physician*, 31, 164–168, 2002.
66. Patel, C. et al. Trial of relaxation in reducing coronary risk: Four year follow up. *Br Med J*, 13, 1103–1106, 1985.

5 The Role of Stress in Mental Illness: The Practice

R.O. Stanley and G.D. Burrows

CONTENTS

INTRODUCTION

The role of stress in mental ill health is a controversial area of study and yet is of considerable importance with implications for the etiology, prevention, course, and treatment of mental illnesses.

For some professionals and laypeople alike, mental ill health arises primarily from the biological predispositions of the individual passed from generation to generation, while for others, life stressors precipitate and perpetuate mental illness. Among those who focus on the biological predispositions, there are alternative perspectives: those who emphasize the impact of genetic inheritance and those who propose that biology is changed by early-childhood experiences. On the other hand, those with a psychological explanation variously propose that current life stresses, accumulated life stresses, or the impacts of developmental or childhood stressors on

0-8493-1820-3/05/$0.00+$1.50

personality and coping mechanisms are the initiators and perpetuators of mental ill health. Not having acquired coping skills or the appropriate coping skills, or having acquired inappropriate ones, can contribute to the stress process.

The sociological viewpoint proposes that stress is a part of social processes and that sociological impacts are translated into personal distress. This approach emphasizes the impact of social roles, role loss, and role conflict on the individual's ability to function. Stress and distress resulting in mental illness are then symptomatic of social processes.

All of these approaches have some truth, and yet all have their shortcomings. Like most aspects of human existence, the processes around mental illness are likely to be multifactorial, and the causality and course of one condition will differ from the cause and process of another. Seeking or expecting a single and uncomplicated connection between genetic inheritance environmental stressors and mental illness is bound to disappoint. The processes initiating mental ill health can differ considerably from the factors that maintain the pathological processes once commenced.

WHAT IS STRESS?

Stress is a process rather than a diagnosis.[1] Stress is demonstrated when individuals experience either physical or psychological distress, as the demands (or perceived demands) being made upon them exceed their ability to cope (or their self-believed ability to cope). The demands can come from external sources or from individuals' perceptions or expectations of themselves or of others. The impact on coping or not coping can result from their available coping skills or their beliefs about their ability to cope, that is, their confidence and hence diligence in putting into effect the coping strategies they have. On both sides of the stress process, the demands or the available coping strategies can be the result of either real or believed-in factors or impacts.

The demands of the situation or stresses come in a variety of forms. There are those that have their impact because they are severe and would distress any human being, such as can occur in wartime, or when exposed to injury or death associated with disaster or accident. Then there are those that are less severe, as can occur in the work environment, but whose duration and persistence eventually exhaust an individual's resources to cope. Then there are those events that are stressful because they represent personal issues and impacts that are not spread across the population. This personal significance is based on previous life events, prior personal trauma, or developmental learning.

The resources available to allow the individual to cope are likely to vary considerably. The impact of the interaction of the severity and duration of stressful event exposure will be dependent at least to some degree on individual coping skills. When the coping skills are exhausted, stress and distress follow. There are coping resources that are common, if not universal, and those that are highly specialized. The majority have the coping skills to deal with a family bereavement, but few develop or are required to develop the coping skills of emergency workers dealing with horrific events on a frequent basis. Such coping skills can by definition allow the individual to cope, but they cannot in themselves be healthy. For example, the abused child who develops a dissociative mechanism to allow himself to cope with the trauma of abuse can find that that very mechanism, as helpful as it was at the time, becomes unhealthy and pathological as it continues beyond the events that precipitated it.

Those who promote a primarily biological/genetic explanation for stress responses and those who promote a psychological/developmental understanding are both in the minority. For most, the relationship of the stress process to the initiation and maintenance of mental illness results from an interaction of biological or genetic sensitivities; premorbid personality; childhood experiences; acquired coping skills; accumulated, contemporary, or recent external demands; current cognitive style; and self-confidence to effect coping strategies. The most influential proposal over the last decade has been the stress-diathesis theory.

THE STRESS-DIATHESIS PROPOSAL

In its simplest form, this model proposes that emotional and psychiatric disorders arise from the interaction of negative life events with preexisting vulnerabilities. To complicate the picture, these vulnerabilities can represent psychological and biological domains and can be either general or specific in focus.

The model proposes that events interacting with vulnerability result in emotional distress and that this distress then becomes the initiator of mental ill health, resulting in psychiatric disorders. The process by which the stress-induced emotional response results in the mental illness is often not clarified.

There are many versions of this stress-diathesis process,[2] with the general psychological vulnerabilities being represented by the mediational model and the moderational model.[2,3] The mediational model proposes that negative or stressful life events stimulate a hypothesized general psychological vulnerability based on a decreased sense of personal control resulting in psychological distress. This represents a process whereby stressful life events activate the emotional or pathological processes directly and additionally activate a general psychological vulnerability to a diminished sense of control. This generalized psychological vulnerability is itself a pathological initiator of the emotional process. Again, the progression from emotional distress to eventual psychiatric disorder is not elucidated.

The moderational approach proposes that the life event directly results in the psychological distress and psychiatric disorder facilitated or amplified by the psychological vulnerability.

While for some disorders, such as posttraumatic stress disorder, stress is a major contributor to the onset of the disorder, the role of stress in mental ill health remains controversial. Methodological difficulties of studies of the role of stress in the onset of depression, summarized by Clark et al.,[4] prevent the wholehearted support of the stress-diathesis proposal, at least in this disorder.

The stress-diathesis model suggests that there is an inverse interaction between stress severity and psychological or biological vulnerability; that is, those with considerable vulnerability require minor stressor exposure to precipitate the stress response, while those with little vulnerability are only distressed by severe stressor events. This relationship remains to be proven. The nature of these vulnerabilities to stress remains to be clarified. Vulnerabilities can represent a general proneness to stress or can represent only a proneness to particular conditions. The vulnerability can be biological or psychological in nature.

It certainly appears that anxious individuals have both a high resting level of cortical arousal sensitive to perceived threat and a high autonomic system reactivity.[2] It may well be that for some individuals or for some conditions, biological vulnerabilities are a key determinant of stress reactivity, and this can vary considerably. For other individuals or conditions, psychological vulnerabilities can be implicated. Then again, it is further complicated by whether the vulnerabilities are a general stress proneness or a proneness to specific psychiatric conditions.

General Vulnerabilities

General psychological vulnerability can revolve around heightened emotionality; the need for apparent control over situations; a perceived inability to influence and control outcomes; perfectionistic expectations; or excessive concerns about others' opinions and evaluations. Those proposing psychological vulnerabilities to emotional disorders have examined a wide variety of psychological variables, including attributional style, perfectionism, interpersonal dependency, self-criticism, sociotropy, and autonomy, among a plethora of personalities. The research findings are equivocal, with there being at best only partial support for the cognitive stress-diathesis hypothesis.[5]

General biological vulnerability to stress can represent a biological emotional reactivity to internal or external causes. Those with a general proneness to emotional instability (i.e., neuroticism) have a high autonomic nervous system activity and very slow rates of habituation to situations. These stress- and anxiety-prone individuals tend to have high resting levels of cortical arousal, high basal autonomic arousal, and high cognitive and autonomic reactivity.[2] Several lines of evidence support the proposal that the tendency to nervousness, emotionality, "neuroticism," negative affect, anxiety, and being "high strung" runs in families and has a strong genetic component, with 50% of these characteristics arising from genetic or biological vulnerabilities.[2] Kendler[6] has proposed on the basis of a substantial number of family and genetic evaluations that both anxiety, in this case general anxiety disorder, and depression share a common genetic-biological vulnerability, with the specific disorder suffered determined by environmental factors.

Specific Vulnerabilities

Specific vulnerabilities to stress responses can result from acquired processes, including learning experiences and conditioning, or from what the stressor events represent, that is, predisposition to interpret situations as challenging. While general cognitive (schematic) vulnerabilities of sociotropy and autonomy have been suggested to relate to proneness to depression,[7] to date sociotropy has been shown to be a more reliable vulnerability factor than has autonomy.[8]

Specific biological vulnerabilities to disorders such as depression based on alterations to neurotransmitters have long been proposed,[7,9] but the evidence is strongest for those depressive disorders characterized by the vegetative symptoms often referred to as the endogenous depressions. Changes in the neurotransmitter systems, particularly serotonin, are implicated, but it remains unclear whether this is a biological vulnerability to or a consequence of the affective changes.[7,10] The strongest evidence for a specific vulnerability to stress-induced depression comes from family genetic studies.[8] Specific biological vulnerabilities for panic responses separate from general biological vulnerabilities to anxiety (i.e., neuroticism) are also reported.[2]

STRESS AND EPISODES OF PSYCHIATRIC ILL HEALTH

Stress is implicated in the development of mental illnesses and in particular in the initiation of symptom episodes of disorders. This is particularly so in the initiation of the early episodes of disorders and can be less so in subsequent episodes. For example, the *Diagnostic and Statistical Manual* (DSM-IV)[11] notes that "Episodes of Major Depressive Disorder often follow a severe psychosocial stressor.... Studies suggest that psychosocial events (stressors) may play a more significant role in the precipitation of the first or second episodes of Major Depressive Disorder" (p. 342). The methodological difficulties of the studies that have been designed to determine the role of stress in the onset of depression are summarized by Clark et al.[4] The evidence to date prevents the wholehearted support of the stress-diathesis proposal.

Most obviously, acute and posttraumatic stress disorders have a significant stressor event as the precipitant for the psychiatric disturbance.[11] For both disorders sufferers must have been exposed to a traumatic event in which they experienced, witnessed, or were confronted with events that involved actual or threatened death or serious injury, and their response involved intense fear, helplessness, or horror.

For other anxiety disorders, the presence of stress precipitants is not universal. Four ways have been proposed for the acquisition of anxiety responses in the anxiety disorders. Anxiety can be acquired through traumatic learning experiences (i.e., conditioning); vicarious learning or modeling; operant learning, associated with reinforcement related to escape and avoidance; and informational, instructional, and symbolic cognitive processes. Traumatic learning experience accounts for only a portion of the acquisition of specific phobias. Rimm et al.[12] found that of their patient population, 36% of patients could not account for the acquisition of their phobia in terms of some past learning or traumatic experience. Öst and Hugdhal[13] found that 48% of animal phobias, 69% of claustrophobias, 61% of blood and dental phobias, 58% of social phobias, and 91% of agoraphobias could identify direct conditioning experiences implicated in the acquisition of the phobic response. The remainder identified vicarious learning (learning by observation of others) or instructional learning as the source of their phobic concern, and 10 to 20% were unable to specify any experience that might account for their phobia. Barlow[2] proposed that the presence of a traumatic event (true-alarm situation) is not necessary for the acquisition of specific phobic responses, but equally, the presence of a false-alarm situation can become associated with the phobic stimulus via conditioning or other forms of learning. He cited the study of Munjack[14] in driving phobias, where only 20% could report an accident or traumatic experience, while 40% could not account for their anxiety in terms of some life- or injury-threatening experience but reported that they had suddenly panicked while driving — what Barlow[2] refers to as a false-alarm response (panic attack).

THE MANAGEMENT OF STRESS AND MENTAL ILLNESS

In managing stress as a factor in psychological and psychiatric ill health there are four aspects to consider.

The first priority is the effective treatment of the disorder the patient is suffering from, using all the psychological, psychiatric, and pharmacological tools available. Vigorous treatment to relieve suffering is a priority. Stress management before the condition is brought under control is likely to be ineffective and inefficient. Such treatment can focus on psychological, pharmacological, or combined treatments of the precipitated anxiety, depression, or whatever disorder is diagnosed. When the psychiatric, psychological, or physical impact of the condition has been somewhat ameliorated, stress management approaches can be instituted.

When it comes to the other three aspects generally subsumed under the framework of stress management, the aim is to restore the balance between the demands of the situation and the available or effective coping resources. The three orientations of stress management are those that focus on the stressors and are problem-focused; those that focus on developing alternative coping strategies, best characterized as response-focused; and those that focus on the processes that interfere with putting effective, existent coping strategies into effect. These approaches will be individualized following an assessment of the predominant sources of the individual's stress process.

When the source of stress is predominantly the external environment — the demands that the family, personal, social, or employment environment make are excessive — the stress management approach can be problem focused. The excessive demands can be excessive to any person or, as a result of environment–individual mismatch, excessive for this particular person. This stage of stress management can focus on changes in family, relationship, employment, or domains to reduce stressor exposure. This can include relationship or family therapy, workplace negotiation and change, and lifestyle or social change.

Alternatively, the stress process can result from an individual's misperception of excessive environmental demands; inadequate personal coping skills having been acquired; adequate coping skills having been acquired, but inadequate confidence to effect the coping techniques; a dominance of avoidance strategies that prevent management of the demands being made by a situation; or secondary interpretations of not coping and the signs of distress that become part of the stress process in their own right. Response-focused stress management therefore focuses on correcting misperceptions and exaggerations, developing coping skills and alternative strategies, and building confidence in effecting already existing coping strategies. Cognitive therapy, graded exposure, imaginative rehearsal, communications skills, assertiveness skills, negotiation skills, and budgeting and financial management can all fall within these response-focused approaches.

The third component of the stress analysis focuses on the management of processes that can interfere or distract from effective stress management. Also a response-focused solution, the management of basal arousal, both cognitive and physiological, and arousability is often an important part of the process. Heightened arousal or responsiveness to stressor exposure can prevent the individual from engaging the management skills he already has, trying new coping skills, or acquiring different approaches to the stressor management.

Treating the Condition That Arises from the Stress Process

Before attempting to manage the stress process, the individual requires assistance with the psychological or psychiatric disorder that the stress has precipitated. As noted, this must be the first priority, and to prevent ongoing, persistent, or future mental illness, vigorous treatment to relieve suffering is required. Depending on the nature of the precipitated condition, treatment can involve medical (pharmacological) or psychological intervention, or a combination thereof.

The treatment of depressive and anxiety disorders can involve either or both interventions. There is no doubt that for the majority of anxiety disorders psychological interventions are extremely important, focused on arousal management, reinterpretation, or reprocessing of anxiety-connected memories, exposure-based treatments, and conditioning-based treatments.[15] Psychological interventions have demonstrated success in treating specific phobias, agoraphobia, social phobia, posttraumatic stress disorder, and panic disorder, as well as the compulsive part of obsessive-compulsive disorder, and contribute successfully to the management of clinical depression. Pharmacological treatments can focus on symptom or arousal management as well as the treatment of underlying anxiety proneness. Particular pharmacological treatments, including minor tranquilizers (e.g., benzodiazepines) and the newer antidepressant medications, have been successfully used in treating panic disorder, social anxiety disorder, and obsessive-compulsive disorder.[10]

The treatment of depression requires vigorous and determined interventions whether it is the first or subsequent depressive episode, as the evidence suggests that each episode makes subsequent episodes more likely. Both psychological and pharmacological interventions have important parts to play in the effective treatment of depression in all its various forms. Given the impairment arising from depression and the seriousness and persistence of the condition, combined psychological and pharmacological therapies are most commonly warranted. Among the psychotherapies, cognitive behavioral (CBT)[4] and interpersonal (IPT)[16] therapies have a significant contribution to make to the management of depression. Effective antidepressant treatment is also extremely important, and particularly so with the more severe depressive conditions as well as any episodes subsequent to the first episode.[15] Hence, while the severity of the depressive episode can influence the treatment modality, vigorous and sustained intervention is warranted.

Physical conditions to which stress responses contribute require the appropriate medical intervention, as they remain real and significant even if primarily a response to stressors. Hence, respiratory, cardiovascular, inflammatory, gastric, and dermatological conditions in which stress can play a part require effective medical management prior to or in parallel with stress management.

THE FOCUS OF CHANGE

Three strategies can be employed in stress management, dependent upon the situation, the resources available, and the realistic options present. They include focusing on:

1. Eliminating the stress or removing it entirely, seldom a realistic focus
2. Isolating the impact of the stress by allowing only limited exposure or ensuring specialized training to deal with the stressors, such as the specialized training offered to military personnel and emergency workers to best prepare them for managing stress by developing their coping skills
3. Minimizing the stress impact by defeating exaggerated stress responses, addressing avoidant and procrastinating behaviors, developing flexible personal coping strategies, teaching problem-solving and arousal management skills, and establishing regular time out from stressor exposure (i.e., recreation, holidays, job rotation, etc.)

ENVIRONMENTAL CHANGE

If after treating or at least managing the consequent condition the individual assessment indicates that the stressor is largely environmental, then the focus of interventions can be environmental. The two most significant areas of environmental stressors are the workplace[17] and the family or relationship situation.

Workplace change can be an important part of stress management. The various alternative foci and negotiations of workplace change are reviewed by Cooper and Cartwright.[17] The ability to negotiate change in the workplace depends upon the characteristics of the workplace, workplace flexibility, workplace relationships and management style, the negotiating skills of the person suffering distress, and in particular their current negotiating capacity influenced by their current mental health. Involvement of an advocate can be a necessary strategy if the individual's capacity to negotiate is interfered with by his or her distress. While not the first choice, resignation can be an appropriate solution to workplace stressors if change cannot be effected or negotiated. One of the requirements in the minimization is appropriate job–person fit, ensuring that the two are not mismatched.

Although the research is incomplete, some jobs have demonstrated high stressor exposure. They include emergency personnel, including ambulance, police, and fire service employees; those in the military, especially at times of conflict; those in the prison services; health care workers, including doctors, dentists, and nursing staff; teachers; and social workers. Shift work and longer than average working hours have also been demonstrated to be stress amplifiers.[18]

If the source of the current stress response is the interpersonal or family relationship, then relationship and family counseling can be an effective intervention.

Relationship counseling focuses on improved interpersonal communications, issues resolution, changing in joint and individual beliefs, and schema that determine expectations and interpersonal behaviors.[19] Similarly, through family therapy issues that are the environmental source of stress can be resolved.[20] As with job-related environmental causes of stress, separation can be an effective solution to the stress process if not resolvable through couples or family therapies.

Environmental interventions can also include any number of environmental foci such as economic and budgeting counseling to ameliorate economic stressors. Problem-solving interventions[21–23] have been demonstrated to be effective in the management of stress, clinical depression, and other stress-related mental ill health.

PERSONAL CHANGE

Stress moderators have been demonstrated to reduce the likely experience of stress responses.[24] High levels of self-esteem, good social support networks, hardiness, good coping skills, mastery and personal control, emotional stability, and good physiological release mechanisms are protectors against stress responses.[24] Interventions to build these positive influences form a useful part of stress management. Self-esteem building, developing social skills to enhance networking, reinforcing internal locus-of-control beliefs, and teaching physiological release through arousal management are effective contributors to stress management.

Apart from assisting with negotiating environmental change, most stress management interventions focus on personal change, including the development and reinforcement of these coping enhancers. Additionally, interventions can focus on overcoming processes that contribute to negative emotional responses. Cognitive behavioral therapy interventions can be used to alter negative affect-inducing automatic thought processes and schema,[15,25] and other interventions can be used to establish more appropriate coping skills and a more effective habitual coping style.

Part of the analysis of the individual stress process is identification of the idiosyncratic personal and unrealistic perceptions of precipitating events and their personal significance. Stress management can involve the traditional cognitive therapy techniques of assisting the individual, challenging his or her irrational, unrealistic, and maladaptive thoughts.[26]

Coping can be viewed as either a trait or a process,[25] both approaches having strengths and weaknesses. There is evidence that individuals indicate a range of preferred habitual ways of coping, but the preference does not necessarily relate to what can be applied in a particular situation, as noted by Lazarus.[25] From the trait view there are habitual ways of coping with stressful situations: problem solving, effective use of social support, problem avoidance, self-blaming, and fantasy coping.[27] These preferences are not mutually exclusive. It is proposed that there is a hierarchy of preferred coping strategies, with the particular strategy chosen dependent on the situation confronted. An individual can prefer two or three of these strategies over the others. Generally, it is accepted that effective stress management involves a shift to adaptive coping approaches, particularly problem solving and the appropriate seeking of social support. Avoidant coping strategies are reported to be associated with higher levels of stress and burnout in occupational settings.[28]

Problem-solving deficits have been shown to reflect both current emotional state and trait or habitual processes.[29] A shift to problem-solving coping strategies can involve not only defeating procrastination and avoidance, but also developing problem identification and analysis skills and stepwise problem solving. Problem-solving training[23,30] involves a number of steps. The stressed individual needs to recognize that a problem exists, be convinced that a solution is possible, and inhibit the temptation to act impulsively or in habitual ways that might not be appropriate to the situation. The specifics of the problem then need to be identified. The process is then to generate as many solutions to this specific problem as possible, rather than seeking the perfect solution, with inappropriate seeking of perfection being defined in terms of predicted or even fantasized outcome or the social approval that is predicted. The advantages and disadvantages and practicality of the alternatives are then evaluated. The most beneficial practical solution is then chosen and a step-by-step plan for effecting that solution worked out. After the stepwise solution, if commenced at each stage, the effectiveness of the steps and finally the whole plan in achieving the solution of the problem are evaluated. If an approach has been successful in dealing with a stressor, it is reviewed briefly and reinforced. If unsuccessful, the next best alternative solution is then addressed in the same stepwise manner. Problem-solving approaches have been shown to be effective in ameliorating a variety of conditions, but the protective effects in stress management remain to be confirmed by prospective studies. While worry about a problem or stressor has been shown to be motivating and positively contribute to problem solving, the presence of actual anxiety concerning the stressor has been suggested to impede problem solving through reduced perceived control, decreased confidence in the ability to solve the problem, and inability to focus effectively on the problem at hand.[2] Anxiety management might be required before problem solving and general stress management can be effected. Teaching effective time management can also play a part in successful stress management, as can communications skills and assertiveness training.

Stress management might also need to specifically address procrastination and avoidance, perfectionistic beliefs, the tendency to seek fantasy solutions, or self-destructive maladaptive behaviors that compromise the management of stressors, including gambling, alcohol, or drugs. These maladaptive behaviors might need to be addressed before realistic stress management approaches can be adopted.

Seeking social support can involve developing personal communications skills and assertiveness. Activating effective problem solving and the seeking of social support can also require programs to develop self-confidence, self-esteem, psychological protection, and hardiness.

AROUSAL MANAGEMENT

Those with a general proneness to emotional instability (i.e., neuroticism) have high autonomic nervous system activity and very slow rates of habituation to situations. These stress- and anxiety-prone individuals tend to have high resting levels of cortical arousal, high basal autonomic arousal, and high cognitive and autonomic reactivity.[2] The management of habitual physiological or cognitive arousal can also benefit stress management. Cognitive and physiological arousal can both interfere with ongoing stress management. Cognitive arousal can interfere with problem solving through distraction. Arousal can distract the individual from the stressor at hand or be a powerful source activating memories of previous distress.[31] Learning effective arousal management has also been noted to reduce avoidance behavior and enhance expectations and confidence in personal control and the ability to deal with the stressor being experienced. Physiological arousal is both a distraction and a potential physical health hazard.

Holidays are a means of unwinding and recharging the stress management resources. They should not only be viewed as an escape from stressor exposure, but also play a part in managing the timing and duration of stressor exposure.[18] Breaks away from the stressor environment serve the purpose not only of restoring basal arousal to a healthy state, but also of restoring focus and confidence in coping strategies. Short-term rotation of staff in a workplace or parents in their parenting roles can also minimize stressor exposure and restore coping strategies.

There are a wide variety of meditation techniques available.[15,32] Meditation approaches have generally not been systematically studied with the exception of transcendental meditation, which has been shown to be superior to other meditation techniques and to general relaxation training in reducing both acute arousal and habitual or trait anxiety.[33,34] Adverse effects of meditation, while rare, are not unknown.[35]

Relaxation approaches have been a prominent part of stress management over the past 30 years, as well as of the treatment of clinical anxiety and depression.[26,36–39] The benefits of relaxation therapy techniques remain to be equivocally demonstrated. Some studies have demonstrated that relaxation approaches are equal to cognitive therapy approaches,[40] while others have not confirmed the benefits.[41] Relaxation techniques can be effective by their influence on basal arousal or, alternatively, through enhanced perceptions of self-control and self-efficacy.

In some individuals prone to panic attacks, relaxation can induce anxiety[2] hypothesized to relate to perceptions of loss of control associated with relaxation.

Hypnosis and self-hypnosis have been demonstrated to be effective techniques of anxiety and stress management[42–44] and can be applied to the management of habitual arousal or to the acute arousal accompanying exposure to a current stressor. Lowering stress or emotional reactivity can be an effective stress prevention,[42] but hypnotic techniques can also be used to enhance expectations of successful coping in addressing stress-inducing problems and the rehearsal of problem-solving strategies, particularly interpersonal ones.[15,44,45] Effective training is essential for the safe use of hypnosis by clinicians engaged in stress management, as complications can arise from hypnosis inexpertly applied.[45,46]

Physical exercise and the maintenance of physical fitness have also been proposed to reduce inappropriate arousal responses to stressful life events.[44] The benefits have been seen in the reduction of both chronic and acute stress responses. The benefits of exercise in stress management are reported immediately after exercise and also following a regular exercise program.[47,48] Both basal and phasic physiological arousal are also reduced as a result of increased physical fitness. Maintaining participants' motivation in physical fitness and exercise programs remains problematic, particularly early in the process of putting in place this stress management technique.

CONCLUSION

Managing stress can protect the individual against ill health and particularly against mental illness. Psychiatric disturbance and its consequences can in themselves become stressors (e.g., stigma). Once the condition precipitated by the stress process is adequately managed, the focus can shift to problem-focused or response-focused stress management. A wide range of environmental negotiations and change, as well as coping skills modification and cognitive therapy approaches, can become part of the individualized package as a preventative of further episodes of psychiatric ill health. Stress management and resilience building are prophylactic to future ill health.

REFERENCES

1. Stanley, RO & Burrows, GD. (2001). Varieties and functions of human emotion. In RL Payne & CL Cooper (Eds.), *Emotions at Work*. Wiley, Chichester, U.K., Chapter 1.
2. Barlow, DH. (2002). *Anxiety and Its Disorders: The Nature and Treatment of Anxiety and Panic*, 2nd ed. Guilford Press, New York.
3. Chorpita, BF & Barlow, DH. (1998). The development of anxiety: The role of control in the early environment. *Psychological Bulletin*, 124, 3–21.
4. Clark, DA, Beck, AT, & Alford, BA. (1999). *Cognitive Theory and Therapy of Depression*. Wiley, New York.
5. Clark, DA & Steer, RA. (1996). Empirical status of the cognitive model of anxiety and depression. In PM Salkovskis (Ed.), *Frontiers of Cognitive Therapy*. Guilford, New York, Chapter 4.
6. Kendler, KS. (1996). Major depression and generalised anxiety disorder: Same genes, (partly) different environments: Revisited. *British Journal of Psychiatry*, 168 (Suppl.), 68–75.
7. Weissenburger, JE & Rush, AJ. (1996). Biology and cognitions in depression: Does the mind know what the brain is doing? In PM Salkovskis (Ed.), *Frontiers of Cognitive Therapy*. Guilford, New York, Chapter 6.
8. Blackburn, IM. (1996). Cognitive vulnerability to depression. In PM Salkovskis (Ed.), *Frontiers of Cognitive Therapy*. Guilford, New York, Chapter 12.
9. Rush, AJ, Cain, JW, Raese, J, Stewart, RS, Waller, DA, & Debus, JD. (1991). Neurological bases for psychiatric disorders. In RN Rosenberg (Ed.), *Comprehensive Neurology*. Raven Press, New York.
10. Olver, JS, Burrows, GD, & Norman, TR. (2002). Third-generation antidepressants: Do they offer advantages over the SSRIs? *Current Therapeutics*, 43(7), 7–13.
11. American Psychiatric Association (APA). (1994). *Diagnostic and Statistical Manual of Diseases*, 4th ed. (DSM-IV). American Psychiatric Association Press, Washington, DC.
12. Rimm, DC, Janda, LH, Lancaster, DW, Nahl, M, & Dittmar, K. (1977). An exploratory investigation of the origin and maintenance of phobias. *Behavior Research and Therapy*, 15, 231–238.
13. Öst, LG & Hugdhal, K. (1983). Acquisition of agoraphobia, mode of onset and anxiety response patterns. *Behavior Research and Therapy*, 21, 27–34.
14. Munjack, DJ. (1984). The onset of driving phobias. *Journal of Behavior Therapy and Experimental Psychiatry*, 15, 305–308.

15. Burrows, GD, Norman, T, & Stanley, RO. (1999). *Stress, Anxiety and Depression.* Addis Press, French's Forest, Australia.
16. Klerman, GL, Weissman, MM, Rounsaville, BJ, & Chevron, E. (1984). *Interpersonal Psychotherapy of Depression.* Basic Books, New York.
17. Cooper, C & Cartwright, S. (2001). Organizational management of stress and destructive emotions at work. In RL Payne & CL Cooper (Eds.), *Emotions at Work.* Wiley, Chichester, U.K., Chapter 11.
18. Occupational Safety & Health Service (OSHS). (2003). *Healthy Work: Managing Stress and Fatigue in the Workplace.* Department of Labour, Wellington, New Zealand.
19. Dattilio, FM, Epstein, NB, & Baucom, DH. (1998). An introduction to cognitive-behavioral therapy with couples and families. In FM Dattilio (Ed.), *Case Studies in Couple and Family Therapy.* Guilford, New York, Chapter 1.
20. Minuchin, S & Nichols, MP. (1998). Structural family therapy. In FM Dattilio (Ed.), *Case Studies in Couple and Family Therapy.* Guilford, New York, Chapter 5.
21. Nezu, AM. (1986). Efficacy of a social problem-solving therapy approach to unipolar depression. *Journal of Consulting and Clinical Psychology,* 54, 196–202.
22. DeRubeis, RJ & Crits-Christoph, P. (1998). Empirically supported individual and group psychological treatments for adult mental disorders. *Journal of Consulting and Clinical Psychology,* 66, 37–52.
23. D'Zurilla, TJ & Nezu, AM. (1999). *Problem-Solving Therapy: A Social Competence Approach to Clinical Intervention.* Springer, New York.
24. Edwards, D, Hannigan, B, Fothergill, A, & Burnard, P. (2002). Stress management for mental health professionals: A review of effective techniques. *Stress and Health,* 18, 203–215.
25. Lazarus, RS. (1999). *Stress and Emotion: A New Synthesis.* Springer, New York.
26. Beck, JS. (1995). *Cognitive Therapy Basics and Beyond.* Guilford, New York.
27. Vitaliano, PP, Russo, J, Carr, JE, Maiuro, RD, & Becker, J. (1985). The ways of coping checklist: Revision and psychometric properties. *Multivariate Behavioral Research,* 20, 3–26.
28. Koske, GF & Kelly, T. (1995). The impact of over involvement on burnout and job satisfaction. *American Journal of Orthopsychiatry,* 65, 282–292.
29. Garland, A, Harrington, J, House, R, & Scott, J. (2000). A pilot study of the relationship between problem-solving skills and outcome in major depressive disorder. *British Journal of Medical Psychology,* 73, 303–309.
30. Brewin, CR. (1988). *Cognitive Foundations of Clinical Psychology.* Laurence Erlbaum, Sussex, U.K.
31. Flack, WF, Litz, BT, & Keane, TM. (1998). Cognitive-behavioral treatment of war-zone-related posttraumatic stress disorder. In VM Follette, JI Ruzek, & FR Abueg (Eds.), *Cognitive-Behavioral Therapies for Trauma.* Guilford, New York, Chapter 4.
32. Seligman, M. (1994). *What Can You Change and What You Can't.* Random House, Sydney, Australia.
33. Eppley, K, Abrams, A, & Shear, J. (1989). Differential effects of relaxation techniques on trait anxiety: A meta-analysis. *Journal of Clinical Psychology,* 45, 957–974.
34. Kabat-Zinn, J, Massion, AO, Kristeller, J, Peterson, LG, Fletcher, KE, Pbert, L, Lenderking, WR, & Santorelli, SF. (1992). Effectiveness of a meditation-based stress reduction program in the treatment of anxiety disorders. *American Journal of Psychiatry,* 149, 936–943.
35. Otis, L. (1984). Adverse effects of transcendental meditation. In D Shapiro & R Walsh (Eds.), *Meditation: Classic and Contemporary Perspectives.* Aldine, New York.

36. Benson, H. (1975). *The Relaxation Response*. William Morrow, New York.
37. Meichenbaum, D. (1977). *Cognitive-Behavior Modification: An Integrative Approach*. Plenum, New York.
38. Beck, AT, Emery, G, & Greenberg, RT. (1985). *Anxiety Disorders and Phobias: A Cognitive Perspective*. Basic Books, New York.
39. Reynold, WM & Coats, KI. (1986). A comparison of cognitive-behavioral therapy and relaxation training for the treatment of depression in adolescents. *Journal of Consulting and Clinical Psychology*, 54, 653–660.
40. Öst, LG & Westling, B. (1995). Applied relaxation vs. cognitive therapy in the treatment of panic disorder. *Behaviour Research and Therapy*, 33, 145–148.
41. Clark, DM. (1996). Panic disorder: From theory to therapy. In PM Salkovskis (Ed.), *Frontiers of Cognitive Therapy*. Guilford, New York, Chapter 15.
42. Edmonston, WE. (1981). *Hypnosis and Relaxation: Modern Verification of an Old Equation*. Wiley, New York.
43. Jackson, A. (1989). *Stress Control through Self-Hypnosis*. Doubleday, Sydney.
44. Stanley, RO, Norman, TR, & Burrows, GD. (2001). Hypnosis in the management of stress and anxiety disorders. In GD Burrows, RO Stanley, & PB Bloom (Eds.), *International Handbook of Clinical Hypnosis*. Wiley, Chichester, U.K., Chapter 8.
45. Stanley, RO. (1994). The use of hypnosis in the treatment of anxiety disorders: General considerations and contraindications. In BJ Evans (Ed.), *Hypnosis in the Management of Anxiety Disorders*. Australian Society of Hypnosis, Melbourne, Chapter 2.
46. Stanley, RO, Rose, L, & Burrows, GD. (1998). Professional training in the practice of hypnosis: The Australian experience. *American Journal of Clinical Hypnosis*, 41, 29–37.
47. Markoff, RA, Ryan, P, & Young, T. (1982). Endorphins and mood changes in long distance running. *Medicine and Science in Sport and Exercise*, 14, 11–15.
48. Ransford, CP. (1982). A role for amines in the antidepressant effect of exercise: A review. *Medicine and Science in Sport and Exercise*, 14, 1–10.

6 Stress, Endocrine Manifestations, and Diseases

Constantine Tsigos, Ioannis Kyrou, and George P. Chrousos

CONTENTS

STRESS, ENDOCRINE MANIFESTATIONS, AND DISEASES: THE CRITICAL RESEARCH

Life exists by maintaining a complex dynamic equilibrium, or *homeostasis*, that is constantly challenged by intrinsic or extrinsic adverse forces or *stressors.* Stress is thus defined as a state of threatened homeostasis or dysharmony and is counteracted by a complex repertoire of physiologic and behavioral responses that reestablish homeostasis. In this overview, we focus on the neuroendocrine, cellular, and molecular infrastructures of the adaptive responses to stress and discuss the altered regulation or dysregulation of these responses in various physiologic and pathophysiologic states.

0-8493-1820-3/05/$0.00+$1.50

TABLE 6.1
Behavioral and Physical Adaptation during Stress

Behavioral Adaptation
Adaptive Redirection of Behavior
Increased arousal and alertness
Increased cognition, vigilance, and focused attention
Suppression of feeding behavior
Suppression of reproductive behavior
Inhibition of gastric motility; stimulation of colonic motility
Containment of the stress response
Physical Adaptation
Adaptive Redirection of Energy
Oxygen and nutrients directed to the CNS and stressed body site(s)
Altered cardiovascular tone; increased blood pressure and heart rate
Increased respiratory rate
Increased gluconeogenesis and lipolysis
Detoxification from toxic products
Inhibition of growth and reproductive systems
Containment of the stress response
Containment of the inflammatory/immune response

Adapted from Chrousos GP and Gold PW, *JAMA*, 267, 1244, 1992.

Stress Syndrome: Phenomenology

The stress system receives and integrates a great diversity of neurosensory (visual, auditory, somatosensory, nociceptive, visceral), blood-borne, and limbic signals, which arrive through distinct pathways. Activation of the stress system leads to behavioral and physical changes that are remarkably consistent in their qualitative presentation (Table 6.1). These changes are normally adaptive and improve the chances of the individual for survival.[1]

Behavioral adaptation includes increased arousal, alertness, vigilance, and cognition, focused attention, and enhanced analgesia, with concurrent inhibition of vegetative functions, such as feeding and reproduction. Concomitantly, physical adaptation occurs principally to promote an adaptive redirection of energy. Thus, oxygen and nutrients are shunted to the central nervous system (CNS) and the stressed body site(s), where they are needed the most. Increases in cardiovascular tone, respiratory rate, and intermediate metabolism (gluconeogenesis, lipolysis) all work in concert to promote availability of vital substrates. Moreover, the ability of the individual to quickly develop the restraining forces that prevent an overresponse is also essential for a successful general adaptive response. If the restraining or counteracting forces of the body fail to control the elements of the stress response in a timely manner, the adaptive responses can turn maladaptive and contribute to the development of pathology.

Often stress is of a magnitude and nature that allows the perception of control by the individual. Thus, stress can be rewarding and pleasant, even exciting, providing positive stimuli to the individual for emotional and intellectual growth and development.[2] It is of note that the activation of the stress system during feeding and sexual activity, both *sine qua non* functions for survival, is also primarily linked to pleasure.

Stress Syndrome: Physiology

Neuroendocrine Effectors of the Stress Response

Modulation of the activity of the hypothalamic-pituitary unit and the central and peripheral components of the autonomic nervous system is central for a successful adaptive response during stress. The central components of the stress system are located in the hypothalamus and the brainstem and include the parvicellular corticotropin-releasing hormone (CRH) and arginine vasopressin (AVP) neurons of the paraventricular nuclei (PVN) of the hypothalamus, and the CRH neurons of the paragigantocellular and parabranchial nuclei of the medulla, as well as the locus ceruleus (LC) and other catecholaminergic cell groups of the medulla and pons (central sympathetic system).[3,4] The hypothalamic-pituitary-adrenal (HPA) axis, together with the efferent sympathetic/adrenomedullary system, represent the peripheral limbs of this system.

Corticotropin-Releasing Hormone/Arginine Vasopressin/Catecholamines

CRH, a 41-amino acid peptide, was first isolated as the principal hypothalamic stimulus to the pituitary-adrenal axis by Vale et al.[5] in 1981. The subsequent availability of synthetic CRH and of inhibitory analogues opened huge vistas for the investigation of stress. Thus, CRH and CRH receptors were found in many extrahypothalamic sites of the brain, including parts of the limbic system, the basal forebrain, the anterior pituitary, and the central arousal–sympathetic systems (LC/sympathetic systems) in the brainstem and spinal cord.[6,7] In addition, central administration of CRH was shown to set into motion a coordinated series of physiologic and behavioral responses, which included activation of the pituitary-adrenal axis and the sympathetic nervous system, as well as characteristic stress-related behaviors.[8,9] CRH appears, therefore, to have a broader role in coordinating the stress response than had been suspected previously.[3,4] In fact, this neuropeptide seems to reproduce the phenomenology of the stress response as it is summarized in Table 6.1.

CRH binds to specific receptors that belong to the class II seven-transmembrane G-protein-coupled receptor superfamily of receptors.[10] In addition to their wide expression throughout the brain, CRH receptors are found in a variety of peripheral sites, such as the adrenal medulla, prostate, gut, spleen, liver, kidney, and testes. To date, two distinct CRH receptor subtypes have been identified in humans, designated CRH-R1 and CRH-R2, which are encoded by distinct genes on human chromosomes 17 and 7, respectively.[11,12] The CRH-R subtypes share a 70% homology of their amino acid sequence, but exhibit unique pharmacologic profiles, are differentially expressed, and appear to mediate selective actions of CRH at different tissues. The CRH-R1 subtype is widely distributed in the brain, mainly in the anterior pituitary, the neocortex, and the cerebellum, as well as in the adrenal gland, skin, ovary, and testis.[13] CRH-R2 receptors are expressed mainly in the peripheral vasculature, the skeletal muscles, the gastrointestinal tract, and the heart, but also exhibit a widespread distribution in subcortical structures of the brain, such as the lateral septum, amygdala, hypothalamus, and brainstem.[14] CRH-R1 is considered the only receptor type present in the locus ceruleus, cerebellar cortex, thalamus, and striatum, while exclusive CRH-R2 expression has been reported in the bed nucleus of the stria terminalis.[15–17] It is noteworthy that both CRH receptor genes have the ability of variant splicing, thus producing different isoforms for each subtype. The CRH-R1 gene appears to have several splice variants, termed R1b, R1c, R1d, R1e, R1f, R1g, and R1h, which encode proteins with altered N-terminal (CRH-R1c, CRH-R1e, CRH-R1h), intracellular (CRH-R1b, CRH-R1f), and transmembrane (CRH-R1g, CRH-R1d) segments compared to the prototypic CRH-R1a, but their expression in native tissues has not been determined yet.[18] Accordingly, the CRH-R2c gene has three splice variants, encoding the CRH-R2a, CRH-R2b, and CRH-R2g isoforms, which differ only at the extracellular N-terminus and have unique tissue distributions. The CRH-R2a receptor is localized to subcortical regions, including the lateral septum and the paraventricular and ventromedial nuclei of the hypothalamus. Conversely, the CRH-R2b receptor is primarily localized to the heart, gastrointestinal tract, skeletal muscles, and in nonneural brain tissues, such as the cerebral arterioles and the choroid plexus, while the CRH2g receptor has recently been identified in human amygdala.[14] The diversity of CRH receptor subtype and isoform expression is considered to play a key role in the modulation of the stress response by implicating locally the actions of different ligands (CRH and CRH-related peptides) and different intracellular second messengers.

The central neurochemical circuitry responsible for activation of the stress system has been studied extensively and is summarized in Figure 6.1. There are apparently multiple sites of interaction among the central components of the stress system. Reciprocal reverberatory neural connections exist between the CRH and catecholaminergic neurons of the central stress system, with CRH and norepinephrine (NE) stimulating each other, the latter primarily through α1-noradrenergic receptors.[19–21] Autoregulatory ultrashort negative feedback loops also exist in both the PVN CRH and brainstem catecholaminergic neurons,[22,23] with collateral fibers inhibiting CRH and catecholamine secretion, respectively, via inhibiting presynaptic CRH and α2-noradrenergic receptors.[24] Both the CRH and catecholaminergic neurons also receive stimulatory innervation from the serotoninergic and cholinergic systems[25,26] and inhibitory input from the γ-aminobutyric acid (GABA)/benzodiazepine (BZD) and the opioid neuronal systems of the brain,[27,28] as well as by the end product of the HPA axis, glucocorticoids.[29]

Arginine vasopressin (AVP) is a nonapeptide also produced by parvicellular neurons of the PVN and secreted into the hypophyseal portal system. While AVP secreted by the magnocellular neurons of neurohypophysis is crucial for fluid and electrolyte homeostasis, AVP of PVN origin holds a key role in the response to stressors, being the second most important modulator of pituitary corticotropin (ACTH) secretion.[30] Whereas CRH appears to directly stimulate ACTH secretion, AVP and other factors, such as angiotensin II, have synergistic or additive effects.[31–33] AVP shows synergy with CRH *in vivo*, when the peptides are co-administered in

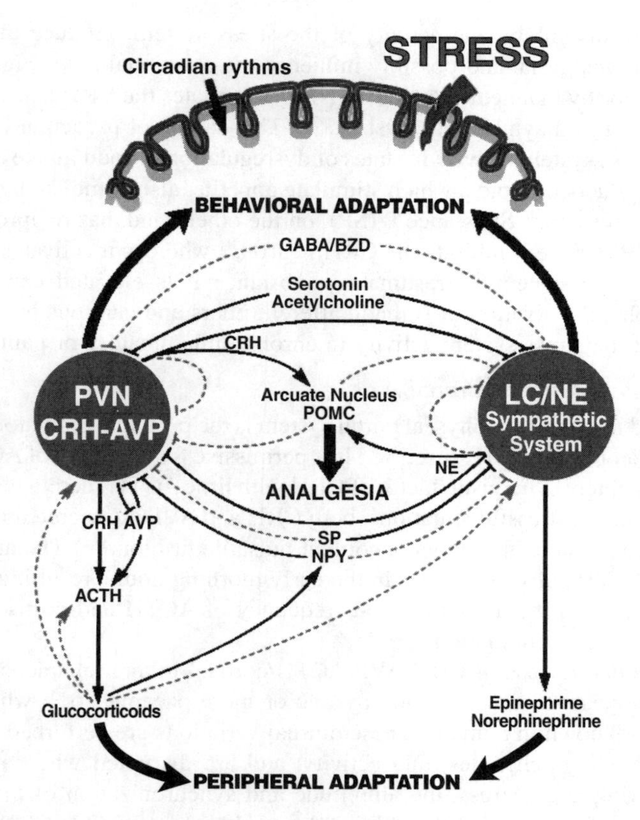

FIGURE 6.1 A simplified representation of the central and peripheral components of the stress system, their functional interrelations, and their relationships to other central nervous systems involved in the stress response. Activation is represented by solid lines and inhibition by dashed lines. (Adapted from Chrousos GP and Gold PW, *JAMA*, 267, 1244, 1992.)

humans.[34] AVP interacts with a V1-type receptor (V1β, also referred to as V3) and exerts its effects through calcium/phospholipid-dependent mechanisms.[35] The synergistic effect of AVP on the pituitary ACTH secretion offers an alternate pathway, mediated by different neuropeptides, to influence the subsequent HPA axis activation at the hypothalamic level, since catecholamines stimulate CRH secretion, while ghrelin, a novel growth hormone (GH) secretagogue factor, appears to stimulate predominantly AVP secretion.[36,37] A subset of parvocellular neurons synthesize and secrete both CRH and AVP. The relative proportion of this subset increases significantly with stress.

Another group of PVN CRH neurons also sends projections to proopiomelanocortin (POMC)-containing neurons in the arcuate nucleus of the hypothalamus, which in turn reciprocally project to the PVN CRH neurons and innervate the catecholaminergic neurons of the central stress system in the brainstem, as well as descending pain control neurons of the hindbrain and spinal cord. Thus, activation of the stress system stimulates hypothalamic β-endorphin and other POMC–peptide secretions, which reciprocally inhibit the activity of the stress system, produce the so-called stress-induced analgesia, and possibly influence the emotional tone (Figure 6.1).

It is noteworthy that neuropeptide Y (NPY) stimulates the CRH neuron, whereas it inhibits the central sympathetic system.[38,39] This can be of particular relevance to changes in stress system activity in states of dysregulation of food intake and obesity. Interestingly, glucocorticoids, which stimulate appetite, also stimulate hypothalamic NPY gene expression.[40] Substance P (SP), on the other hand, has reciprocal actions to those of NPY, since it inhibits the CRH neuron,[41] whereas it activates the central catecholaminergic system.[42] Presumably, substance P is elevated centrally when there is peripheral activation of somatic afferent fibers and can thus have relevance to changes in the stress system activity in chronic inflammatory or painful states.[43]

Hypothalamic-Pituitary-Adrenal Axis

CRH released into the hypophyseal portal system is the principal regulator of anterior pituitary corticotroph ACTH secretion.[4] It is permissive for secretion of ACTH, while AVP acts as a potent synergistic factor of CRH with little ACTH secretagogue activity by itself.[44–46] In nonstressful situations, both CRH and AVP are secreted in the portal system in a circadian and highly concordant pulsatile fashion.[47,48] The amplitude of the CRH and AVP pulses increases in the early morning hours, resulting eventually in increases of both the amplitude and frequency of ACTH and cortisol secretory bursts in the general circulation.[49,50]

The circadian release of CRH/AVP/ACTH/cortisol in their characteristic pulsatile manner appears to be controlled by one or more pacemakers,[51] whose precise location is not known in humans. These diurnal variations are perturbed by changes in lighting, feeding schedules, and activity, and are disrupted when a stressor is imposed. During acute stress, the amplitude and synchronization of the CRH and AVP pulsations increases, with additional recruitment of PVN, CRH, and AVP secretion. Especially in conditions of strong hypovolemic stress, such as created by marked hypotension or hemorrhage, additional AVP of magnocellular neuron origin is secreted into both the hypophyseal portal system, via collateral neuraxon terminals, and the systemic circulation. In addition, depending on the stressor, angiotensin II as well as various cytokines and lipid mediators of inflammation are secreted and act on hypothalamic, pituitary, and adrenal components of the HPA axis, mostly to potentiate its activity.

The adrenal cortex is the principal target organ of the pituitary-derived circulating ACTH. The latter is the key regulator of glucocorticoid and adrenal androgen secretion by the *zonae fasciculata* and *reticularis*, respectively, while it also participates in the control of aldosterone secretion by the *zona glomerulosa*.[52] Moreover, there is evidence suggesting that the regulation of cortisol secretion is also influenced by other hormones and cytokines, originating from the adrenal medulla or coming from the systemic circulation, and by neuronal signals from the autonomic innervation of the adrenal cortex.

Glucocorticoids are the final effectors of the HPA axis. These hormones are pleiotropic and exert their effects through their ubiquitously distributed intracellular receptors.[53] The nonactivated glucocorticoid receptor resides in the cytosol in the form of a hetero-oligomer with heat-shock proteins and immunophilin.[54] Upon ligand binding, the glucocorticoid receptors dissociate from the rest of the hetero-oligomer, homodimerize, and translocate into the nucleus, where they interact with specific glucocorticoid-responsive elements (GREs) within the DNA to transactivate or transrepress appropriate hormone-responsive genes.[55]

In addition, the activated receptors inhibit, by protein–protein interactions, important transcriptional factors, such as the c-jun/c-fos heterodimer, which promotes the transcription of several genes involved in the activation of immune and other cells,[56,57] and the NF-κB[58] heterodimer, which is of particular importance in immune and inflammatory responses. They also change the stability of mRNAs and hence the translation rates of several glucocorticoid-responsive proteins. Furthermore, glucocorticoids influence the secretion rates of specific proteins and alter the electrical potential of neuronal cells, through mechanisms that have not yet been precisely defined.

Glucocorticoids play a key regulatory role in the basal control of HPA axis activity and in the termination of the stress response, by acting at extrahypothalamic regulatory centers, the hypothalamus, and the pituitary gland.[59] The inhibitory glucocorticoid feedback on the ACTH secretory response acts to limit the duration of the total tissue exposure to glucocorticoids, thus minimizing the catabolic, lipogenic, antireproductive, and immunosuppressive effects of these hormones. Interestingly, a dual receptor system exists for glucocorticoids in the CNS, including the glucocorticoid receptor type I, or mineralocorticoid receptor, which responds to low levels of glucocorticoids and is primarily activational, and the classic glucocorticoid receptor (type II), which responds to higher levels of glucocorticoids, stress-related or not, and is dampening in some systems and activational in others. The negative feedback control of the CRH and ACTH secretions is mediated through type II glucocorticoid receptors.

Sympathetic/Adrenomedullary and Parasympathetic Systems

The autonomic nervous system provides a rapidly responsive mechanism to control a wide range of functions. Cardiovascular, respiratory, gastrointestinal, renal, endocrine, and other systems are regulated by either the sympathetic nervous system or the parasympathetic system or both.[60] Generally, the parasympathetic system can equally assist sympathetic functions by withdrawing or antagonize them by increasing its activity.

Sympathetic innervation of peripheral organs is derived from the efferent preganglionic fibers whose cell bodies lie in the intermediolateral column of the spinal cord. These nerves synapse in the bilateral chain of sympathetic ganglia with postganglionic sympathetic neurons, which innervate widely the smooth muscle of the vasculature, the skeletal muscles, heart, kidney, gut, adipose tissue, and many other organs.[61] The preganglionic neurons are primarily cholinergic, whereas the postganglionic neurons release mostly noradrenaline. The sympathetic system also has a humoral contribution from circulating epinephrine and, to a lesser extent, norepinephrine released from the adrenal medulla, which can be considered a modified sympathetic ganglion.

In addition to the classic neurotransmitters acetylcholine and norepinephrine, both sympathetic and parasympathetic subdivisions of the autonomic nervous system contain several subpopulations of target-selective and neurochemically coded neurons that express a variety of neuropeptides and, in some cases, adenosine triphosphate (ATP), nitric oxide, or lipid mediators of inflammation.[62] Thus, CRH, NPY, somatostatin, and galanin are colocalized in noradrenergic vasoconstrictive neurons, whereas vasoactive intestinal polypeptide (VIP) and, to a lesser extent, substance P (SP) and calcitonin gene-related peptide (CGRP) are colocalized in cholinergic neurons. Transmission in sympathetic ganglia is also modulated by neuropeptides released from preganglionic fibers and short interneurons (e.g., enkephalin, neurotensin) and primary afferent (e.g., substance P, VIP) collaterals.[63] Thus, the particular combination of neurotransmitters in sympathetic neurons is strongly influenced by central and local factors, which can trigger or suppress specific genes.

Stress System Interactions with Other CNS Components

In addition to setting the level of arousal and influencing the vital signs, the stress system also interacts with two other major CNS elements, the mesocorticolimbic dopaminergic system and the amygdala/hippocampus.[64–66] Both of these systems are activated during stress and, in turn, influence the activity of the stress system.

Mesocorticolimbic Dopaminergic System

The mesocortical and mesolimbic components of the dopaminergic system are innervated by PNV CRH neurons and the LC-NE/sympathetic noradrenergic system. Both components are activated by catecholamines, CRH, and glucocorticoids during stress. The mesocortical system contains dopaminergic neurons of the ventral tegmentum that send projections to the prefrontal cortex. The activation of these neurons is thought to centrally suppress the response of the stress system and is implicated in anticipatory phenomena and cognitive functions.[65] The mesolimbic system, which consists of dopaminergic neurons, also of the ventral tegmentum, that innervate the nucleus accumbens, is believed to play a principal role in motivational/reinforcement/reward phenomena.[67]

Amygdala/Hippocampus

The amygdala/hippocampus complex is activated during stress primarily by ascending catecholaminergic neurons originating in the brainstem or by inner emotional stressors, such as conditioned fear, possibly from cortical association areas.[66] The amygdala nuclei are the principal brain locus for fear-related behaviors, and their activation is important for retrieval and emotional analysis of all the relevant stored information for any given stressor. In response to emotional stressors, the amygdala can directly stimulate both central components of the stress system and the mesocorticolimbic dopaminergic system. Interestingly, there are CRH peptidergic neurons in the amygdala that respond positively to glucocorticoids and whose activation leads to stimulation of the stress system and anxiety. CRH neurons in the central nucleus of the amygdala send projections to the parvicellular regions of the PVN and the parabrachial nucleus of the brainstem, which are considered crucial for the CRH neuroendocrine, autonomic, and behavioral effects. CRH fibers also interconnect the amygdala with the bed nucleus of the stria terminalis and the hypothalamus.[68,69] Conversely to the stimulatory influence of norepinephrine and CRH, the hippocampus exerts an important inhibitory influence on the activity of the amygdala, as well as of the PVN/CRH and LC/sympathetic systems.

Stress System: Endocrine Interactions

Reproductive Axis

The reproductive axis is inhibited at all levels by various components of the HPA axis (Figure 6.2). CRH suppresses the gonadotropin hormone-releasing hormone (GnRH) neuron both directly and indirectly, via enhancing β-endorphin secretion by the arcuate POMC neurons. Glucocorticoids, on the other hand, exert inhibitory effects at the level of the GnRH neuron, the pituitary gonadotroph, and the gonads themselves, and additionally render target tissues of sex steroids resistant to these

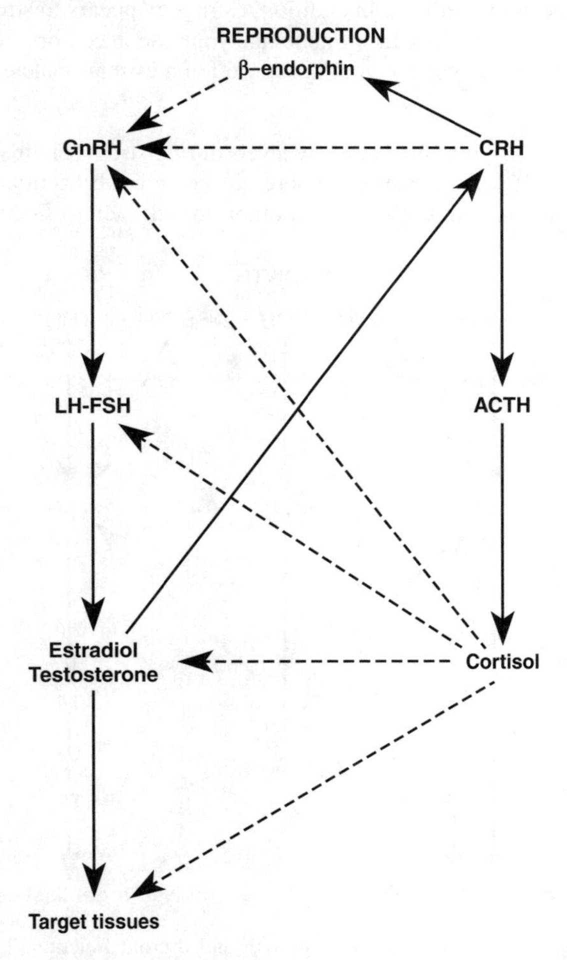

FIGURE 6.2 A simplified representation of the interactions between the HPA axis and the reproductive axis. Activation is represented by solid lines and inhibition by dashed lines. (Adapted from Chrousos GP and Gold PW, *JAMA*, 267, 1244, 1992.)

hormones.[70–72] Cytokines also suppress reproductive function at several levels.[73] Thus, steroidogenesis is directly inhibited at both ovaries and testes, with concomitant inhibition of the pulsatile secretion of the gonadotropin-releasing hormone from the hypothalamus. The latter effect is exerted both directly and by activating hypothalamic neural circuits that contain CRH and POMC.

The interaction between CRH and the gonadal axis appears to be bidirectional. The presence of estrogen response elements in the promoter area of the CRH gene and direct stimulatory estrogen effects on CRH gene expression have been shown.[74] This finding implicates the CRH gene, and therefore the HPA axis, as a potentially important target of ovarian steroids and a potential mediator of gender-related differences in the stress response/HPA axis activity.[75] On the other hand, the activated estrogen receptor interacts with and, on occasion, potentiates the c-jun/c-fos heterodimer, which mediates several cytokine effects. In addition, estrogen appears to stimulate adhesion molecules and their receptors in immune and immune accessory cells. This might explain why autoimmune diseases afflict more females than males.

Growth Axis

The growth axis is also inhibited at many levels during stress (Figure 6.3). Prolonged activation of the HPA axis leads to suppression of growth hormone secretion and inhibition of somatomedin C (SmC) and other growth factor effects on their target

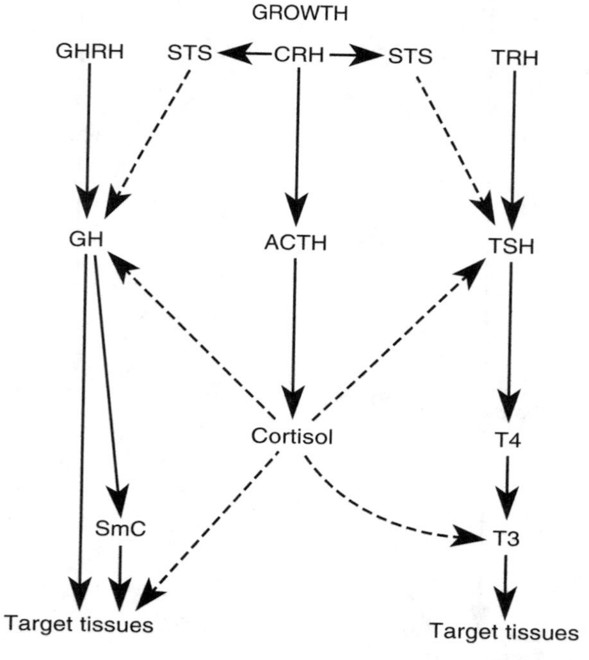

FIGURE 6.3 Effects of the HPA axis on growth and thyroid function. T4, thyroxine; T3, triiodothyronine. Activation is represented by solid lines and inhibition by dashed lines. (Adapted from Chrousos GP and Gold PW, *JAMA*, 267, 1244, 1992.)

tissues by glucocorticoids,[76–78] the latter presumably via inhibition of the c-jun/c-fos heterodimer. However, acute elevations of growth hormone concentration in plasma can occur at the onset of the stress response in man and after acute administration of glucocorticoids, presumably through stimulation of the growth hormone gene by glucocorticoids through its GREs.[79] In addition to direct effects of glucocorticoids, which are pivotal in the suppression of growth observed in prolonged stress, increases in somatostatin secretion caused by CRH, with resultant inhibition of growth hormone secretion, have also been implicated as a potential mechanism of stress-related suppression of growth hormone secretion.[80] The redirection of nutrients and vital substrates to the brain and other areas where they are needed most during stress is the apparent teleology for the adverse effects of chronic stress on growth.

Thyroid Axis

A corollary phenomenon to growth axis suppression is the stress-related inhibition of thyroid axis function (Figure 6.3). Activation of the HPA axis is associated with decreased production of thyroid-stimulating hormone (TSH) and inhibition of conversion of the relatively inactive thyroxine to the more biologically active triiodothyronine in peripheral tissues (the "euthyroid sick" syndrome).[81,82] Although the exact mechanism(s) for these phenomena is not known, both phenomena might be caused by the increased levels of glucocorticoids and can serve to conserve energy during stress. Inhibition of TSH secretion by CRH-stimulated increases in somatostatin might also participate in the central component of thyroid axis suppression during stress. In the case of inflammatory stress, inhibition of TSH secretion and enhancement of somatostatin production can be in part through the action of cytokines on the hypothalamus and pituitary.[83,84]

Metabolism

Glucocorticoids, the hormonal end product of the HPA axis, exert primarily catabolic effects as part of a generalized effort to utilize every available energy resource against the challenge posed by intrinsic or extrinsic stressors. Thus, glucocorticoids increase hepatic gluconeogenesis and plasma glucose concentration, induce lipolysis (although they favor abdominal and dorsocervical fat accumulation), and cause protein degradation at multiple tissues (e.g., muscle, bone, skin) to provide amino acids that would be used as an additional substrate at oxidative pathways. In addition to their direct catabolic actions, glucocorticoids also antagonize the beneficial anabolic actions of GH, insulin, and sex steroids on their target tissues.[85] This shift of the metabolism toward a catabolic state under the control of the activated HPA axis normally reverses upon retraction of the enforced stressor. Thus, chronic activation of the HPA axis would be damaging, as it is expected to increase visceral adiposity, decrease lean body (muscle and bone) mass, suppress osteoblastic activity, and cause insulin resistance (Figure 6.4). Interestingly, the phenotype of Cushing's syndrome, characterized by abdominal and trunk fat accumulation and decreased lean body mass, in combination with manifestations of the metabolic syndrome (visceral adiposity, insulin resistance, dyslipidemia, hypercoagulability, hypercytokinemia, hypertension), is present in a variety of pathophysiologic conditions, collectively described as pseudo-Cushing's states. The pseudo-Cushing's states are presumably

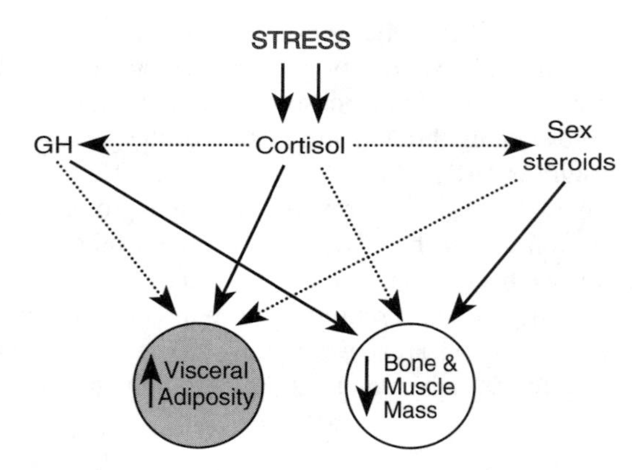

FIGURE 6.4 Detrimental effects of chronic stress on adipose tissue metabolism and bone and muscle mass. Stimulation is represented by solid lines and inhibition by dashed lines.

attributed to HPA-induced mild hypercortisolism or to adipose tissue-specific hypersensitivity to glucocorticoids.[85–87]

The balance of metabolic homeostasis is also centrally affected by the neuroendocrine integration of the HPA axis and the central stress pathways to the CNS centers that control appetite/satiety and energy expenditure.[88] It is a common observation that stressful situations are associated with anorexia and profound suppression of food intake. Indeed, CRH stimulates the POMC neurons of the arcuate nucleus, which via α-melanocyte-stimulating hormone (α-MSH) release elicit antiorexigenic signals and increase thermogenesis.[89] Suppression of neuropeptide Y secretion is likely to be involved in stress-induced anorexia. It should also be noted, however, that glucocorticoids enhance the intake of carbohydrates and fat and inhibit energy expenditure by stimulating the secretion of NPY at the hypothalamus, which is a potent appetite stimulator[90] that additionally inhibits the locus ceruleus–norepinephrine system and activates the parasympathetic system, thus facilitating digestion and storage of nutrients.[91,92]

Gastrointestinal Function

An increasing body of evidence suggests that CRH is involved in the central mechanisms by which stress influences gastrointestinal function (Figure 6.5). During acute stress, PVN CRH induces both inhibition of gastric emptying and stimulation of colonic motor function, independently of the associated stimulation of the HPA axis, by alterations in the autonomic nervous system activity. It is considered that inhibition of the vagus nerve activity at the dorsal vagal complex results in selective inhibition of gastric motility, while stimulation of the sacral parasympathetic system activity, possibly through CRH projections of the Barrington nucleus,[93] which is part of the locus ceruleus complex, results in selective stimulation of colonic motility.[94] It is believed that inhibition of gastric emptying involves the medullary CRH-R2 receptors and possibly the peripheral CRH-R2 receptors at the gastrointestinal track, while the CRH-R1 subtype appears to mediate the colonic motor responses. Thus, CRH might be implicated in the gastric stasis that is asso-

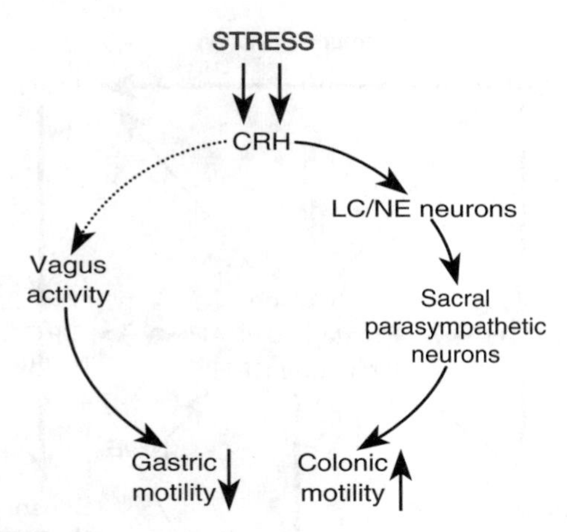

FIGURE 6.5 Effects of stress on gastrointestinal function. Stimulation is represented by solid lines and inhibition by dashed lines.

ciated with the stress of surgery or with high levels of central interleukin-1,[95] as well as in the stress-induced colonic hypermotility of irritable bowel syndrome (IBS). Interestingly, the colonic contraction in patients with IBS can activate the LC/sympathetic neurons, thus forming a vicious cycle, which can help explain the chronicity of the condition. In addition to altering the motility pattern, stressors exert profound influences in several other aspects of the gastrointestinal function, as it has been found that the stress-induced activation of central and peripheral CRH receptors causes dysfunction of the intestinal barrier, increases gastrointestinal permeability, and can enhance relapses of inflammatory bowel disease.[96–98]

Stress System: Immune System Interactions

Effects of the Immune System on the Stress System

The immune system exerts its surveillance–defense function constantly and mostly unconsciously for the individual. It has been known for several decades that immune/inflammatory insults in the form of an infectious disease, an active autoimmune inflammatory process, or an accidental or operative trauma are associated with concurrent activation of the HPA axis. More recently, it also became apparent that immune cytokines and other humoral mediators of inflammation are potent activators of central stress-responsive neurotransmitter systems, constituting the afferent limb of the feedback loop through which the immune/inflammatory system and the CNS communicate (Figure 6.6). Through this pathway, the peripheral immunologic apparatus signals the brain to participate in maintaining immunological and behavioral homeostasis.[99,100]

The three main inflammatory cytokines, tumor necrosis factor-alpha (TNF-α), interleukin-1 (IL-1), and interleukin-6 (IL-6), are produced at inflammatory sites and elsewhere in a cascade-like fashion, with TNF-α appearing first, followed by IL-1 and IL-6 in tandem, and can cause stimulation of the HPA axis *in vivo*, alone, or in synergy with each other.[101,102] This can be blocked significantly with CRH-

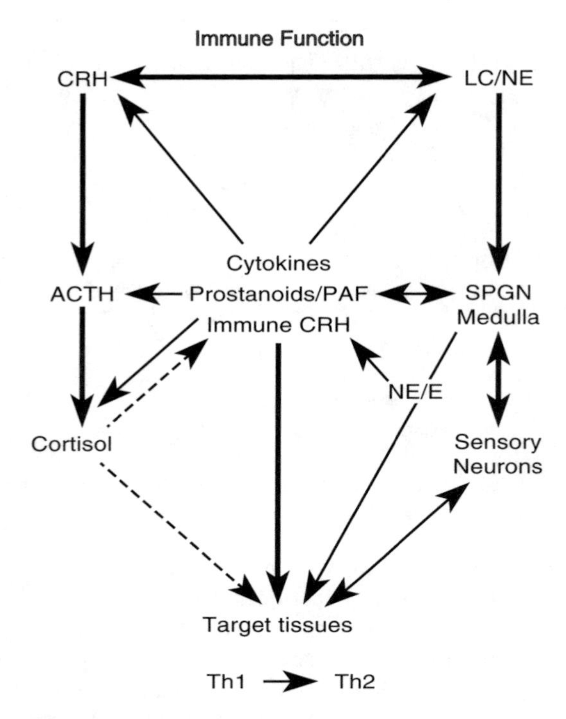

FIGURE 6.6 Interactions between stress and the immune system. SPGN, sympathetic post-gaglionic neuron. Stimulation is represented by solid lines and inhibition by dashed lines.

neutralizing antibodies, prostanoid synthesis inhibitors, and glucocorticoids. In addition, all three cytokines directly stimulate hypothalamic CRH secretion *in vitro*, an action also suppressed by glucocorticoids and prostanoid synthesis inhibitors.[103–105]

There is evidence to suggest that IL-6, the main endocrine cytokine, plays the primary role in the immune stimulation of the human HPA axis, especially in the long term. Thus, in humans, IL-6 is an extremely potent activator of the axis, importantly without the vascular leak-promoting and hypotensive side effects of the other two inflammatory cytokines.[83,106] The elevations of ACTH and cortisol attained by IL-6 are well above those observed with maximal stimulatory doses of CRH, suggesting that parvicellular AVP and other ACTH secretagogues are also stimulated by this cytokine. At high doses, IL-6 also stimulates peripheral elevations of AVP, presumably as a result of a stimulatory effect on magnocellular AVP-secreting neurons.[107] This suggests that IL-6 might be involved in the genesis of the syndrome of inappropriate antidiuretic hormone secretion (SIADH), which is observed during the course of infectious/inflammatory disease or during trauma.

Some of the activating effects of inflammation on the HPA axis can be exerted indirectly, via stimulation of the central catecholaminergic pathways by the inflammatory cytokines and other humoral mediators of inflammation. Also, activation of peripheral nociceptive, somatosensory, and visceral afferent fibers would lead to stimulation of both the catecholaminergic and CRH neuronal systems via ascending spinal pathways. Interestingly, in chronic inflammatory states, where chronic central elevations of substance P might take place, an impairment of HPA axis responsiveness to stimuli or stress is observed, probably because of the suppressive effect of substance P on the CRH neuron.[41] Such an impairment has been observed in African trypanosomiasis and extensive burns in humans and in chronic animal models of inflammation.[43,108]

Other inflammatory mediators can also participate in the activation of the HPA axis, in addition to the three inflammatory cytokines. Thus, several eicosanoids, platelet-activating factor (PAF), and serotonin show potent CRH-releasing properties.[26,109,110] It is not clear, however, which of the above effects are endocrine and which are paracrine. Direct effects, albeit delayed, of most of the above cytokines and mediators of inflammation on pituitary ACTH secretion, on the other hand, have also been shown,[83,111,112] and direct effects of these substances on adrenal glucocorticoid secretion appear to be present as well.[113]

An interesting aspect of the immune response is that CRH is also secreted peripherally at inflammatory sites (peripheral or immune CRH) by postganglionic sympathetic neurons and by cells of the immune system (e.g., macrophages, tissue fibroblasts).[114] The secretion of immune CRH has been examined in both experimental animal models of inflammation[114] and patients with rheumatoid arthritis,[115] Hashimoto thyroiditis, and other inflammatory illnesses.[116] Immune CRH secretion is suppressed by glucocorticoids and somatostatin.[114] Mast cells are considered the primary target of immune CRH, where, along with substance P, it acts via CRH-R1 receptors causing degranulation. Subsequently, histamine is released, causing vasodilation, increased vascular permeability, and other manifestations of local inflammation. Thus, locally secreted CRH triggers a peripheral CRH-mast cell-histamine axis, which has potent pro-inflammatory properties, whereas central CRH alleviates the immune response.[99,117]

Effects of the Stress System on the Immune/Inflammatory Reaction

Activation of the HPA axis has profound inhibitory effects on the inflammatory/immune response, because virtually all the components of the immune response are inhibited by cortisol (Figure 6.6). At the cellular level, alterations of leukocyte traffic and function, decreases in production of cytokines and mediators of inflammation, and inhibition of their effects on target tissues are among the main anti-inflammatory effects of glucocorticoids.[53] These effects are exerted both at the resting, basal state and during inflammatory stress, when the circulating concentrations of glucocorticoids are elevated. Thus, a circadian activity of several immune functions has been demonstrated in reverse-phase synchrony with that of plasma glucocorticoid levels.

A large infrastructure of anatomical, chemical, and molecular connections allows communication not only within, but also between the neuroendocrine and the immune system. The efferent sympathetic/adrenomedullary system apparently participates in a major fashion in the interactions of the HPA axis and the immune/inflammatory stress by being reciprocally connected with the CRH system, by receiving and transmitting humoral and nervous immune signals from the periphery, by densely innervating both primary and secondary lymphoid organs, and by reaching all sites of inflammation via the postganglionic sympathetic neurons.[118,119] Thus, leukocytes and macrophages contain specific receptors for neurotransmitters, neuropeptides, and neurohormones that influence their functions, while the immune cells themselves are also capable of producing many of these substances. When activated during stress, the autonomic system exerts its own direct effects on immune organs, which can be immunosuppressive (e.g., inhibition of natural killer cell activity) or both immunopotentiating and immunosuppressive by inducing secretion of IL-6 in the systemic circulation.[120]

It should be underlined that the effects of stress on the immune system are better characterized as immunomodulating, rather than immunosuppressing. Both glucocorticoids and catecholamines directly inhibit the production of type 1 cytokines, such as IL-12, IL-2, TNF-α, and interferon-γ(INF-γ), which enhance cellular immunity and T-helper 1 (Th1) formation, and conversely favor the production of type 2 cytokines, such as IL-10, IL-4, and IL-13, which induce humoral immunity and T-helper 2 (Th2) formation.[121] Thus, during an immune challenge, stress causes an adaptive Th1-to-Th2 shift to protect the tissues from the potentially destructive actions of the pro-inflammatory type 1 cytokines and other products of activated macrophages. The homeostatic role of stress-induced Th2 shift against overshooting of cellular immunity often complicates pathologic conditions where either cellular immunity is beneficial (e.g., carcinogenesis, infections) or humoral immunity is deleterious (e.g., allergy, autoimmune diseases).

STRESS, ENDOCRINE MANIFESTATIONS, AND DISEASES: THE PRACTICE

Generally, the stress response with the resultant activation of the HPA axis is meant to be acute or at least of limited duration. The time-limited nature of this process renders its accompanying catabolic, antireproductive, antigrowth, and immunosuppressive effects temporarily beneficial and of no adverse consequences. Chronicity of stress system activation, on the other hand, would lead to the syndromal state that Selye described in 1936.[1] Since CRH coordinates behavioral, neuroendocrine, autonomic, and immunologic adaptation during stressful situations, increased and prolonged production of CRH could explain the pathogenesis and all the manifestations of the chronic stress syndrome, including the psychiatric, circulatory, metabolic, and immune components.

INCREASED HYPOTHALAMIC-PITUITARY-ADRENAL AXIS ACTIVITY: PATHOPHYSIOLOGY

Dysregulation of the generalized stress response is typically described in the syndrome of melancholic depression, which leads to dysphoric hyperarousal and chronic activation of the HPA axis and the sympathetic nervous system.[122,123] Indeed, cortisol excretion is elevated and plasma ACTH response to exogenous CRH is decreased.[124,125] These abnormalities are state related and resolve coincident to waning psychopathology. Hypersecretion of CRH has been shown in depression and suggests that CRH might participate in the initiation or perpetuation of a vicious cycle. It is

TABLE 6.2
States Associated with Altered Hypothalamic-Pituitary-Adrenal Axis Activity and Dysregulation of Behavioral and Peripheral Adaptation

Increased HPA Axis	Decreased HPA Axis
Chronic stress	Adrenal insufficiency
Melancholic depression	Atypical/seasonal depression
Anorexia nervosa	Chronic fatigue syndrome
Obsessive-compulsive disorder	Fibromyalgia
Panic disorder	Hypothyroidism
Excessive exercise (obligate athleticism)	Nicotine withdrawal
Chronic active alcoholism	Postglucocorticoid therapy
Alchohol and narcotic withdrawal	Post-Cushing's syndrome cure
Diabetes mellitus	Postpartum period
Central obesity (pseudo-Cushing's syndrome)	Postchronic stress
Childhood sexual abuse	Rheumatoid arthritis
Hyperthyroidism	Premenstrual tension syndrome
Cushing's syndrome	Climacteric depression
Pregnancy	

Updated from Chrousos GP and Gold PW, *JAMA*, 267, 1244, 1992.

noteworthy that depressed patients were found on autopsy to have increased numbers of PVN CRH neurons.[126] Whether this is genetically determined, environmentally induced, or both is unclear at the present time.

In addition to melancholic depression, a spectrum of other conditions can be associated with increased and prolonged activation of the HPA axis (Table 6.2). These include anorexia nervosa and malnutrition,[127–129] obsessive-compulsive disorder,[130] panic anxiety,[131] excessive exercising,[132] chronic active alcoholism,[133] alcohol and narcotic withdrawal,[134,135] diabetes mellitus, especially when complicated by diabetic neuropathy,[136,137] central (visceral) obesity,[87,138] childhood sexual abuse,[139] and perhaps hyperthyroidism[140] and the premenstrual tension syndrome.[141] In addition, Cushing's syndrome is characterized by autonomous excess production of glucocorticoids, which interrupts the integrity of the HPA axis by suppressing PVN CRH and by increasing the exposure of tissues to glucocorticoids. It is of interest that anorexia nervosa and malnutrition are characterized by increased levels of CSF NPY, which could provide an explanation as to why the HPA axis in these subjects is activated, while the LC/sympathetic system shows clear evidence of profound hypoactivity. Glucocorticoids, by stimulating NPY and by inhibiting the NE/sympathetic system, would produce the hyperphagia and visceral obesity observed in Cushing's syndrome.

Pregnancy is another condition characterized by hypercortisolism of a degree similar to that observed in severe depression, anorexia nervosa, and mild Cushing's syndrome, and is the only known physiologic state in humans in which CRH circulates in plasma at levels high enough to cause activation of the HPA axis.[142,143] Although circulating CRH, which is of placental origin, is bound with high affinity to CRH-binding protein,[144,145] it appears that the circulating free fraction is sufficient to explain the observed escalating hypercortisolism when the concentration of CRH-binding protein starts to gradually decrease in plasma after the 35th week of pregnancy.[146]

Hyperactivation of the HPA axis is associated with increased susceptibility of the individual to a host of infectious agents and tumors. An excessive response of the HPA axis and a prolonged Th2 shift has been associated with relapse of mycobacterial infections, progression of HIV infection, and infections that follow major traumatic injuries or burns. In addition, several studies report a higher incidence of tumor growth and metastases in correlation to stress, highlighting the role of cellular immunity in surveillance and eradication of tumor cells.[147]

Decreased Hypothalamic-Pituitary-Adrenal Axis Activity: Pathophysiology

Hypoactivation of the stress system, in which chronically reduced secretion of CRH can result in pathological hypoarousal, characterizes another group of states (Table 6.2). Patients with seasonal depression and chronic fatigue syndrome fall in this category.[148,149] In the depressive (winter) state of the former and in the period of fatigue in the latter, there is chronically decreased activity of the HPA axis. Similarly, patients with fibromyalgia have decreased urinary free cortisol excretion and frequently complain of fatigue.[150] Hypothyroid patients also have clear evidence of CRH hyposecretion.[140] Interestingly, one of the major manifestations of hypothyroidism is depression of the atypical type. Withdrawal from smoking has also been associated with decreased cortisol and catecholamine secretion.[151,152] Decreased CRH secretion in the early period of nicotine abstinence could explain the contemporary hyperphagia and weight gain frequently associated with smoking withdrawal. It is interesting that in Cushing's syndrome, the clinical picture of hyperphagia and weight gain, as well as fatigue and anergia, is consistent with the suppression of the CRH neuron by the associated hypercortisolism.[85,153] The period after cure of hypercortisolism, the postpartum period, and periods following cessation of stress are also associated with suppressed PVN CRH secretion and decreased HPA axis activity.[154]

A defective HPA axis response to inflammatory stimuli would reproduce the glucocorticoid deficient state and would lead to relative resistance to infections and neoplastic disease, but increased susceptibility to autoimmune/inflammatory disease.[155,156] Indeed, such properties were unraveled in an interesting pair of near-histocompatible, highly inbred rat strains, the Fischer and Lewis rats, both genetically selected out of Sprague-Dawley rats for their resistance or susceptibility, respectively, to inflammatory disease.[157,158] Setting off from the findings in this animal model, there is increasing evidence that patients with rheumatoid arthritis have a mild form of central hypocortisolism, as they have reduced 24-h cortisol excretion, less pronounced diurnal rhythm of cortisol secretion, and blunted adrenal responses to surgical stress.[159,160] Thus, dysfunction of the HPA axis can actually play a role in the development or perpetuation of autoimmune disease, rather than being an epiphenomenon.

Potential Role of CRH Antagonists in Clinical Practice

The association of a wide spectrum of disease with dysregulation of the stress system response suggests that low-molecular-weight CRH-R1 and CRH-R2 antagonists, which could be absorbed orally and cross the blood–brain barrier, might have a potential role in the treatment of disorders characterized by pathogenetic disturbances of the CRH pathways.[18]

Antalarmin is a nonpeptidic prototype CRH antagonist that binds with high affinity to CRH-R1. This small lipophilic pyrrolopyrimidine compound decreases the activity of the HPA axis and LC-NE, and blocks a variety of manifestations associated with anxiety, as well as the development and expression of conditioned fear.[161] In addition, antalarmin suppresses stress-induced peptic ulcer, colonic hyperfunction, and neurogenic inflammation and blocks CRH-induced skin mast cell degranulation.[18,162–166] Importantly, the chronic administration of antalarmin is not associated with glucocorticoid or catecholamine deficiency and permits HPA axis and LC-NE responses to severe stress.[167] The data from several studies that tested the efficacy of such CRH-R1 antagonists indicate a potential therapeutic role in human pathologic states, such as melancholic depression, chronic anxiety, narcotic withdrawal, irritable bowel syndrome, allergic reactions, and autoimmune inflammatory disorders.

Experimental data from the use of selective CRH-R2 antagonists are limited.[18] The identification of the specific CRH-R2 neuronal pathways that are implicated in pathologic conditions in humans and a better understanding of the physiologic role of CRH-related peptides, such as urocortin (Ucn) I, UcnII, UcnIII, and urotensin I, will clarify the therapeutic potential of these agents. CRH-R2 antagonists are expected to be useful in the treatment of atypical depression, chronic fatigue syndrome, fibromyalgia, and stress-induced anorexia.[18,168–170]

ABBREVIATIONS

α-MSH	α-Melanocyte-stimulating hormone
AVP	Arginine vasopressin
ACTH	Corticotropin
BZD	Benzodiazepine
cAMP	Cyclic adenosine monophosphate
CNS	Central nervous system
CRH	Corticotropin-releasing hormone
CRH-R	Corticotropin-releasing hormone receptor
DNA	Deoxyribonucleic acid
FSH	Follicle-stimulating hormone
GABA	γ-Aminobutyric acid
GH	Growth hormone
GHRH	Growth hormone-releasing hormone
GnRH	Gonadotropin-releasing hormone
GREs	Glucocorticoid-responsive elements
HPA axis	Hypothalamic-pituitary-adrenal axis

IL-1	Interleukin-1
IL-6	Interleukin-6
LC-NE	Locus ceruleus–norepinephrine/sympathetic system
LH	Luteinizing hormone
PAF	Platelet-activating factor
POMC	Proopiomelanocortin
PVN	Paraventricular nucleus
SmC	Somatomedin C
STS	Somatostatin
T-helper lymphocyte	Th lymphocyte
TRH	Thyrotropin-releasing hormone
TNF-α	Tumor necrosis factor-α
TSH	Thyroid-stimulating hormone

REFERENCES

1. Chrousos GP, Gold PW. (1992). The concepts of stress system disorders: Overview of behavioral and physical homeostasis. *JAMA* 267:1244–1252.
2. Dorn LD, Chrousos GP. (1993). The endocrinology of stress and stress system disorders in adolescence. *Endocrinol Metab Clin North Am* 22:685–700.
3. Chrousos GP. (1992). Regulation and dysregulation of the hypothalamic-pituitary-adrenal axis: The corticotropin-releasing hormone perspective. *Endocrinol Metab Clin North Am* 21:833–858.
4. Tsigos C, Chrousos GP. (1994). Physiology of the hypothalamic-pituitary-adrenal axis in health and dysregulation in psychiatric and autoimmune disorders. *Endocrinol Metab Clin North Am* 23:451–466.
5. Vale W, Spiess J, Rivier C, et al. (1981). Characterization of a 41-residue ovine hypothalamic peptide that stimulates secretion of corticotropin and beta-endorphin. *Science* 213:1394–1397.
6. Aguilera G, Millan MA, Hauger RL, et al. (1987). Corticotropin-releasing factor receptors: Distribution and regulation in brain, pituitary, and peripheral tissues. *Ann NY Acad Sci* 512:48–66.
7. DeSouza EB, Insel TR, Perrin MH, et al. (1985). Corticotropin-releasing factor receptors are widely distributed within the rat central nervous system. *J Neurosci* 5:3189–3203.
8. Cole B, Koob GF. (1991). Corticotropin-releasing factor, stress and animal behavior. In *Stress, Neuropeptides and Systemic Disease*, McCubbin JA, Kauffman PG, Nemeroff CB (Eds.). Academic Press, New York, p. 119.
9. Dunn AJ, Berrigde CW. (1990). Physiological and behavioral responses to corticotropin-releasing factor administration: Is CRF a mediator of anxiety or stress response? *Brain Res Rev* 15:71–100.
10. Perrin MH, Vale WW. (1999). Corticotropin releasing factor receptors and their ligand family. *Ann NY Acad Sci* 20:312–328.
11. Polymeropoulos MH, Torres R, Yanovski JA, et al. (1995). The human corticotrophin releasing factor receptor gene maps to chromosome 17q12-q22. *Genomics* 1:123–124.

12. Meyer AH, Ullmer C, Schmuck K, et al. (1997). Localization of the human CRF2 receptor to 7p21-p15 by radiation hybrid mapping and FISH analysis. *Genomics* 15:189–190.
13. Chen R, Lewis KA, Perrin MH, Vale WW. (1993). Expression cloning of a human corticotropin-releasing-factor receptor. *Proc Natl Acad Sci USA* 90:8967–8971.
14. Lovenberg TW, Halmers DT, Liu C, et al. (1995). CRF2a and CRF2b receptor mRNAs are differentially distributed between the rat central nervous system and peripheral tissues. *Endocrinology* 136:4139–4142.
15. Chalmers DT, Lovenberg TW, De Souza EB. (1995). Localization of novel corticotropin-releasing factor receptor (CRF2) mRNA expression to specific subcortical nuclei in rat brain: Comparison with CRF1 receptor mRNA expression. *J Neurosci* 15:6340–6350.
16. Sanchez MM, Young LJ, Plotsky PM, et al. (1999). Autoradiographic and *in situ* hybridization localization of corticotropin-releasing factor 1 and 2 receptors in the nonhuman primate brain. *J Comp Neurol* 408:365–377.
17. Wong ML, Licinio J, Pasternak KI, Gold PW. (1994). Localization of corticotropin-releasing hormone receptor mRNA in adult rat brain by *in situ* hybridization histochemistry. *Endocrinology* 135:2275–2278.
18. Grammatopoulos DK, Chrousos GP. (2002). Functional characteristics of CRH receptors and potential clinical applications of CRH-receptor antagonists. *Trends Endocrinol Metab* 13:436–444.
19. Calogero AE, Gallucci WT, Gold PW, et al. (1988). Multiple regulatory feedback loops on hypothalamic CRH secretion. Potential clinical implications. *J Clin Invest* 82:767–774.
20. Valentino RJ, Foote SL, Aston-Jones G. (1983). Corticotropin-releasing hormone activates noradrenergic neurons of the locus ceruleus. *Brain Res* 270:363–367.
21. Kiss A, Aguilera G. (1992). Participation of α_1-adrenergic receptors in the secretion of hypothalamic corticotropin-releasing hormone during stress. *Neuroendocrinology* 56:153–160.
22. Calogero AE, Gallucci WT, Chrousos GP, et al. (1988). Effect of the catecholamines upon rat hypothalamic corticotropin releasing hormone secretion *in vitro*. *J Clin Invest* 82:839–846..
23. Silverman A, Hou-Yu A, Chen WP. (1989). Corticotropin-releasing factor synapses within the paraventricular nucleus of the hypothalamus. *Neuroendocrinology* 49:291–299.
24. Aghajanian GK, Van der Maelen CP. (1982). α_2-Adrenoreceptor-mediated hyperpolarization of locus ceruleus neurons: Intracellular studies *in vivo*. *Science* 215:1394–1396.
25. Calogero AE, Bagdy G, Szemeredi K, et al. (1990). Mechanisms of serotonin agonist-induced activation of the hypothalamic-pituitary-adrenal axis in the rat. *Endocrinology* 126:1888–1894.
26. Fuller RW. (1992). The involvement of serotonin in regulation of pituitary-adrenocortical function. *Front Neuroendocrinol* 13:250–270.
27. Calogero AE, Gallucci WT, Chrousos GP, et al. (1988). Interaction between GABAergic neurotransmission and rat hypothalamic CRH *in vitro*. *Brain Res* 463:28–36.
28. Overton JM, Fisher LA. (1989). Modulation of central nervous system actions of corticotropin-releasing factor by dynorphin-related peptides. *Brain Res* 488:233–240.
29. Keller-Wood ME, Dallman MF. (1984). Corticosteroid inhibition of ACTH secretion. *Endocr Rev* 5:1–24.

30. Antoni FA. (1993). Vasopressinergic control of pituitary adrenocorticotropin secretion comes of age. *Front Neuroendocrinol* 14:76–122.
31. Gillies GE, Linton EA, Lowry PJ. (1982). Corticotropin-releasing activity of the new CRF is potentiated several times by vasopressin. *Nature* 299:355–357.
32. Rivier C, Rivier J, Mormede P, et al. (1984). Studies on the nature of the interaction between vasopressin and corticotropin-releasing factor on adrenocorticotropin release in the rat. *Endocrinology* 115:882–886.
33. Vale W, Vaughan J, Smith M, et al. (1983). Effects of synthetic ovine corticotropin-releasing factor, glucocorticoid, catecholamines, neuro-hypophyseal peptides, and other substances on cultured corticotropic cells. *Endocrinology* 113:1121–1131.
34. Lamberts SW, Verleun T, Oosterom R, et al. (1984). Corticotropin-releasing factor and vasopressin exert a synergistic effect on adrenocorticotropin release in man. *J Clin Endocrinol Metab* 58:298–303.
35. Antoni FA. (1987). Receptors mediating the CRH effects of vasopressin and oxytocin. *Ann NY Acad Sci* 512:195–204.
36. Al-Damluji S, Cunnah D, Grossman A, et al. (1987). Effect of adrenaline on basal and ovine corticotropin-releasing factor-stimulated ACTH secretion in man. *J Endocrinol* 112:145–150.
37. Korbonits M, Kaltsas G, Perry LA, et al. (1999). The growth hormone secretagogue hexarelin stimulates the hypothalamo-pituitary-adrenal axis via arginine vasopressin. *J Clin Endocrinol Metab* 84:2489–2495.
38. Egawa M, Yoshimatsu H, Bray GA. (1991). Neuropeptide Y suppresses sympathetic activity to interscapular brown adipose tissue in rats. *Am J Physiol* 260(Pt 2):R328–R334.
39. Oellerich WF, Schwartz DD, Malik KU. (1994). Neuropeptide Y inhibits adrenergic transmitter release in cultured rat superior cervical ganglion cells by restricting the availability of calcium through a pertussis toxin-sensitive mechanism. *Neuroscience* 60:495–502.
40. White BD, Dean RG, Edwards GL, Martin RJ. (1994). Type II corticosteroid receptor stimulation increases NPY gene expression in basomedial hypothalamus of rats. *Am J Physiol* 266(Pt 2):R1523–R1529.
41. Larsen PJ, Jessop D, Patel H, et al. (1993). Substance P inhibits the release of anterior pituitary adrenocorticotrophin via a central mechanism involving corticotrophin-releasing factor-containing neurons in the hypothalamic paraventricular nucleus. *J Neuroendocrinol* 5:99–105.
42. Culman J, Tschope C, Jost N, et al. (1993). Substance P and neurokinin A induced desensitization to cardiovascular and behavioral effects: Evidence for the involvement of different tachykinin receptors. *Brain Res* 15:75–83.
43. Jessop DS, Chowdrey HS, Larsen PJ, et al. (1992). Substance P: Multifunctional peptide in the hypothalamo-pituitary system? *J Endocrinol* 132:331–337.
44. Abou-Samra AB, Harwood JP, Catt KJ, et al. (1987). Mechanisms of action of CRF and other regulators of ACTH release in pituitary corticotrophs. *Ann NY Acad Sci* 512:67–84.
45. Gillies GE, Linton EA, Lowry PJ. (1982). Corticotropin-releasing activity of the new CRF is potentiated several times by vasopressin. *Nature* 299:355–357.
46. Antoni FA. (1993). Vasopressinergic control of pituitary adrenocorticotropin secretion comes of age. *Front Neuroendocrinol* 14:76–122.
47. Engler D, Pham T, Fullerton MJ, et al. (1989). Studies on the secretion of corticotropin releasing factor and arginine vasopressin into hypophyseal portal circulation of the conscious sheep. *Neuroendocrinology* 49:367–381.

48. Redekopp C, Irvine CH, Donald RA, et al. (1990). Spontaneous and stimulated adrenocorticotropin and vasopressin pulsatile secretion in the pituitary venous effluent of the horse. *Endocrinology* 118:1410–1416.
49. Horrocks PM, Jones AF, Ratcliffe WA, et al. (1990). Patterns of ACTH and cortisol pulsatility over twenty-four hours in normal males and females. *Clin Endocrinol (Oxf)* 32:127–134.
50. Iranmanesh A, Lizarralde G, Short D, et al. (1990). Intensive venous sampling paradigms disclose high-frequency adrenocorticotropin release episodes in normal men. *J Clin Endocrinol Metab* 71:1276–1283.
51. Veldhuis JD, Iranmanesh A, Johnson ML, et al. (1990). Amplitude, but not frequency, modulation of adrenocorticotropin secretory bursts gives rise to the nyctohemeral rhythm of corticotropic axis in man. *J Clin Endocrinol Metab* 71:452–463.
52. Aguilera G. (1993). Factors controlling steroid biosynthesis in the zona glomerulosa of the adrenal. *J Steroid Biochem Molec Biol* 45:147–151.
53. Munck A, Guyre PM, Holbrook NJ. (1984). Physiological functions of glucocorticoids in stress and their relation to pharmacological actions. *Endocr Rev* 5:25–44.
54. Smith DF, Toft DO. (1993). Steroid receptors and their associated proteins. *Mol Endocrinol* 7:4–11.
55. Pratt WB. (1990). Glucocorticoid receptor structure and the initial events in signal transduction. *Prog Clin Biol Res* 322:119–320.
56. Jonat C, Rahmsdorf HJ, Park KK, et al. (1990). Antitumor promotion and anti-inflammation: Down modulation of AP-1 (fos/jun) activity by glucocorticoid hormone. *Cell* 62:1189–1204.
57. Yang-Yen HF, Chambard JC, Sun YL, et al. (1990). Transcriptional interference between c-jun and the glucocorticoid receptor: Mutual inhibition of DNA binding due to direct protein-protein interaction. *Cell* 62:1205–1215.
58. Matsusaka T, Fujikawa K, Nishio Y, et al. (1993). Transcription factors NF-IL6 and NF-kappa B synergistically activate transcription of the inflammatory cytokines, interleukin 6 and interleukin 8. *Proc Natl Acad Sci USA* 1:10193–10197.
59. deKloet ER. (2000). Stress in the brain. *Eur J Pharmacol* 29:187–198.
60. Gilbey MP, Spyer KM. (1990). Essential organization of the sympathetic nervous system. *Baillieres Clin Endocrinol Metab* 7:259–278.
61. Burnstock G, Miller P. (1989). Structural and chemical organization of the autonomic nervous system with special reference to noradrenergic non-cholinergic transmission. In *Autonomic Failure. A Textbook of Clinical Disorders of the Autonomic Nervous System*, Bannister R, Mathias CJ (Eds.). Oxford Medical Press, Oxford, p. 107.
62. Benarroch EE. (1994). Neuropeptides in the sympathetic system: Presence, plasticity, modulation, and implications. *Ann Neurol* 36:6–13.
63. Elfvin LC, Lindh B, Hokfelt T. (1993). The chemical neuroanatomy of sympathetic ganglia. *Annu Rev Neurosci* 16:471–507.
64. Nikolarakis KE, Almeida OF, Herz A. (1986). Stimulation of hypothalamic beta-endorphin and dynorphin release by corticotropin-releasing factor (*in vitro*). *Brain Res* 3:152–155.
65. Roth RH, Tam SY, Ida Y, et al. (1988). Stress and the mesocorticolimbic dopamine systems. *Ann NY Acad Sci* 537:138–147.
66. Gray TS. (1989). Amygdala, role in autonomic and neuroendocrine responses to stress. In *Stress, Neuropeptides and Systemic Disease*, McCubbin JA, Kauffman PG, and Nemeroff C (Eds.). Academic Press, New York, p. 37.
67. Chrousos GP. (1998). Stressors, stress, and neuroendocrine integration of the adaptive response. The 1997 Hans Selye Memorial Lecture. *Ann NY Acad Sci* 30:311–335.

68. Grigoriadis D, Heroux J, De Souza EB. (1993). Characterization and regulation of corticotropin-releasing factor receptors in the central nervous, endocrine and immune systems. *Ciba Found Symp* 72:85–101.
69. Millan MJ. (1981). Stress and endogenous opioid peptides. *Mod Probl Pharmacopsychiatry* 17:49–67.
70. MacAdams MR, White RH, Chipps BE. (1986). Reduction in serum testosterone levels during chronic glucocorticoid therapy. *Ann Intern Med* 140:648–651.
71. Rabin D, Schmidt P, Gold PW, et al. (1990). Hypothalamic-pituitary-adrenal function in patients with the premenstrual syndrome. *J Clin Endocrinol Metab* 71: 1158–1162.
72. Rivier C, Rivier J, Vale W. (1986). Stress-induced inhibition of reproductive function: Role of endogenous corticotropin releasing factor. *Science* 231:607–609.
73. Tsigos C, Papanicolaou DA, Kyrou I, et al. (1999). Dose-dependent effects of recombinant human interleukin-6 on the pituitary-testicular axis. *J Interferon Cytokine Res* 19:1271–1276.
74. Vamvakopoulos NC, Chrousos GP. (1993). Evidence of direct estrogen regulation of human corticotropin releasing hormone gene expression: Potential implications for the sexual dimorphism of the stress response and immune/inflammatory reaction. *J Clin Invest* 92:1896–1902.
75. Vamvakopoulos NC, Chrousos GP. (1994). Hormonal regulation of human corticotropin-releasing hormone gene expression: Implications for the stress response and immune/inflammatory reaction. *Endocr Rev* 15:409–420.
76. Burguera B, Muruais C, Penalva A, et al. (1990). Dual and selective actions of glucocorticoids upon basal and stimulated growth hormone release in man. *Neuroendocrinology* 51:51–58.
77. Dieguez C, Page MD, Scanlon MF. (1988). Growth hormone neuroregulation and its alterations in disease states. *Clin Endocrinol (Oxf)* 28:109–143.
78. Unterman TG, Phillips LS. (1985). Glucocorticoid effects on somatomedins and somatomedin inhibitors. *J Clin Endocrinol Metab* 61:618–626.
79. Casanueva FF, Burguera B, Muruais C, et al. (1990). Acute administration of corticosteroids: A new and peculiar stimulus of growth hormone secretion in man. *J Clin Endocrinol Metab* 70:234–237.
80. Rivier C, Vale W. (1985). Involvement of corticotropin-releasing factor and somatostatin in stress induced inhibition of growth hormone secretion in the rat. *Endocrinology* 117:2478–2482.
81. Benker G, Raida M, Olbricht T, et al. (1990). TSH secretion in Cushing's syndrome: Relation to glucocorticoid excess, diabetes, goiter, and the "the sick euthyroid syndrome." *Clin Endocrin* 133:779–786.
82. Duick DS, Wahner HW. (1979). Thyroid axis in patients with Cushing's syndrome. *Arch Intern Med* 139:767–772.
83. Tsigos C, Papanicolaou DA, Defensor R, et al. (1997). Dose effects of recombinant human interleukin-6 on pituitary hormone secretion and energy expenditure. *Neuroendocrinology* 66:54–62.
84. Torpy DJ, Tsigos C, Lotsikas AJ, et al. (1998). Acute and delayed effects of a single-dose injection of interleukin-6 on thyroid function in healthy humans. *Metabolism* 47:1289–1293.
85. Chrousos GP. (2000). The role of stress and the hypothalamic-pituitary-adrenal axis in the pathogenesis of the metabolic syndrome: Neuro-endocrine and target tissue-related causes. *Int J Obes Relat Metab Disord* 24 (Suppl 2):S50–S55.

86. Tsigos C, Papanicolaou DA, Kyrou I, et al. (1997). Dose-dependent effects of recombinant human interleukin-6 on glucose regulation. *J Clin Endocrinol Metab* 1997:4167–4170.
87. Pasquali R, Cantobelli S, Casimirri F, et al. (1993). The hypothalamic-pituitary-adrenal axis in obese women with different patterns of body fat distribution. *J Clin Endocrinol Metab* 77:341–346.
88. Kalra SP, Dube MG, Pu S, et al. (1999). Interacting appetite-regulating pathways in the hypothalamic regulation of body weight. *Endocr Rev* 20:68–100.
89. Richard D, Lin Q, Timofeeva E. (2002). The corticotropin-releasing factor family of peptides and CRF receptors: Their roles in the regulation of energy balance. *Eur J Pharmacol* 12:189–197.
90. Cavagnini F, Croci M, Putignano P, et al. (2000). Glucocorticoids and neuroendocrine function. *Int J Obes* 24 (Suppl 2):S77–S79.
91. Kaye WH, Berrettini W, Gwirtsman H, et al. (1990). Altered cerebrospinal fluid neuropeptide Y and peptide YY immunoreactivity in anorexia and bulimia nervosa. *Arch Gen Psychiatry* 47:548–556.
92. Munglani R, Hudspith MJ, Hunt SP. (1990). The therapeutic potential of neuropeptide Y: Analgesic, anxiolytic and antihypertensive. *Drugs* 52:371–389.
93. Valentino RJ, Kosboth M, Colflesh M, et al. (2000). Transneuronal labeling from the rat distal colon: Anatomic evidence for regulation of distal colon function by a pontine corticotropin-releasing factor system. *J Comp Neurol* 417:399–414.
94. Monnikes H, Schmidt BG, Tebbe J, et al. (1994). Microinfusion of corticotropin releasing factor into the locus coeruleus/subcoeruleus nuclei stimulates colonic motor function in rats. *Brain Res* 25:101–108.
95. Suto G, Kiraly A, Tache Y. (1994). Interleukin 1 beta inhibits gastric emptying in rats: Mediation through prostaglandin and corticotropin-releasing factor. *Gastroenterology* 106:1568–1575.
96. Soderholm JD, Perdue MH. (2001). Stress and the gastrointestinal tract. II. Stress and intestinal barrier function. *Am J Physiol Gastrointest Liver Physiol* 280:G7–G13.
97. Tache Y, Martinez V, Million M, et al. (2001). Stress and the gastrointestinal tract. III. Stress-related alterations of gut motor function: Role of brain corticotropin-releasing factor receptors. *Am J Physiol Gastrointest Liver Physiol* 280:G173–G177.
98. Collins SM. (2001). Stress and the gastrointestinal tract. IV. Modulation of intestinal inflammation by stress: Basic mechanisms and clinical relevance. *Am J Physiol Gastrointest Liver Physiol* 280:G315–G318.
99. Chrousos GP. (1995). The hypothalamic-pituitary-adrenal axis and immune-mediated inflammation. *N Engl J Med* 332:1351–1362.
100. Reichlin S. (1993). Neuroendocrine-immune interactions. *N Engl J Med* 329:1246–1253.
101. Akira S, Hirano T, Taga T, et al. (1990). Biology of multifunctional cytokines: IL-6 and related molecules (IL-1 and TNF). *FASEB J* 4:2860–2867.
102. Besedovsky HO, del Rey A. (1992). Immune-neuroendocrine circuits: Integrative role of cytokines. *Front Neuroendocrinol* 13:61–94.
103. Bernardini R, Kamilaris TC, Calogero AE, et al. (1990). Interactions between tumor necrosis factor-alpha, hypothalamic corticotropin-releasing hormone, and adrenocorticotropin secretion in the rat. *Endocrinology* 126:2876–2881.
104. Busbridge NJ, Grossman AB. (1991). Stress and the single cytokine: Interleukin modulation of the pituitary-adrenal axis. *Mol Cell Endocrinol* 82:C209–C214.
105. Sapolsky R, Rivier C, Yamamoto G, et al. (1987). Interleukin-1 stimulates the secretion of hypothalamic corticotropin releasing factor. *Science* 238:522–524.

106. Mastorakos G, Chrousos GP, Weber J. (1993). Recombinant interleukin-6 activates the hypothalamic-pituitary-adrenal axis in humans. *J Clin Endocrinol Metab* 77:1690–1694.
107. Mastorakos G, Weber JS, Magiakou MA, et al. (1994). Hypothalamic-pituitary-adrenal axis activation and stimulation of systemic vasopressin secretion by recombinant interleukin-6 in humans: Potential implications for the syndrome of inappropriate vasopressin secretion. *J Clin Endocrinol Metab* 79:934–939.
108. Reincke M, Heppner C, Petzke F, et al. (1994). Impairment of adrenocortical function associated with increased plasma tumor necrosis factor-alpha and interleukin-6 concentrations in African trypanosomiasis. *Neuroimmunomodulation* 1:14–22.
109. Bernardini R, Calogero AE, Ehrlich YH, et al. (1989). The alkyl-ether phospholipid platelet-activating factor is a stimulator of the hypothalamic-pituitary-adrenal axis in the rat. *Endocrinology* 125:1067–1073.
110. Bernardini R, Chiarenza A, Calogero AE, et al. (1989). Arachidonic acid metabolites modulate rat hypothalamic corticotropin releasing hormone *in vitro*. *Neuroendocrinology* 50:708–715.
111. Bernton EW, Beach JE, Holaday JW, et al. (1987). Release of multiple hormones by a direct action of interleukin-1 on pituitary cells. *Science* 23:519–521.
112. Fukata J, Usui T, Naitoh Y, et al. (1988). Effects of recombinant human interleukin-1α, IL-1β, IL-2 and IL-6 on ACTH synthesis and release in the mouse pituitary tumor cell line AtT-20. *J Endocrinol* 122:33–39.
113. Salas MA, Evans SW, Levell MJ, et al. (1990). Interleukin-6 and ACTH act synergistically to stimulate the release of corticosterone from adrenal gland cells. *Clin Exp Immunol* 79:470–473.
114. Karalis K, Sano H, Redwine J, et al. (1991). Autocrine or paracrine inflammatory actions of corticotropin-releasing hormone *in vivo*. *Science* 254:421–423.
115. Crofford LJ, Sano H, Karalis K, et al. (1993). Corticotropin-releasing hormone in synovial fluids and tissues of patients with rheumatoid arthritis and osteoarthritis. *J Immunol* 151:1587–1596.
116. Webster EL, Torpy DJ, Elenkov IJ, Chrousos GP. (1998). Corticotropin releasing hormone and inflammation. *Ann NY Acad Sci* 1:21–32.
117. Elenkov IJ, Webster EL, Torpy DJ, Chrousos GP. (1999). Stress, corticotropin-releasing hormone, glucocorticoids, and the immune/inflammatory response: Acute and chronic effects. *Ann NY Acad Sci* 876:1–11; discussion, 11–13.
118. Ottaway CA, Husband AJ. (1992). Central nervous system influences on lymphocyte migration. *Brain Behav Immun* 6:97–116.
119. Bellinger DL, Lorton D, Felten SY, et al. (1992). Innervation of lymphoid organs and implications in development, aging, and autoimmunity. *Int J Immunopharmacol* 14:329–344.
120. Hirano T, Akira S, Taga T, et al. (1990). Biological and clinical aspects of interleukin 6. *Immunol Today* 11:443–449.
121. Elenkov IJ, Chrousos GP. (2002). Stress hormones, proinflammatory and antiinflammatory cytokines, and autoimmunity. *Ann NY Acad Sci* 966:290–303.
122. Gold PW, Goodwin F, Chrousos GP. (1988). Clinical and biochemical manifestations of depression: Relationship to the neurobiology of stress, part 1. *N Engl J Med* 319:348.
123. Gold PW, Goodwin F, Chrousos GP. (1988). Clinical and biochemical manifestations of depression: Relationship to the neurobiology of stress, part 2. *N Engl J Med* 319:413–420.

124. Gold PW, Chrousos GP. (2002). Organization of the stress system and its dysregulation in melancholic and atypical depression: High vs. low CRH/NE states. *Mol Psychiatry* 7:254–275.
125. Tsigos C, Chrousos GP. (2002). Hypothalamic-pituitary-adrenal axis, neuroendocrine factors and stress. *J Psychosom Res* 53:865–871.
126. Raadsheer F, Hoogendijk W, Stam FC, et al. (1994). Increased numbers of corticotropin-releasing hormone expressing neurons in the hypothalamic paraventricular nucleus of depressed patients. *Neuroendocrinology* 60:436–444.
127. Gold PW, Gwirtsman H, Avgerinos P, et al. (1986). Abnormal hypathalamic-pituitary-adrenal function in anorexia nervosa: Pathophysiologic mechanisms in underweight and weight-corrected patients. *N Engl J Med* 314:1335–1342.
128. Kaye WH, Gwirtsman HE, George DT, et al. (1987). Elevated cerebrospinal fluid levels of immunoreactive corticotropin-releasing hormone in anorexia nervosa: Relation to state of nutrition, adrenal function, and intensity of depression. *J Clin Endocrinol Metab* 64:203–208.
129. Malozowski S, Muzzo S, Burrows R, et al. (1990). The hypothalamic-pituitary-adrenal axis in infantile malnutrition. *Clin Endocrinol (Oxf)* 32:461–465.
130. Insel TR, Kalin NH, Guttmacher LB, et al. (1982). The dexamethasone suppression test in obsessive-compulsive disorder. *Psychiatry Res* 6:153–160.
131. Gold PW, Pigott TA, Kling MK, et al. (1988). Basic and clinical studies with corticotropin releasing hormone: Implications for a possible role in panic disorder. *Psychiatr Clin North Am* 11:327–334.
132. Luger A, Deuster P, Kyle SB, et al. (1987). Acute hypothalamic-pituitary-adrenal responses to the stress of treadmill exercise: Physiologic adaptations to physical training. *N Engl J Med* 316:1309–1315.
133. Wand GS, Dobs AS. (1991). Alterations in the hypothalamic-pituitary-adrenal axis in actively drinking alcoholics. *J Clin Endocrinol Metab* 72:1290–1295.
134. Bardeleben U, Heuser I, Holsboer F. (1989). Human CRH stimulation response during acute withdrawal and after medium-term abstention from alcohol abuse. *Psychoneuroendocrinology* 14:441–449.
135. Risher-Flowers D, Adinoff B, Ravitz B, et al. (1988). Circadian rhythms of cortisol during alcohol withdrawal. *Adv Alcohol Subst Abuse* 7:37–41.
136. Roy MS, Roy A, Gallucci WT, et al. (1993). The ovine corticotropin-releasing hormone test in type I diabetic patients and controls: Suggestion of mild chronic hypercortisolism. *Metabolism* 42:696.
137. Tsigos C, Young RJ, White A. (1993). Diabetic neuropathy is associated with increased activity of the hypothalamic-pituitary-adrenal axis. *J Clin Endocrinol Metab* 76:554–558.
138. Streeten DH. (1993). Is hypothalamic-pituitary-adrenal hyperactivity important in the pathogenesis of excessive abdominal fat distribution? *J Clin Endocrinol Metab* 77:339–340.
139. DeBellis M, Chrousos GP, Dorn LD, et al. (1994). Hypothalamic-pituitary-adrenal axis dysregulation in sexually abused girls. *J Clin Endocrinol Metab* 78:249–255.
140. Kamilaris TC, DeBold CR, Pavlou SN, et al. (1987). Effect of altered thyroid hormone levels on hypothalamic-pituitary-adrenal function. *J Clin Endocrinol Metab* 65:994–999.
141. Rabin D, Gold PW, Margioris A, et al. (1988). Stress and reproduction: Interactions between the stress and reproductive axis. In *Mechanisms of Physical and Emotional Stress*, Chrousos GP, Loriaux DL, Gold PW (Eds.). Plenum Press, New York, p 377–390.

142. Margioris A, Grino M, Gold PW, et al. (1988). Human placenta and the hypothalamic-pituitary-adrenal axis. *Adv Exp Med Biol* 245:389–398.
143. Sasaki A, Shinkawa O, Margioris AN, et al. (1987). Immunoreactive corticotropin releasing hormone in human plasma during pregnancy, labor and delivery. *J Clin Endocrinol Metab* 64:224–229.
144. Behan DP, Linton EA, Lowry PJ. (1989). Isolation of the human plasma corticotropin-releasing factor-binding protein. *J Endocrinol* 122:23–31.
145. Potter E, Behan DP, Fischer WH, et al. (1991). Cloning and characterization of the cDNAs for human and rat corticotropin-releasing factor-binding proteins. *Nature* 349:423–426.
146. Linton E, Perkins A, Woods R, et al. (1993). Corticotropin releasing hormone-binding protein (CRH-BP): Plasma levels decrease during the third trimester of normal human pregnancy. *J Clin Endocrinol Metab* 76:260–262.
147. Elenkov IJ, Chrousos GP. (1999). Stress hormones, Th1/Th2 patterns, pro/anti-inflammatory cytokines and susceptibility to disease. *Trends Endocrinol Metab* 10:359–368.
148. Demitrack M, Dale J, Straus S, et al. (1991). Evidence of impaired activation of the hypothalamic-pituitary-adrenal axis in patients with chronic fatigue syndrome. *J Clin Endocrinol Metab* 73:1224–1234.
149. Vanderpool J, Rosenthal N, Chrousos GP, et al. (1991). Abnormal pituitary-adrenal responses to corticotropin-releasing hormone in patients with seasonal affective disorder: Clinical and pathophysiological implications. *J Clin Endocrinol Metab* 72:1382–1387.
150. Griep EN, Boersma JW, de Kloet ER. (1993). Altered reactivity of the hypothalamic pituitary adrenal axis in the primary fibromyalgia syndrome. *J Rheumatol* 20:469–474.
151. Elgerot A. (1978). Psychological and physiological changes during tobacco-abstinence in habitual smokers. *J Clin Psychol* 34:759–764.
152. Puddey JB, Vandongen R, Neilin LJ, et al. (1984). Haemodynamic and neuroendocrine consequences of stopping smoking. A controlled study. *Clin Exp Pharmacol Physiol* 11:423–426.
153. Kling MA, Roy A, Doran, et al. (1991). CSF levels of CRH, ACTH, and SRIF in Cushing's syndrome, major depression, and normal volunteers: Physiological and pathophysiological interrelationships. *J Clin Endocrinol Metab* 72:260–271.
154. Doherty GM, Nieman LK, Cutler GB Jr, et al. (1990). Time to recovery of the hypothalamic pituitary adrenal axis following curative resection of adrenal tumors in patients with Cushing's syndrome. *Surgery* 108:1085–1090.
155. Sternberg EM, Glowa J, Smith MA. (1992). Corticotropin-releasing hormone-related behavioral and neuroendocrine responses to stress in Lewis and Fischer rats. *Brain Res* 570:54–60.
156. Sternberg EM, Chrousos GP, Wilder RL, et al. (1992). The stress response and the regulation of inflammatory disease. *Ann Intern Med* 117:854–866.
157. Sternberg EM, Hill JM, Chrousos GP, et al. (1989). Inflammatory mediator-induced hypothalamic-pituitary-adrenal axis activation is defective in streptococcal cell arthritis in Lewis rats. *Proc Natl Acad Sci USA* 86:2374–2378.
158. Sternberg E, Young W Jr, Bernardini R, et al. (1989). A central nervous defect in the stress response is associated with susceptibility to streptococcal cell wall arthritis in Lewis rats. *Proc Natl Acad Sci USA* 86:4771–4775.
159. Chikanza IC, Petrou P, Chrousos GP, et al. (1992). Defective hypothalamic response to immune/inflammatory stimuli in patients with rheumatoid arthritis. *Arthritis Rheum* 35:1281–1288.

160. Chikanza IC, Chrousos GP, Panayi GS. (1992). Abnormal neuroendocrine-immune communications in patients with rheumatoid arthritis. *Eur J Clin Invest* 22:635–637.
161. Habib KE, Weld KP, Rice KC, et al. (2000). Oral administration of a corticotropin-releasing hormone receptor antagonist significantly attenuates behavioral, neuroendocrine, and autonomic responses to stress in primates. *Proc Natl Acad Sci USA* 23:6079–6084.
162. Webster EL, Lewis DB, Torpy DJ, et al. (1996). *In vivo* and *in vitro* characterization of antalarmin, a nonpeptide corticotropin-releasing hormone (CRH) receptor antagonist: Suppression of pituitary ACTH release and peripheral inflammation. *Endocrinology* 137:5747–5750.
163. Bornstein SR, Webster EL, Torpy DJ, et al. (1998). Chronic effects of a nonpeptide corticotropin-releasing hormone type I receptor antagonist on pituitary-adrenal function, body weight, and metabolic regulation. *Endocrinology* 139:1546–1555.
164. Deak T, Nguyen KT, Ehrlich AL, et al. (1999). The impact of the nonpeptide corticotrophin releasing hormone antagonist antalarmin on behavioral and endocrine responses to stress. *Endocrinology* 140:79–86.
165. Webster EL, Barrientos RM, Contoreggi C, et al. (2002). Corticotropin releasing hormone (CRH) antagonist attenuates adjuvant induced arthritis: Role of CRH in peripheral inflammation. *J Rheumatol* 29:1252–1261.
166. Gabry KE, Chrousos GP, Rice KC, et al. (2002). Marked suppression of gastric ulcerogenesis and intestinal responses to stress by a novel class of drugs. *Mol Psychiatry* 7:474–483.
167. Wong ML, Webster EL, Spokes H, et al. (1999). Chronic administration of the non-peptide CRH type 1 receptor antagonist antalarmin does not blunt hypothalamic-pituitary-adrenal axis responses to acute immobilization stress. *Life Sci* 65:PL53–PL58.
168. Lawrence AJ, Krstew EV, Dautzenberg FM, et al. (2002). The highly selective CRF(2) receptor antagonist K41498 binds to presynaptic CRF(2) receptors in rat brain. *Br J Pharmacol* 136:896–904.
169. Sajdyk TJ, Gehlert DR. (2000). Astressin, a corticotropin releasing factor antagonist, reverses the anxiogenic effects of urocortin when administered into the basolateral amygdala. *Brain Res* 877:226–234.
170. Mackay KB, Stiefel TH, Ling N, et al. (2003). Effects of a selective agonist and antagonist of CRF(2) receptors on cardiovascular function in the rat. *Eur J Pharmacol* 23:111–115.

7 Stress, Immunity, and Disease

Cinnamon Stetler, Rama Murali, Edith Chen, and Gregory E. Miller

CONTENTS

Although once believed to have an exclusively negative effect on the immune system, stress is now seen as a multifaceted concept that impacts immune function in a variety of ways. Current research reveals that stress's impact often varies according to its intensity, duration, or modality. This chapter will outline the complex nature of the relationship between stress and the immune system by highlighting the empirical research examining these two concepts. To facilitate understanding, we begin with a brief primer on components of the immune system that are most often measured in studies of stress. Then we provide definitions and examples of how the immune system is affected for each category of stress, in hopes of giving readers a sense of the complex nature of the stress–immune relationship. Next we examine the role of stress in the context of disease, to determine which diseases have the strongest evidence to support a relationship with stress, and what immunologic path

0-8493-1820-3/05/$0.00+$1.50

this relationship might take. Last, we discuss what conclusions can be drawn from our reading of the literature and what directions future research should take.

IMMUNE SYSTEM

The human immune system is a complex network of cells and proteins that seek to protect the body from foreign organisms, or pathogens. As part of its defensive function, the immune system must be able to determine whether the substances it encounters (e.g., proteins, bacteria, parasites) are self or nonself. Once the immune system recognizes a protein or other molecule as nonself, an immune response is initiated. Immune responses to pathogens fall into two broad categories: natural and specific responses. A natural immune response involves white blood cells such as monocytes, granulocytes, and neutrophils accumulating at sites of injury and infection, where they act to provide early, nonspecific defense against invading pathogens and to alert the specific components of the immune system. Specific immunity, comprised of cellular and humoral immunity, involves lymphocytes that generate responses specific to particular types of antigens. Cellular immune responses are directed against intracellular pathogens such as viruses and involve T cells recognizing and destroying the infected cell. There are two general classes of T cells: helper (CD4+) and cytotoxic (CD8+) cells. Humoral immune responses are directed against extracellular pathogens such as bacteria and involve B cells secreting antibodies that specifically bind to the pathogen. Although one type of immune response usually predominates during any given infection, a complex network of signaling pathways exists between each arm of the immune system. A detailed discussion of each type of immune response is beyond the scope of this chapter. However, we will provide a brief overview of how they are modeled in the study of stress.

Although a wide range exists, researchers know that the body needs a certain amount of T and B cells in circulation in order for the immune system to be effective. Thus, quantifying the presence of these lymphocytes has been employed as a rough measure of immune system function. This is done by using antibodies to the B and T cells themselves; these antibodies are coupled with a fluorescent dye that can be measured by an instrument called a flow cytometer. The greater the levels of dye, the higher the levels of T or B cells. Because antibodies are specific and will only bind to one type of cell, researchers can assess the presence of more than one type of lymphocyte, as well as determine what percentage of the total lymphocyte population in circulation they comprise. Under normal conditions, B cells comprise 10 to 15% of total lymphocytes circulating in the blood, while T cells make up 50 to 60% (CD4+) and 20 to 25% (CD8+) of lymphocytes in the blood (Abbas et al., 1997). Within the normal range, the clinical significance of a small change in lymphocyte levels is unclear. Vastly elevated levels of lymphocytes can indicate that the body might be responding to some type of infection. On the other hand, a T cell count below 200 indicates a progression to AIDS in persons infected with HIV.

In addition to getting a sense of their numbers, researchers want to know how well lymphocytes function. Although lymphocyte function can be assessed in the body, *in vitro* models have also been developed. The *in vitro* approach involves incubating lymphocytes with mitogens, substances (usually plant derived) that elicit a broad, nonspecific response from lymphocytes. This response, called blastogenesis, is essentially cellular replication. The amount of cellular replication measured is taken as an indicator of lymphocyte functioning; the greater the replication, the better functioning the immune system is believed to be. While this *in vitro* model is generally seen as indicative of what happens inside the body when lymphocytes encounter a pathogen, researchers should keep in mind that lymphocyte proliferation inside the body is initiated by a single, specific antigen that generates a response from only particular T or B cells, unlike the general response generated by the mitogen. Lymphocyte proliferation *in vivo* is a very complex chain of events, and we cannot say for certain how well those events are represented in the *in vitro* model. Researchers often employ measures of antibody production after a stimulus such as vaccination to gain a sense of specific immune function *in vivo*. The greater the numbers of antibodies produced or the longer these numbers are sustained over time, the healthier the immune response is thought to be.

Natural killer (NK) cells are large lymphocytes that kill virus-infected cells as well as certain types of neoplastic cells. They comprise less than 10% of the lymphocytes circulating in the blood under normal, healthy circumstances. Natural killer cells can play an important role in containing some infections before T cells have a chance to respond, as they are able to recognize and destroy infected cells without the help of antibodies. NK cells do their killing by releasing molecules that punch holes in the infected or cancerous cell's outer membrane, allowing fluids to rush in and causing the cell to burst or lyse. Researchers take advantage of this process when they want to assess *in vitro* how effective NK cells are at their job, or how responsive they are to cytokines. The NK cells are placed in a dish with target (often cancerous) cells that have incorporated a radioactive molecule (usually chromium) into their cytosol. When the target cells are lysed by the NK cells, researchers measure the amount of chromium that has been released. The more radioactive the molecule present, the better the function of the NK cells.

When one arm of the immune system encounters injured tissues or pathogens, those cells will communicate the need for action to the rest of the immune system by way of cytokines. Cytokines are proteins, produced by lymphocytes as well as other cells in the body, that promote or inhibit an immune or inflammatory response. Many cells in the body, including T cells, B cells, and macrophages, have receptors for cytokines. Cytokine secretion is a brief, self-limited event, and their baseline levels in circulation are often very low. Thus, valid baseline levels of some cytokines are difficult, if not impossible, to obtain with even highly sensitive assays. Researchers will often stimulate lymphocytes with lipopolysaccharides (LPS) or other generally recognized pathogens to measure stimulated levels of a cytokine. Interpretation of these measures is complex and often depends upon the cytokine assayed. Although robust production of cytokine following stimulation might mean a healthier immune system in some cases, in other cases it can indicate a hyperresponsive immune system or an inability to quell the response once the pathogen has been contained.

Although presented in a brief overview here, the immune system is a highly complex network of proteins, cells, and tissues whose components often have redundant or opposing functions. As such, no one measure can be said to represent global immune functioning; broad interpretations from specific assessments should be avoided. Because the system is quite redundant with an array of built-in compensatory mechanisms, specific changes in immune system functioning rarely translate into disease vulnerability. Thus, readers are cautioned against extrapolating any changes in one specific immune measure out to disease risk.

THE EFFECT OF STRESS ON THE IMMUNE SYSTEM

One of the interesting challenges in the study of the relationship between stress and the immune system is defining the complex construct of stress. Research in the arena of stress and the immune system has flourished over the last several decades; however, ambiguous and conflicting definitions are present in the literature. The concept of stress has evolved from a definition based primarily on physiological responses, as discussed in Hans Seyle's early stress research (Seyle, 1950), to one that grasps the important psychological components of appraisal and coping in the processing of environmental stressors (Lazarus & Folkman, 1984). In this chapter, we highlight the environmental component of stressors — events that elicit behavioral or physiological responses — because it is the component emphasized in most of the data and literature regarding stress and immunity. We also consider the importance of the psychological response component in thoroughly understanding stress responses. Thus, we define stress as a "relationship between the person and the environment that is elicited by a stressor event and is subsequently appraised by the person as taxing or exceeding his or her resources and endangering his or her well-being" (Lazarus & Folkman, 1984). It is important to highlight the concept of appraisal as it is mentioned in the above definition, and its integral role in stressor perception and response. Appraisal, in this context, is the subjective judgment of the individual regarding whether the stressor he encounters poses a threat and can be managed through personal resources. Once the individual judges, or appraises, the stressor to be threatening and unmanageable, a behavioral and biological response is elicited. This idea of appraisal is indeed an important one, as it can help us understand why different individuals might perceive the same events as stressful or harmless, and consequently respond in a distinct psychological and biological manner. Thus, this definition, emphasizing appraisal, takes into account individual differences in response to a stressor, which are evident as people differ in their interpretations, sensitivities, and reactions to stressors (Lazarus & Folkman, 1984).

TYPES OF STRESSORS

Surveying the stress–immune literature reveals a multitude of stressors that are studied, such as caregiver's stress, academic exams, electric shocks, marital conflict, bereavement, job loss, lab-based stressors (i.e., public-speaking tasks, mirror-tracing tasks), noise, concealing homosexual identity, and daily life events (Kiecolt-Glaser et al., 1995; Marshall et al., 1998; Laudenslager et al., 1983; Miller et al., 1999; Irwin et al., 1988; Arnetz et al., 1987; Chen & Matthews, 2001; Evans et al., 1997; Cohen et al., 1998; Stone et al., 1994). These diverse stressors vary along many dimensions, including the duration of the stressor, the duration it is perceived as threatening, the frequency with which it occurs, and the overall severity — which is usually some combination of these dimensions (Baum et al., 1993).

Although there is no taxonomy that adequately considers all of these dimensions, the Panel on Psychosocial Assets and Modifiers of Stress proposed four types of stressors that are primarily characterized by duration and exposure frequency (Elliott & Eisdorfer, 1982): acute, chronic unrelenting, chronic intermittent, and stressful event. For the purposes of this chapter, we will divide the construct of acute stress into laboratory acute stressors and brief naturalistic stressors, as they are distinct subcategories that are not acknowledged as such in the Elliott and Eisdorfer (1982) categorization. Before we begin our discussion of the immune trends associated with each stressor, it is important to note that the taxonomy we are describing here is far from comprehensive. Frequency and duration of the stressor events are important elements; however, this categorization fails to include the response component of stress. That is, the event (stressor) can be short in duration, but it could be responded to over a long period. The event can be chronic and long lasting, but the response could be short-lived and the individual can adapt to the stressor. The response component is vital to understanding the potential effects of the stressor, but it is a highly variable component that is often mediated by subjective appraisals. Thus, the responses are difficult to categorize and quantify and are rarely considered in experimental study designs. To conduct studies, a rough and often inadequate (in that it rarely addresses the appraisal component) qualitative taxonomy is often employed because it is the most convenient way to test hypotheses. Our choice to use these stressor groups is bound by the literature, but is not to be considered a complete representation of stressor types. For the purposes of this chapter, we will discuss the general immune outcomes associated with each type of stressor and suggest reevaluation of stressor subgroups when there are significantly differential immune changes across studies that regard the same stressor type (i.e., stressful event sequences).

Acute Stressors

Acute stressors (as discussed in this taxonomy) are time-limited in duration, perception, *and the response they elicit* (Gump & Matthews, 1999; Baum et al., 1993). It is important to make the distinction that they are perceived *and* responded to in a time-limited fashion, as later we will discuss certain cases of acute stress that are perceived and responded to over time. Acute stressors are studied in both laboratory-based and naturalistic, or naturally occurring, settings. The distinction between these groups goes beyond their stressor origin, as they each have specific effects on the immune parameters and functioning.

Laboratory Stressors

To study acute stress in the laboratory, researchers will often develop paradigms that will allow simulation of a short-lived stressful event, such as a public-speaking task or a time-pressured puzzle-solving task (Elliott & Eisdorfer, 1982). Aside from those typical psychological stressors, actual physical acute stressors such as loud noises or a cold-pressor task (where an individual submerges and briefly holds his arm under freezing water) can be administered in a lab setting (Delahanty et al., 1996;

Weisse et al., 1990). Following these acute stressors, the investigators can measure aspects of natural immunity by performing cell counts of different cell subtypes, or they can measure the function of cells in response to the acute stressor (Herbert et al., 1994).

Over 100 studies have been conducted that consider the effects of acute lab stress on immune functioning. In a recent meta-analysis on stress and immunity in humans, Segerstrom and Miller (2003) present a comprehensive discussion of the natural and functional immune alterations due to acute laboratory stressors. We will describe their findings here as this meta-analysis quantitatively synthesizes the results of the many acute lab stress studies and presents the general immune trends due to acute lab stress. They find that the effects of acute lab stress include increases in natural immunity, such as increases in the counts of NK and suppressor/cytotoxic T cells, as well as neutrophils in the peripheral blood. They also find that acute lab stress affects functional measures of immunity such that there are significant increases in NK cell cytotoxicity and production of interleukin-6 (IL-6) and interferon-γ (IFN-γ) cytokines, and decreases in mitogen-stimulated proliferative responses (markers of decreased specific immunity). These findings suggest that acute lab stress upregulates natural immunity and downregulates specific immunity. The functional significance of these acute stress-induced immune alterations can be understood in the evolutionary context. An upregulation in natural immunity indicates a pattern of response that shifts or prepares the immune system to respond in a nonspecific, but immediate manner. This pattern of immune alteration mimics the evolutionary fight-or-flight response in duration and similarly in effect. Thus, acute laboratory stressors induce a response similar to a fight-or-flight stressor and seem to serve an adaptive function to prepare the immune system's first and immediate line of defense to fight off potential "invaders" and prepare the immune system to heal potential wounds.

Brief Naturalistic Stressors

Brief naturalistic stressors are often used in studies because they provide a glimpse of immune changes in response to events we can actually encounter in life (as most of us do not usually indulge in cold-pressor type tasks), and consequently can reveal whether immune changes or shifts occur in response to acute stressors in the context of our daily lives. In the current literature, naturalistic acute stressors such as academic exams and brief hospitalization are studied, as substantial populations of individuals are exposed to these types of stress (Elliott & Eisdorfer, 1982; Marshall et al., 1998). Exam stress models are considered reliable, and the stress associated with taking exams has been associated with reductions in NK cell cytotoxicity and increased activation of latent viruses, which is manifest in greater antibody production (Kiecolt-Glaser et al., 1984; Glaser et al., 1987). The last decade has seen a substantial group of academic exam studies that illustrate cytokine level shifts in response to the brief naturalistic stressors (Marshall et al., 1998; Kang & Fox, 2001; Liu et al., 2002).

The Segerstrom and Miller (2003) meta-analysis helps to synthesize and understand the above-mentioned immune changes associated with brief naturalistic stressors. They find that this stressor has an effect on cytokine production that involves a shift away from T-helper 1 (Th1) (cellular) immunity and toward Th2 (humoral) immunity. They go on to say that this shift explains the decrease in NK cell cytotoxicity (cellular immunity) and the increased reactivation of latent viruses (humoral immunity) in terms of suppression of cellular immunity and enhancement of humoral immunity. This type of shift toward humoral immunity could be potentially harmful. If individuals encountering brief naturalistic stressors are challenged by viruses or bacteria that are defended by Th1 or cellular immunity, it could be more difficult for the immune system to fend off these pathogens. It is interesting to note the very different immune implications of this brief naturalistic type of acute stress and acute lab stressors. The immune shift to natural immunity described in acute lab stress situations is more adaptive, as it prepares the immune system's first line of defense against an immediate threat. The brief naturalistic acute stressor seems to create another type of shift that is more maladaptive, as it could compromise comprehensive immune responsiveness by decreasing cellular immunity.

Chronic Unrelenting Stressors

Chronic unrelenting stressors take place over time, often have an unknown endpoint, and elicit prolonged psychological and biological responses. Chronic stressors are most often studied in naturalistic settings; however, there is a considerable body of animal research that uses sleep deprivation, prolonged confinement, and prolonged shaking to simulate the effects of chronic stress (Elliott & Eisdorfer, 1982). In humans, for obvious ethical reasons, chronic stressors are studied in naturalistic settings. A common naturalistic chronic stressor paradigm is caregiver stress, wherein a spouse or relative is caring for a chronically ill relative (Kiecolt-Glaser et al., 1995; Cacioppo et al., 1998). In the Kiecolt-Glaser et al. study (1995), caregivers of relatives suffering from dementia were investigated to assess the effects of chronic stress on wound healing and healing-related immune parameters. In this controlled study design involving female caregivers and matched controls, all subjects underwent a punch biopsy wound. The subjects were then monitored to determine how long it took the wound to heal and immune measures were assessed. They found that wound healing took significantly longer in caregivers, compared to controls, and that the caregivers also produced less interleukin-1β (a cytokine that can be important for healing and the regulation of other cytokines that can aid healing) in response to *in vitro* mitogen stimulation (Kiecolt-Glaser et al., 1995).

Other chronic stress caregiver studies have found lower percentages of NK cell cytotoxicity, decreased proliferative responses of peripheral blood leukocytes to mitogens, and impaired immune responses to influenza virus vaccination in caregivers vs. control groups (Cacioppo et al., 1998; Kiecolt-Glaser et al., 1991, 1996; Vedhara et al., 1999).

Segerstrom and Miller (2003) synthesized the above-mentioned studies and summarized the effects of chronic stress on immune functioning. They found that chronic stress negatively affects most functional measures of the immune system. Specifically, chronic stressors are associated with declines in both natural and specific immune responses. Also, both Th1 (mitogen-stimulated lymphocyte proliferation) and Th2 (antibody response to influenza vaccine antibody) responses were decreased in chronically stressed individuals. Chronic unrelenting stress seems to be most illustrative of the traditional idea of stress-induced immunosuppression. This global immune suppression has a great potential for increased disease susceptibility, as both natural and specific immunity are downregulated. Interestingly, some recent work has found that chronic unrelenting stress might contribute to increased disease susceptibility via upregulation of some immune parameters. For example, in a recent study by Miller et al. (2002), chronic caregiver stress actually upregulated some aspects of the pro-inflammatory response. Miller et al. (2002) found that caregiver stress impairs the immune system's ability to respond to anti-inflammatory signals, specifically the suppression of production of IL-6 (a pro-inflammatory cytokine) by the synthetic glucocorticoid hormone dexamethasone. This increased pro-inflammatory cytokine expression seems to counter the findings reported above that illustrate general immunosuppression associated with chronic unrelenting stress. However, Miller et al. (2002) present a model of glucocorticoid (the hormones that suppress pro-inflammatory cytokine) resistance to explain how one immune component can be elevated in a system that is mostly downregulated due to chronic stress (this model is discussed further in the autoimmune diseases section below). This work illustrates that chronic stress does not necessarily downregulate all aspects of immune response; however, it contributes to a type of suppression of ability to respond to anti-inflammatory signals. It is important to note that the type of immune dysregulation associated with chronic stress can play a detrimental role in diseases, such as asthma and autoimmune disorders and cardiac disease, that already involve excessive inflammation. Thus, whether downregulating the natural and specific immunities or harmfully altering cytokine regulatory systems, chronic unrelenting stressors have the potential to pose the greatest threat to overall immune function and regulation.

Chronic Intermittent Stressors

Chronic intermittent stressors are discrete stressors that take place repeatedly over time and consist of specific events with start and endpoints. Some examples are having to visit one's in-laws once a month or daily hassles such as traffic on the commute to work (Elliott & Eisdorfer, 1982; Lazarus & Folkman, 1984). Chronic intermittent stressors in humans are only studied in naturalistic settings. Most commonly, the chronic intermittent stressors that are evaluated in the literature are daily hassles (Stone et al., 1994; Brosschot et al., 1994).

In a study of daily events and immune function, Stone et al. (1994) found that reporting more desirable daily events was associated with increased daily levels of secretory immunoglobulin A (IgA). This study uses an elegant paradigm that elicits an actual *in vivo* immune response and involves IgA, an immune parameter that can be modulated by less acute and lasting events, to ascertain the effects of daily hassles on immunity. They explain that secretory IgA is an antibody associated with host defense and respiratory infection and is secreted as it is created, so it can readily respond to daily hassles or events (Stone et al., 1994). In their procedure, the body's immune response to a pathogen was ascertained by having the subjects ingest a novel protein (rabbit albumin). This protein acted as an invading pathogen (similar to the viruses that cause respiratory infections and elicit a secretory IgA response) and was conceptualized by Stone et al. (1994) to induce a similar pattern of immune processing. Thus, they were able to monitor the *in vivo* response to this pathogen and measure secretory IgA in the context of both response and daily hassles. They found that reporting more undesirable events was associated with decreased daily levels of secretory IgA (Stone et al., 1994). This study illustrates the importance of studying chronic intermittent stressors as unique stressors with direct immune implications outside of the context of acute and chronic stressors. However, this type of stressor is not well studied in the literature. It will be important for the field of stress and immunity to build upon this study and conduct additional research on this stressor, as it pervades our daily lives and is ecologically valid.

Stressful Event Sequences

Stressful event sequences are best described as series of events, occurring as the result of an initiating event, that take place over time and have a likely resolution (Lazarus & Folkman, 1984). This stressor is only studied in naturalistic settings in humans. Some examples of stressful event sequences are divorce, bereavement, or loss of employment (Lazarus & Folkman, 1984). For example, when an individual is getting a divorce, the legal action of the divorce is the initiating event, and as a result of that, other events such as relocation, child custody battles, asset redistribution, and overall psychological adjustment to loss of companionship and dissolution of a family unit often take place. Arnetz et al. (1987) looked at women in Sweden who were unemployed and receiving benefits from the state. When an individual loses her job, the loss of employment is the initiating event that can prompt other events, such as an inability to pay utility bills, loss of psychological security, loss of housing, and an inability to meet the basic needs of oneself or one's family. In this study Arnetz et al. found that even though their basic needs were met due to the benefits they were receiving, the unemployed women showed a reduced lymphocyte response to phytohemaglutinin (PHA) and purified protein derivative of tuberculin (PPD), presumably due to the psychological stress of being unemployed. Irwin et al. (1988) looked at populations of bereaved and anticipatory bereaved women and found reduced NK activity in these populations compared with controls. Kiecolt-Glaser et al. (1988) looked at separated/divorced men and found that they reported more recent illness and decreased antibody titers to herpes virus than did married men. Segerstrom and Miller (2003) discuss immune responses to natural disasters and perceived health threats as other types of stressful event sequences. They found that following a disaster, there was a nonsignificant increase in immune response and no immune changes in response to perceived health threats. They conclude that compared with the other stressors we have discussed, it is difficult to present a straightforward and consistent pattern of immune alteration that is associated with stressful event sequences. The decline in immune response that is associated with bereavement, job loss, and divorce shows a pattern regarding these three types of stressful event sequences. However, perceived health threats and natural disasters did not produce alterations in immune parameters. Aside from illustrating that stressful event sequences as a type of stressor do not yield consistent findings, the studies suggest that perhaps subdivisions within this stressor category need to be investigated. That is, thus far we have noticed patterns of immune responsiveness/alteration to each stressor. If we continue with the idea that different types of stressors have specific and differential effects on immune functioning, then it will be important to delve into potential implications of specific stressful event sequences, as bereavement, divorce, and job loss seem to suggest one immune pattern, and threats to health and natural disasters suggest another.

Subjective Appraisal of Stressors

The above-mentioned categories based on the Elliott and Eisdorfer (1982) stressor taxonomy describe a great deal of stressors and stress paradigms that are discussed in the literature. However, stressors are not comprehensively described by their occurrence. There is also the important idea of the subjective (perceived) component of stress. At the onset of this section on the stress–immune link, we highlighted the appraisal component of evaluating whether a situation is considered stressful. Subjective appraisal is a psychological construct that is integral to understanding how stress "gets into the body" and affects health. That is, understanding how one sees a particular situation will provide insight into whether the situation will be perceived as stressful and induce particular psychological and biological responses.

In a paper by Baum et al. (1993), stress is described as a construct that consists of both the duration of the threat (stressor) *and* the duration of the psychological/biological response. The literature we have discussed has focused on the duration-of-threat dimension of Baum et al.'s stress model, but has not considered the duration-of-response dimension. Baum et al. describe a traumatic acute event in their study and evaluate it on both dimensions of their model. That is, the event is acute in duration, but is appraised as threatening and responded to biologically for a longer period. They go on to theorize that subjective appraisal plays an important role in the persistence of threat seen in chronic stress perception. In an area affected by a nuclear accident, they found in their longitudinal study of chronic stress that up to 5 years after the event, and in some cases even longer, residents of the area reported significantly more intrusive thoughts and memories of the traumatic event than individuals in a control group. In addition, the persistent intrusive memories were positively associated with measures of cortisol, norepinephrine, systolic blood pressure, and somatic complaints, suggesting that consistent appraisal of the event activates biological indicators of the stress response. This suggests that the actual occurrence of the event, or the stressor, might not be the best indicator of stress response, as it does not capture the important component of appraisal. Subjective appraisal accounts for unresolved stress affecting one's current psychological state, which might not be captured by focusing on the categorization or measurement of the stressor. In a recent study by Chen et al. (in press), children of varying socioeconomic status (SES) with asthma were studied to determine if appraisal of stressors played a role in immune alterations associated with asthma exacerbation. They found that children from low SES neighborhoods had higher production of cytokines implicated in asthma (e.g., IL-5), and that stress appraisals mediated the relationship between SES and immune responses. Specifically, through mediational analysis, they found that psychological stress (measured by both a subjective appraisal method and objective life events) was a potential link between low SES status and heightened inflammatory markers such as the cytokine IL-5. Although we will not thoroughly delve into the complex issue of appraisal here, it is important to note its integral role in fully conceptualizing stress.

Combined Effect of Acute and Chronic Stress

Another important idea that has emerged in the stress–health literature is that of the combined effects of different types of stress. Specifically, some researchers have posed the question of what happens when an individual under chronic stress encounters a new acute stressor. Much of the work on acute stressor reactivity in the presence of chronic stress has focused on cardiovascular and neuroendocrine reactivity. For example, Gump and Matthews (1999) reviewed 19 studies that investigated the effects of pervasive chronic stressors on reactivity to acute stressors and reported that the majority of the studies found greater acute stressor reactivity with heightened background stressors, although a considerable minority of the studies revealed reduced acute stressor reactivity. This review exemplifies the standing debate about whether acute reactivity in the presence of chronic stress supports a habituation (reduced reactivity) or sensitization (heightened reactivity) hypothesis. Understanding this pattern of response in the immunological context will reveal whether an acute stressor will enhance or reduce immune parameters during the period of general immune downregulation that is the result of chronic unrelenting stress. This is a relatively unexplored area in the field of psychoneuroimmunology (PNI). In a study by Cohen et al. (1998), the influence of chronic and acute stressors on cold susceptibility was studied. There was a marginally significant finding that acute stress was protective for those experiencing chronic stress. That is, those that reported chronic stress with an acute event were at less risk to get a cold than those that solely reported chronic stress. The combined effects of the two stressors in this study is provocative, as they suggest that acute stress still has an immunoenhancement effect in the presence of chronic stress, and consequently has positive implications for disease protection during a time of general immune downregulation. However, this is a single study, and much more research needs to be conducted in this area to understand whether acute stress has a global positive, negative, or unsubstantial effect on immune functioning. It will also be important to identify the types of acute stress that are investigated in this combined stress paradigm, as we have already illustrated in this chapter that acute stress has differential immune effects when presented in the laboratory or in naturalistic settings.

Stress is a difficult construct to define, and the definition one chooses also shapes one's synthesis of the enormous number of studies that examine stress and the immune system. The definition used in this chapter is one that embraces both the objective qualities of the stressor and the individual's appraisal of the stressor. However, appraisal has rarely been incorporated in previous empirical research, and the duration of the stressor, rather than the duration of the response, is the primary way that stress has traditionally been conceptualized. How long a stressor lasts and how long someone stands to be affected by that stressor are important factors to consider because the immune system is a dynamic entity. It adjusts its level of functioning considerably over time, as the body attempts to not only confront the pathogenic threats from the external environment, but also to maintain homeostasis. A full-on immune response is an expensive undertaking for the body in terms of energy and resources, and it cannot afford to maintain such a response longer than necessary. If a stressor requires a sustained immunological response, then immune system functioning might be compromised in some way, as evidenced by the suppressive and dysregulating effects seen in studies of chronic stress. Much like an elastic band that will spring back to its original shape after it is stretched the first hundred times, but gradually loses its elasticity after being extensively and repeatedly stretched over time, stress eventually impairs the immune system's ability to regulate itself and return to its normal level of functioning (McEwen, 1998). Whether this has implications for disease is the topic of the second half of this chapter.

STRESS AND DISEASE: LINKED BY THE IMMUNE SYSTEM?

Given that various types of stressors do seem to have an effect on the immune system, the question that arises is whether these alterations are of sufficient duration and magnitude to influence the onset or progression of disease. Many researchers have hypothesized that the immune system represents one pathway from stress to disease. In the remaining sections of this chapter, we first review evidence for associations between stress and specific disease outcomes. First and foremost, we examine the literature to determine whether a relationship exists between stress and disease outcomes. When disparate findings arise, we give greater weight to methodologically sound studies whose results are tempered with fewer alternate explanations. For diseases in which stress plays a role in etiology or course, we next evaluate the literature regarding the pathways that might link these two factors. We seek to understand by what mechanism(s) stress is getting inside the body to affect biology. Often the research here is scarce or in its early stages; much remains to be determined.

CANCER

The link between stressful life events and cancer risk is unclear. Most of the work has been done in breast cancer, and the studies have been of variable quality. Two separate groups of researchers have performed meta-analyses to synthesize the wide range of methods and results. McKenna et al. (1999) examined a broader range of studies in their analysis under the heading of psychosocial factors than did Petticrew et al. (1999), who limited their analysis to only studies that examined the role of stressful life events. To make the comparison of their findings as clear as possible, we will focus on the findings of McKenna et al. that relate to stressful life events. Their analysis included 12 studies, 10 of which were also included in Petticrew et al.'s analysis of 29 prospective, case-control studies. Petticrew et al. also gave each of their studies a methodological quality score, based on nine methodological standards, such as inclusion of newly diagnosed cases only, descriptions of baseline characteristics, and adjustment for confounders. The two reports generated disparate results and reached very different conclusions.

McKenna et al. (1999) find that their studies generated a statistically significant effect size estimate, indicating that there is an association between stressful life events and the development of breast cancer. Petticrew et al. (1999), using the 15 studies that provided sufficient data, found that the odds of developing breast cancer were higher for women who report more stressful life events than for women who report fewer events. However, the authors recalculated their results using only those studies that had a methodological quality score at or above the median. Studies with sound methodologies do one or more of the following: enroll enough participants to have the statistical power to detect a modest effect; clearly define the criteria employed for diagnosing breast cancer; use population-based rather than hospital-based controls; keep the interviewer or researchers blind to the participants' breast cancer status; and adjust for potential confounders such as age, race, and socioeconomic status. Including only the methodologically sound studies produced much different results. The studies with the best methods found no evidence for a significant link between stressful life events and breast cancer. These findings suggest that when large, well-controlled studies are conducted, there is no link between the experience of stressful events in one's life and the later development of breast cancer. However, this does not rule out a link between stress appraisals or coping responses and breast cancer or other forms of cancer (see Petticrew et al., 2002).

Given that there is little good evidence for stressful life events leading to the development of cancer, the question then becomes whether stress plays a role in disease progression once cancer has been diagnosed. Correlational studies of varying quality have been conducted; the best studies seem to indicate that stressful life events do not increase risk of recurrence or cancer-related mortality. High-quality studies include a prospective design, a standardized, validated, interview-based stressor assessment, and controls for medical variables. Barraclough et al. (1992) interviewed 204 women with localized breast cancer at 4, 24, and 42 months postoperation and determined that experiencing stressful life events did not place women at a greater risk for recurrence. Unlike other studies in this area, this study enrolled enough women and followed them for enough time to have the statistical power to detect an association, if one existed in their sample. A more recent study used similar methods and found a similar pattern of results (Graham et al., 2002). They measured stress from a year before breast cancer diagnosis up to 5 years postdiagnosis and did not find any link between stressful life events and cancer recurrence. Experiencing life events such as divorce, death of a close family member, or unemployment does not appear to place a woman at greater risk for developing or experiencing a relapse of breast cancer. However, these studies have typically used a narrow definition of stress: whether a stressful event has occurred. When stress is operationalized that way, no association is found. Intervention studies suggest that other dimensions of stress, such as one's coping mechanisms, can affect cancer outcomes.

Interventional research has typically involved randomizing cancer patients to either receive some type of stress-related group intervention or receive "usual care" as a part of the control group. Patients in the control group are usually free to pursue adjuvant treatments on their own if they wish. Results in this area of research have been promising, but each positive finding seems to be followed by a failure to replicate. As Edelman et al. (2000) point out, psychological interventions do not uniformly increase patients' survival time. One early study involved women with advanced breast cancer (Speigel et al., 1989). Approximately half (50) were randomly assigned to attend a weekly support group where they were encouraged to express their feelings about their cancer, process the ordeal that they were facing, and learn self-hypnosis for pain management. The support group lasted for 1 year. Women who were assigned to the control group (36) received their usual medical care. Although the support groups were originally designed to positively influence the quality of life, the results showed that women in the support groups lived an average of 18 months longer than the women in the control group. The survival outcome was measured as time (in months) from when the women were enrolled in the study until they died (or the conclusion of the 10-year follow-up). Because the women were randomly assigned, the groups did not differ on many variables thought to be important to prognosis, although some have suggested that the control group in this study died at a faster rate than normal, or differed on some important but unmeasured variable (Fox, 1998).

Several follow-up studies have failed to replicate this pattern of results (Cunningham et al., 1998; Edelman et al., 1999; Goodwin et al., 2001). These studies have been of high quality, with large sample sizes, lengthy follow-up periods, and interventions similar to the one used by Spiegel and colleagues, so methods are probably not to blame for the failure to replicate. Other possible explanations remain. Breast cancer at the time of the Spiegel study was a stigmatized condition that largely went undiscussed in larger society. The intervention could have had an effect when offered against that background that it would not necessarily have today, when breast cancer has by and large lost its stigma and access to information and support is much easier for women. In addition, advances in diagnosis and treatment might put women on much firmer ground medically, reducing the influence of a psychosocial intervention. The study by Spiegel and colleagues sparked great interest in the role of support groups in the health of medical patients. Unfortunately, the failure to find a similar pattern of results in other studies has cast doubts on the validity of this effect.

In a later study, patients with a different type of cancer, malignant melanoma, were randomly assigned to a group intervention more structured than the breast cancer study's treatment or to usual medical care (Fawzy et al., 1993). Researchers measured the patients' survival after 6 years. They also assessed psychological and immune parameters before and after the group intervention to further investigate how such groups might have their influence. The group intervention in this study consisted of educational as well as supportive components; instead of just expressing emotions, the group members were taught about the basics of their disease and proper nutrition, relaxation, problem solving, and other coping techniques. This intervention met weekly for only 6 weeks. Their results showed that the group intervention patients had better NK cell functioning, had reduced psychological distress, and were more likely to be cancer-free and alive at the 6-year follow-up point. This survival advantage was still present even after accounting for the invasiveness of the melanoma at baseline, an important medical predictor of prognosis.

Of note, NK cell functioning, although it differed between groups, was not correlated with survival, and therefore is not responsible for the improved outcomes seen in the intervention group.

Researchers have not consistently found that psychosocial interventions improve survival outcomes in breast cancer, nor do they consistently find a relationship between life stress and breast cancer outcomes. The equivocal findings can be due to the fact that the hypothesized relationship rests upon the idea that stress inhibits the immune system, whose role in breast cancer development is limited. Chronic or life event stressors can affect immune function, but not in a way that would influence whether a woman develops or recovers from breast cancer, a disease that has strong genetic and environmental determinants. Traditionally, researchers have referenced the immunosurveillance hypothesis as a putative mechanism linking stress and cancer. In short, this hypothesis maintains that the immune system, specifically cytotoxic T cells and NK cells, continually scans the tissues of the body for neoplastic cells to eliminate them. While the role of the immune system in tumor elimination has been well documented in animals (see Ben-Eliyahu, 2003 for a review), the evidence in humans is more equivocal. Indirect evidence can be found in the studies that report a higher incidence of cancers in persons who are dramatically immunosuppressed (e.g., following a transplant, due to a congenital deficiency). However, the types of cancer that immunosuppressed persons develop are rarely the lung, breast, or GI cancers seen in the general population; they are rarer forms of cancer, often non-Hodgkins lymphomas (Stutman, 1985; Bovbjerg & Valdimarsdottir, 1998). Thus, the immune system can play a role in preventing a few, but not the most common, forms of cancer. It is probably most relevant for virus-induced cancers, such as most cervical cancers, Burkitt's lymphoma, or hepatocellular carcinoma. Infectious disease research has convincingly demonstrated that stress influences host resistance to viral infection (see "Infectious Disease" section below). Thus, it might be advantageous for researchers to begin considering the role of stress in virally induced cancers. Evidence for this proposition derives from studies by Pereira and colleagues (2003), who found a link between life stress and the occurrence of precancerous changes in the cervix a year later. HIV-positive women who reported higher levels of stressful life events were at a greater risk of developing cervical lesions than those who reported fewer events.

Other alternatives to the immunosurveillance hypothesis exist, as outlined by Forlenza & Baum (2000). Many studies have shown that damage to DNA, the failure of DNA repair mechanisms, inhibition of apoptosis, and somatic mutations increase the rate of cancer development. Future research could focus on how these intracellular pathways are affected by psychosocial stress, to achieve a more complete picture regarding the complex pathways linking stress and cancer. Given that NK cell functioning did not explain longer survival in the Fawzy et al. study, one must consider other potential mechanisms through which psychosocial interventions might have their effects on cancer patients. Because the immunosurveillance hypothesis is not well supported in humans, researchers might consider shifting their focus from immune-based measures (e.g., NK cell function) to other measures of the intracellular processes that can lead to cancer.

Infectious Disease

Infectious disease represents a broad category of diseases whose pathogenesis is mediated by a bacteria or virus. In the past, research in this area has been plagued by a retrospective assessment of stress or a failure to control for potential confounds such as level of exposure or strain of the pathogen. Recent research has avoided these methodological pitfalls and generated a consistent link between high psychosocial stress and susceptibility to infectious disease (Cohen et al., 1991, 1998, 1999). Perhaps the link between stress and infectious disease has been easier to conclusively demonstrate because it is within ethical bounds to deliberately expose people to a cold or flu virus, unlike a carcinogenic agent. Thus, many potentially confounding factors can be controlled for in studies of infectious disease, where all participants in the study are exposed to the same quantity and strain of virus or bacteria. Once exposed, disease signs and symptoms usually develop fairly quickly, often a matter of days or weeks, unlike cancer, whose etiology probably takes years or decades.

Humans are constantly exposed to pathogens in the environment, but not every incidence of exposure results in an infection. Also, some people will go on to develop symptoms of an illness, whereas others who are exposed to the same pathogen will not. To help explain the role that stress plays in infection and the development of symptoms, researchers exposed a group of participants to identical quantities and strains of the virus that is responsible for the common cold (Cohen et al., 1998). These participants were housed in quarantine and monitored for signs of a cold. Infection was verified by the presence of viral proteins in nasal secretions or virus-specific antibodies in the blood. The participants were also asked for self-reports of symptoms such as runny nose, congestion, sneezing, and coughing and had cold symptoms rated by a physician. Prior to viral exposure, participants completed a semistructured interview to assess life stressors, both acute (lasting less than 1 month) and chronic (lasting longer than 1 month). Researchers found that which subjects developed a cold was not related to the presence of acute stressors, but was instead related to experiencing a chronic stressor. In fact, there was a direct linear relationship where the longer one experienced a chronic stressor, the greater one's risk was for developing a cold. This pattern of results has been replicated across several different contexts (Cohen et al., 1991, 1998, 1999). Interestingly, the results also showed that experiencing an acute stressor on top of a chronic stressor gave a participant slightly *less* risk of developing a cold than just experiencing a chronic stress by itself. The relationship between chronic stress and colds was not fully accounted for by any of the immune factors that the researchers measured, such as helper T cell count, neutrophil count, or NK cell cytotoxicity. So again, stress seems to be playing a role in disease outcome, but its precise immune system effects remain unknown.

A similar study gives more information for answering that question (Cohen et al., 1999). Most cold symptoms (e.g., runny nose, sneezing, congestion) are not caused by the presence of the cold virus per se, but instead are the consequences of the immune system's production of cytokines as it attempts to combat the virus. Perceived stress at the time of the study was associated not only with flu symptoms in participants exposed to an influenza virus, but also with levels of the cytokine interleukin-6 in nasal lavage samples. Also, the higher the levels of IL-6, the more flu symptoms subjects exhibited. Furthermore, when researchers statistically controlled for IL-6 levels, the relationship between stress and flu symptoms was diminished, suggesting that this cytokine might be one pathway through which stress has its effects on the development of flu symptoms, perhaps through glucocorticoid-induced upregulation (Miller et al., 2002).

HIV

HIV is an infectious disease that has received a lot of attention from PNI researchers. In persons infected with the HIV virus, the amount of time that elapses before symptomatic AIDS develops varies greatly. Although medical factors such as effective antiretroviral drugs can extend this time, there is much variability left to explain. Several studies suggest that factors such as stressful life events, bereavement, and coping also impact symptom-free survival time with HIV. HIV-positive gay men who experienced the chronic stress of concealing their homosexuality experienced a more rapid decline in CD4 count and less time until death than HIV-positive men who were not concealing their sexual orientation (Cole et al., 1996). Findings from an HIV-positive cohort in North Carolina link stress with several disease outcomes. Evans and colleagues (1997) reported that severe stress was associated with the faster development of clinical symptoms early in the disease. As these patients were followed over time, the effects of stress seemed to accumulate to predict faster progression to AIDS and AIDS-related mortality (Lesserman et al., 1999, 2000, 2002). These studies do a nice job of taking biological (CD4 count) and self-report (e.g., symptoms) measures of progression to AIDS and measuring stress independent of subject appraisal. Like most studies of HIV-positive individuals, these studies did not control for length of infection, since the timing of HIV exposure is often impossible to determine. However, these studies, unlike many others, consistently find effects because they have the largest sample sizes, longest follow-up periods, and most reliable measures of stress and disease.

Plausible mechanisms for a relationship between stress and HIV progression have been proposed but are just beginning to be systematically examined *in vivo* (Cole & Kemeny, 1997). Glucocorticoids and hormones such as epinephrine and norepinephrine might be a link between stress and HIV outcomes. Glucocorticoids have been shown to increase levels of HIV replication *in vitro* (Markham et al., 1986, as discussed in Cole et al., 2001), although the concentrations used were greater than typically found in the body. Glucocorticoids can also shift cytokine profiles from Th1 to Th2, preparing the immune system to respond inappropriately to a viral infection such as HIV (Spellberg and Edwards, 2001). In addition, the autonomic nervous system (ANS) is activated during times of challenge or stress, and hormonal products of the autonomic nervous system can also influence the immune system. Its effects include alterations in lymphocyte trafficking (potentially exposing more T cells to the HIV virus), alterations in cytokine production, and decreasing control over latent viruses and opportunistic infections (Cole & Kemeny, 1997; Cole et al., 1998). Researchers recently demonstrated a linear correlation between ANS activity, assessed during an acute stressor, and HIV disease markers in HIV patients receiving antiretroviral therapy (Cole et al., 2001). The drug treatment was much more effective in reducing viral load and increasing CD4+ count in patients who had low levels of ANS activity than in patients with elevated ANS activity. Differences in demographic characteristics, health behaviors, or treatment adherence did not explain the superior response to the drug treatment in low ANS patients. We anticipate that future research in this area will investigate whether ANS activity differences influence disease outcomes or survival time in persons with HIV.

Autoimmune Disease

Autoimmune diseases, such as rheumatoid arthritis and multiple sclerosis, arise when the body's healthy tissues are mistakenly recognized as foreign by the immune system. The signal of "foreign" then sets off a complex cascade of events in the immune system, usually resulting in the destruction of the mistakenly identified cells, but damage to other nearby tissues. As we have seen in the studies above, stress is generally thought to play a disruptive or inhibitory role on the immune system, leaving a person more vulnerable to disease onset or progress. But if autoimmune disease is a case of overactive immunity (the immune system is attacking cells it should ignore), then it follows that stress might have beneficial effects on autoimmune outcomes. We shall see that the reality is more complex than what should be true theoretically.

Multiple sclerosis (MS) is a devastating disease in which the cells that line the neurons and aid in the conduction of nerve impulses are the targets of an immune system attack (Mohr & Cox, 2001). When these cells are destroyed, the functioning of the central nervous system becomes impaired, leading to a variety of symptoms. Often the disease has a variable course, in which symptoms will flare up for a period and then remit, or nerve function will be affected in one part of the body (e.g., optic nerve) and then another (skeletal muscles). Doctors and researchers have wondered if there is any link between stress and these disease flare-ups. Recently, a few prospective studies have demonstrated that there is a link between stress and MS flare-ups, but the nature of the relationship has been hard to characterize. It seems that all stressors are not the same when it comes to MS outcomes, although some studies disagree. Ackerman et al. (2002) found that there was a rather immediate (average of 14 days in between) link between experiencing a stressor and an MS flare-up, but that the severity or the source of the stressor did not matter. Mohr and colleagues (2000) found that moderate stressors (increased conflict and disruption in routine) but not severe stressors predicted the development of new MS-related brain lesions 8 weeks later. The lesions were verified using magnetic resonance imaging (MRI) scans. Similarly, Sibley (1997) found that marital and job-related stress was followed by clinical exacerbation, while more severe negative life events, like a death in the family, were not. And under the highly stressful conditions of threatened missile attack during a war, MS patients actually experienced a decreased rate of flare-ups (Nisipeanu & Korczyn, 1993).

A similar pattern of findings appears to exist for rheumatoid arthritis (RA), a painful condition in which the tissues around one or more joints trigger an inflammatory response, affecting joint mobility. In general, studies that look prospectively at daily hassles (minor stressors) find that there is a positive association between these types of stresses and disease activity in RA (Thomason et al., 1992; Zautra et al., 1998), whereas studies that look at major stressors tend to find either no association or improved disease states (Potter & Zautra, 1997).

Although little research has been done that focuses on the mechanisms behind these associations, these findings suggest that acute/moderate stressors, inasmuch as they increase the inflammatory response, can play a role in disease exacerbations perhaps via augmentation of natural immunity. Severe stressors, on the other hand, can be potent enough to activate the HPA axis, leading to immune system inhibition by glucocorticoids and a temporary improvement in disease state. However, the effects of exposure to chronic stress have not directly been examined in the context of autoimmune disease. Several studies (see summary in Walker et al., 1999) indicate that a disruption in the normal neuroendocrine–immune system signaling pathways might exist in chronic inflammatory diseases such as MS and RA. Chronic stress can exacerbate these disruptions by chronically elevating cortisol levels. Over time, the immune system can downregulate its receptors for glucocorticoids, leading to a loss of anti-inflammatory regulation, or glucocorticoid resistance. Once glucocorticoids are less able to regulate immune function, inflammation can continue unabated, leading to an exacerbation of existing disease or increased risk for disease development. Support for the development of glucocorticoid resistance has been found in a healthy sample of chronically stressed adults (Miller et al., 2002) but remains to be examined within the context of autoimmune disease.

CONCLUSION

Our review of the literature shows that different types of stressors have distinct immune implications. Acute stress generally produces an adaptive upregulation in immune function. Brief naturalistic stressors produce a mildly dysregulated immune response, while chronic unrelenting stressors tend to invoke diminished immune responses, perhaps leading to increased disease risk in some cases. Regarding the link between stress and disease, solid empirical support for stress's causative role is not present for all diseases reviewed. Infectious diseases such as colds, flu, and HIV are one area where the link between stress and disease is strongest, while breast cancer seems to have the least support for an immune system-mediated impact of stress. Autoimmune diseases such as multiple sclerosis and rheumatoid arthritis appear to be affected by stress, but the exact nature of this relationship has been hard to characterize. In general, minor stressors seem to exacerbate symptoms while major stressors have either no effect or tend to improve disease outcomes.

The reason that a stress–disease link has not been found for breast cancer is perhaps due to the limited role that the immune system plays in the etiology of breast cancer, presumably a disease that develops over many years. Researchers should shift their focus to virally mediated cancers such as cervical cancer, because the immune system's role in defending against viruses is better established. More generally, researchers should seek a firm understanding of a given disease's pathophysiology and work backward from there regarding what aspects of the immune system (e.g., humoral immunity, cytokines, inflammation) might be serving as a mechanism for stress. Furthermore, stressors can have different effects at different stages of disease. For example, in the case of infectious diseases, stress can have one effect on the immune system following pathogen exposure and another effect when the immune system is trying to control a burgeoning infection. With autoimmune diseases such as MS and RA, the duration and intensity of the stressor can have predictive value regarding the disease's response to stress. However, further research is needed to clarify this question.

In addition, a more complete understanding of stress, immunity, and disease will only come with a more refined strategy for conceptualizing and assessing stressful experiences. The majority of studies in this area have focused on an environmental conceptualization of stress as an event that happens to an individual, but have failed to consider other dimensions such as duration, frequency of exposure, coping strategies, and, most importantly, subjective appraisals. Given the dramatic individual differences in people's emotional, behavioral, and immunologic responses to stressful experiences, a long-needed step forward in this domain of research will involve incorporating the role of subjective appraisals of stress into conceptual models.

On the whole, remarkable progress has been made in recent years in this area of research. The challenge that remains is to carefully examine and understand the immune mechanisms at a microlevel while still holding on to the bigger picture regarding a human's experience of stress and the development of disease. For many diseases, medical or biological predictors do not explain all the disparities that exist regarding morbidity and mortality. A better understanding of stress's impact on the body can help science gain further insight into why some people get sick and others do not.

ACKNOWLEDGMENT

Preparation of this chapter was supported by grants from the National Alliance for Research on Schizophrenia and Depression, the William T. Grant Foundation, and the Michael Smith Foundation for Health Research.

REFERENCES

Abbas, A.K., Lichtman, A.H., & Pober, J.S. (1997). *Cellular and Molecular Immunology*, 3rd ed. Philadelphia: W.B. Saunders.

Ackerman, K., Heyman, R., Rabin, B., Anderson, B., Houck, P., Frank, E., et al. (2002). Stressful life events precede exacerbations of multiple sclerosis. *Psychosomatic Medicine*, 64, 916–920.

Anderson, B., Farrar, W., Golden-Kreutz, D., Kutz, L., MacCallum, R., Courtney, M., et al. (1998). Stress and immune responses after surgical treatment for regional breast cancer. *Journal of the National Cancer Institute*, 90, 30–36.

Arnetz, B.B., Wasserman, J., Petrini, B., & Brenner, S.O. (1987). Immune function in unemployed women. *Psychosomatic Medicine*, 49, 3–12.

Barraclough, J., Pinder, P., Cruddas, M., Osmond, C., Taylor, I., & Perry, M. (1992). Life events and breast cancer prognosis. *British Medical Journal*, 304, 1078–1081.

Baum, A., Cohen, L., & Hall, M. (1993). Control and intrusive memories as possible determinants of chronic stress. *Psychosomatic Medicine*, 55, 274–286.

Ben-Eliyahu, S. (2003) The promotion of tumor metastasis by surgery and stress: Immunological basis and implications for psychoneuroimmunology. *Brain, Behavior and Immunity*, 17, S27–36.

Bovbjerg, D., & Valdimarsdottir, H. (1998). Psychoneuroimmunology: Implications for psycho-oncology. In J.C. Holland (Ed.), *Psycho-oncology* (pp. 125–134). New York: Oxford University Press.

Brosschot, J.F., Benschop, R.J., Godaert, G.L.R., & Olff, M. (1994). Influence of life stress on immunological reactivity to mild psychological stress. *Psychosomatic Medicine*, 56, 216–224.

Byrnes, D., Antoni, M., Goodkin, K., Efantis-Potter, J., Asthana, D., Simon, T., Munajj, J., Ironson, G., & Fletcher, M. (1998). Stressful events, pessimism, natural killer cell cytotoxicity, and cytotoxic/suppressor T cells in HIV+ black women at risk for cervical cancer. *Psychosomatic Medicine*, 60, 714–722.

Cacioppo, J.T., Poehlmann, K.M., Kiecolt-Glaser, J.K., Malarkey, W.B., Burleson, M.H., Berntson, G.G., et al. (1998). Cellular immune responses to acute stress in female caregivers of dementia patients and matched controls. *Health Psychology*, 17, 182–189.

Chen, E., Fisher, E.B., Bacharier, L.B., & Strunk R.C. (2003). Socioeconomic status, stress, and immune markers in adolescents with asthma. *Psychosomatic Medicine*, 65, 984–992.

Chen, E., & Matthews, K.A. (2001). Cognitive appraisal biases: An approach to understanding the relation between socioeconomic status and cardiovascular reactivity in children. *Annals of Behavioral Medicine*, 23, 101–111.

Cohen, S., Doyle, W.J., & Skoner, D.P. (1999). Psychological stress, cytokine production, and severity of upper respiratory illness. *Psychosomatic Medicine*, 61, 175–180.

Cohen, S., Doyle, W., Skoner, D., Frank, E., Rabin, B., & Gwaltney, J. (1998). Types of stressors that increase susceptibility to the common cold in healthy adults. *Health Psychology*, 17, 214–223.

Cohen, S., Tyrrell, D., & Smith, A. (1991). Psychological stress and susceptibility to the common cold. *New England Journal of Medicine*, 325, 606–612.

Cole, S., & Kemeny, M. (1997). Psychobiology of HIV infection. *Critical Reviews in Neurobiology*, 11, 289–321.

Cole, S., & Kemeny, M. (2001). Psychosocial influences on the progression of HIV infection. In R. Ader, D. Felten, & N. Cohen (Eds.), *Psychoneuroimmunology* (pp. 583–612). New York: Academic Press.

Cole, S., Kemeny, M., Taylor, S., Visscher, B., & Fahey, J. (1996). Accelerated course of human immunodeficiency virus infection in gay men who conceal their homosexual identity. *Psychosomatic Medicine*, 58, 219–231.

Cole, S., Korin, Y., Fahey, J., & Zack, J. (1998). Norepinephrine accelerates HIV replications via protein kinase A dependent effects on cytokine production. *Journal of Immunology*, 161, 610–616.

Cole, S., Naliboff, B., Kemeny, M., Griswold, M., Fahey, J., & Zack, J. (2001). Impaired response to HAART in HIV-infected individuals with high autonomic nervous system activity. *Proceedings of the National Academy of Sciences of the United States of America*, 98, 12695–12700.

Cunningham, A., Edmonds, C., Jenkins, G., Pollack, H., Lockwood, G., & Warr, D. (1998). A randomized controlled trial of the effects of group psychological therapy on survival in women with metastatic breast cancer. *Psycho-oncology*, 7, 508–517.

Delahanty, D.L., Dougall, A.L., Hawken, L., & Tratowski, J.H. (1996). Time course of natural killer cell activity and lymphocyte proliferation in response to two acute stressors in healthy men. *Health Psychology*, 15, 48–55.

Dhabhar, F.S., & McEwen, B. (1997). Acute stress enhances while chronic stress suppresses cell-mediated immunity *in vivo*: A potential role for leukocyte trafficking. *Brain, Behavior, and Immunity*, 11, 286–306.

Edelman, S., Craig, A., & Kidman, A.D. (2000). Can psychotherapy increase the survival time of cancer patients? *Journal of Psychosomatic Research*, 49, 149–156.

Edelman, S., Lemon, J., Bell, D., & Kidman, A. (1999). Effects on group CBT on the survival time of patients with metastatic breast cancer. *Psycho-oncology*, 8, 474–481.

Elliott, G.R., & Eisdorfer, C. (1982). *Stress and Human Health: An Analysis and Implications of Research. A Study by the Institute of Medicine, National Academy of Sciences*. New York: Springer.

Evans, D.L., Leseman, J., Perkins, D.O., Stern, R.A., Murphy, C., Zheng, B., Gettes, D., Longmate, J.A., Silva, S.G., van der Horst, C.M., Hall, C.D., Folds, J.D., Golden, R.N. & Petitto, J.M. (1997). Severe life stress as a predictor of early disease progression in HIV infection. *American Journal of Psychiatry*, 154, 630–634.

Fawzy, F., Fawzy, N., Hyun, C., Elashoff, R., Guthrie, D., Fahey, J., et al. (1993). Malignant melanoma: Effects of an early structured psychiatric intervention, coping and affective state on recurrence and survival 6 years later. *Archives of General Psychiatry*, 50, 681–689.

Forlenza, M., & Baum, A. (2000). Psychosocial influences on cancer progression: Alternative cellular and molecular mechanisms. *Current Opinion in Psychiatry*, 13, 639–645.

Fox, B. (1998). Psychosocial factors in cancer incidence and prognosis. In J.C. Holland (Ed.), *Psycho-oncology* (pp. 110–123). New York: Oxford University Press.

Glaser, R., Rice, J., Sherridan, J., & Fertel, R. (1987). Stress-related immune suppression: Health implications. *Brain, Behavior and Immunity*, 1, 7–20.

Goodwin, P., Leszcz, M., Ennis, M., Koopmans, J., Vincent, L., Guther, H., et al. (2001). The effect of group psychosocial support on survival in metastatic breast cancer. *New England Journal of Medicine*, 345, 1719–1726.

Graham, J., Ramirez, A., Love, S., Richards, M., & Burgess, C. (2002). Stressful life experiences and risk of relapse of breast cancer: Observation cohort study. *British Medical Journal*, 324, 1420–1424.

Gump, B.B., & Matthews, K.A. (1999). Do background stressors influence reactivity to and recovery from acute stressors? *Journal of Applied Social Psychology*, 29, 469–494.

Herbert, T.B., Cohen, S., Marsland, A.L., & Bachen, E.A. (1994). Cardiovascular reactivity and the course of immune response to an acute psychological stressor. *Psychosomatic Medicine*, 56, 337–344.

Irwin, M., Daniels, M., Risch, S.C., & Bloom, E. (1988). Plasma cortisol and natural killer cell activity during bereavement. *Biological Psychiatry*, 24, 173–178.

Kang, D., & Fox, C. (2001). Th1 and Th2 cytokine responses to academic stress. *Research in Nursing and Health*, 24, 245–257.

Kiecolt-Glaser, J.K., Dura, J.R., Speicher, C.E., Trask, J., & Glaser, R. (1991). Spousal caregivers of dementia victims: Longitudinal changes in immunity and health. *Psychosomatic Medicine*, 53, 345–362.

Kiecolt-Glaser, J.K., Garner, W., Speicher, C., Penn, G.M., Holliday, J., & Glaser, R. (1984). Psychosocial modifiers of immunocompetence in medical students. *Psychosomatic Medicine*, 46, 7–14.

Kiecolt-Glaser, J.K., Glaser, R., Gravenstein, S., Malarkey, W.B., & Sheridan, J. (1996). Chronic stress alters the immune response to influenza virus vaccine in older adults. *Proceedings of the National Academy of Sciences of the United States of America*, 93, 3043–3047.

Kiecolt-Glaser, J.K., Kennedy, S., Malkoff, S., & Fisher, L. (1988). Marital discord and immunity in males. *Psychosomatic Medicine*, 50, 213–229.

Kiecolt-Glaser, J.K., Marucha, P.T., Malarkey, W.B., Mercado, A.M., & Glaser, R. (1995). Slowing of wound healing by psychological stress. *Lancet*, 346, 1194–1196.

Laudenslager, M.L., Ryan, S.M., Drugan, R.C., Hyson, R.L., & Maier, S.F. (1983). Coping and immunosuppression: Inescapable but not escapable shock suppresses lymphocyte proliferation. *Science*, 221, 568–570.

Lazarus, R.S., & Folkman, S. (1984). *Stress, Appraisal, and Coping*. New York: Springer Publishing Company.

Lesserman, J. (2003). The effects of stressful life events, coping and cortisol on HIV infection. *CNS Spectrums*, 8, 25–30.

Leserman, J., Jackson, E., Petitto, J., Golden, R., Silva, S., Perkins, D., et al. (1999). Progression to AIDS: The effects of stress, depressive symptoms, and social support. *Psychosomatic Medicine*, 61, 397–406.

Leserman, J., Petitto, J., Golden, R., Gaynes, B., Gu, H., Perkins, D., et al. (2000). Impact of stressful life events, depression, social support, coping and cortisol on progression to AIDS. *American Journal of Psychiatry*, 157, 1221–1228.

Leserman, J., Petitto, J., Gu, H., Perkins, D., Silva, S., Folds, J., et al. (2002). Progression to AIDS, a clinical AIDS condition and mortality: Psychosocial and physiological predictors. *Psychological Medicine*, 32, 1059–1073.

Liu, L.Y., Coe, C.L., Swenson, C.A., Kelly, E.A., Kita, H., & Busse, W.W. (2002). School examinations enhance airway inflammation to antigen challenge. *American Journal of Respiratory Critical Care Medicine*, 165, 1062–1067.

Marshall, G.D., Agarwal, S.K., Lloyd, C., Cohen, L., Henniger, E.M., & Morris, G.J. (1998). Cytokine dysregulation associated with exam stress in healthy medical students. *Brain, Behavior and Immunity*, 12, 297–307.

McEwen, B. (1998). Protective and damaging effects of stress mediators. *New England Journal of Medicine*, 338, 171–179.

McKenna, M., Zevon, M., Corn, B., & Rounds, J. (1999). Psychosocial factors and the development of breast cancer: A meta-analysis. *Health Psychology*, 18, 520–531.

Miller, G., & Cohen, S. (2001). Psychological interventions and the immune system: A meta-analytic review and critique. *Health Psychology*, 20, 47–63.

Miller, G., Cohen, S., & Ritchey, A. (2002). Chronic psychological stress and the regulation of pro-inflammatory cytokines: A glucocorticoid-resistance model. *Health Psychology*, 21, 531–541.

Miller, G.E., Dopp, J.M., Myers, H.F., Stevens, S.Y., & Fahey, J.L. (1999). Psychosocial predictors of natural killer cell mobilization during marital conflict. *Health Psychology*, 18, 262–271.

Mohr, D., & Cox, D. (2001). Multiple sclerosis: Empirical literature for clinical health psychologist. *Journal of Clinical Psychology*, 57, 479–499.

Mohr, D., Goodkin, D., Bacchetti, P., Boudewyn, A., Huang, L., Marrietta, P., et al. (2000). Psychosocial stress and the subsequent appearance of new brain MRI lesions in MS. *Neurology*, 55, 55–61.

Nisipeanu, P., & Korczyn, A. (1993). Psychological stress as risk factor for exacerbations in multiple sclerosis. *Neurology*, 43, 1311–1312.

Nott, K., Vedhara, K., & Spickett, G. (1995). Psychology, immunology and HIV. *Psychoneuroendocrinology*, 20, 451–474.

Pereira, D., Antoni, M., Danielson, A., Simon, T., Efantis-Potter, J., Carver, C., et al. (2003). Life stress and cervical squamous intraepithelial lesions in women with human papillomavirus and human immunodeficiency virus. *Psychosomatic Medicine*, 65, 427–434.

Petticrew, M., Bell, R., & Hunter, D. (2002). Influence of psychological coping on survival and recurrence in people with cancer: A systematic review. *British Medical Journal*, 325, 1066–1075.

Petticrew, M., Fraser, J., & Regan, M. (1999). Adverse life-events and risk of breast cancer: A meta-analysis. *British Journal of Health Psychology*, 4, 1–17.

Potter, P., & Zautra, A. (1997). Stressful life events' effects on rheumatoid arthritis disease activity. *Journal of Consulting and Clinical Psychology*, 65, 319–323.

Segerstrom, S.C., & Miller, G.E. (in press). Psychological stress and the immune system in humans: A meta-analytic review of 30 years of inquiry, *Psychological Bulletin*.

Seyle, H. (1950). *Stress*. Montreal: Acta.

Sibley, W. (1997). Risk factors in multiple sclerosis. In C. Raine, H. McFarland, & W. Tourtellotte (Eds.), *Multiple Sclerosis: Clinical and Pathogenetic Basis* (pp. 141–148). London: Chapman & Hall.

Speigel, D., Bloom, J., Kraemer, H., & Gottheil, E. (1989). Effect of psychosocial treatment on survival of patients with metastatic breast cancer. *Lancet*, 2, 888–891.

Spellberg, B., & Edwards, J. (2001). Type 1/type 2 immunity in infection disease. *Clinical Infectious Disease*, 32, 76–102.

Stone, A.A., Neale, J.M., Cox, D.S., Napoli, A., Valdimarsdottir, H., & Kennedy-Moore, E. (1994). Daily events are associated with secretory immune response to an oral antigen in men. *Health Psychology*, 13, 440–446.

Stutman, O. (1985). Immunological surveillance revisited. In A. Rest & M. Mitchell (Eds.), *Immunity to Cancer* (pp. 323–345). New York: Academic Press.

Thomason, B., Brantley, P., Jones, G., Dyer, H., & Morris, J. (1992). The relation between stress and disease activity in rheumatoid arthritis. *Journal of Behavioral Medicine*, 15, 215–220.

Vedhara, K., Cox, N.K., Wilcock, G.K., Perks, P., Hunt, M., Anderson, S., et al. (1999). Chronic stress in elderly carers of dementia patients and antibody response to influenza vaccination. *Lancet*, 353, 1969–1979.

Walker, J., Littlejohn, G., McMurray, N., & Cutolo, M. (1999). Stress system response and rheumatoid arthritis: A multilevel approach. *Rheumatology*, 38, 1050–1057.

Weisse, C.S., Pato, C.N., McAllister, C.G., & Littman, R. (1990). Differential effects of controllable and uncontrollable acute stress on lymphocyte proliferation and leukocyte percentages in humans. *Brain, Behavior and Immunity*, 4, 339–351.

Zautra, A.J., Hoffman, J.M., & Matt, K.S. (1998). An examination of individual differences in the relationship between interpersonal stress and disease activity among women with rheumatoid arthritis. *Arthritis Care and Research*, 11, 271–279.

8 Stress and Burnout: The Critical Research

Christina Maslach and Michael P. Leiter

CONTENTS

Job burnout is a psychological syndrome that involves a prolonged response to chronic interpersonal stressors on the job. The three key dimensions of this response are overwhelming exhaustion, feelings of cynicism and detachment from the job, and a sense of ineffectiveness and lack of accomplishment. The significance of this three-dimensional model is that it clearly places the individual stress experience within a social context and involves the person's conception of both self and others. Although there have been a few attempts to extend the burnout model to other domains of life, such as marriage and parenting, burnout has been identified primarily as a phenomenon in the world of work.

Work plays a central role in people's physical and psychological well-being. The physical hazards of work, in terms of injuries and diseases caused by the job, have long been the concern of the field of occupational health, but now more attention

0-8493-1820-3/05/$0.00+$1.50

has been given to social and psychological risk factors. Much of this attention has focused on job stress, which is a general rubric referring to the impact of external job demands (stressors) on the worker's internal experience (stress response), and to the subsequent outcomes of this process. Stress impairs job performance by reducing people's capacity for complex physical skills and by impairing cognitive functioning. Stress compromises the immune system, increasing the risk of viral and bacterial infections, and thus leading to higher rates of absenteeism and sick leave. The chronic tension associated with stress increases vulnerability to musculoskeletal problems. Empirical evidence has been found for the negative effects of job stress on physical health (especially cardiovascular problems), as well as on psychological well-being (e.g., job dissatisfaction, negative affect). Job stress is also predictive of various behavioral responses, such as lowered job performance, problems with family relationships, and self-damaging behaviors (see Kahn & Byosiere, 1992; Sauter & Murphy, 1995).

Unlike acute stress reactions, which develop in response to specific critical incidents, burnout is a cumulative reaction to ongoing occupational stressors. To put it in the terms of Selye's (1967) general adaptation syndrome, burnout is the exhaustion phase, following those of alarm and resistance. However, unlike more traditional stress research, which has focused on the physical damage that can occur, the emphasis in burnout research has been on the process of psychological erosion, and the psychological and social outcomes of this chronic exposure. Because burnout is a prolonged response to chronic interpersonal stressors on the job, it tends to be fairly stable over time.

A BRIEF HISTORY OF BURNOUT RESEARCH

For many years, burnout has been recognized as an occupational hazard for various people-oriented professions, such as human services, education, and health care. The therapeutic or service relationships that such providers develop with recipients require an ongoing and intense level of personal, emotional contact. Although such relationships can be rewarding and engaging, they can also be quite stressful. Within such occupations, the prevailing norms are to be selfless and put others' needs first; to work long hours and do whatever it takes to help a client or patient or student; to go the extra mile and to give one's all. Moreover, the organizational environments for these jobs are shaped by various social, political, and economic factors (such as funding cutbacks or policy restrictions) that result in work settings that are high in demands and low in resources. Recently, as other occupations have become more oriented to "high-touch" customer service, the phenomenon of burnout has become relevant for these jobs as well (Maslach & Leiter, 1997). Although research is beginning to be done with participant samples in this wider range of occupations, the bulk of the research findings on burnout are still based on samples in health care, education, and human services.

Despite the fact that practitioners had identified burnout as an important social problem in the workplace, it was a long time before it became a focus of systematic study by researchers (Maslach & Schaufeli, 1993). The development of a model of burnout was more of a grassroots, bottom-up process, grounded in the realities of people's experiences in the workplace, rather than a top-down derivation from a scholarly theory. Thus, the initial challenge was to identify existing concepts and theories that might help explain the phenomenon. Because the earliest researchers came from social and clinical psychology, they gravitated toward relevant ideas from these fields. The social perspective utilized concepts involving interpersonal relations, i.e., how people perceive and respond to others; these included detached concern, dehumanization in self-defense, and attribution processes. It also brought in concepts of motivation and emotion (and especially coping with emotional arousal). The clinical perspective also dealt with motivation and emotion, but framed these more in terms of psychological disorders, such as depression. Subsequent researchers came from industrial-organizational psychology, and this perspective emphasized work attitudes and behaviors. It was also at this point that burnout was conceptualized as a form of job stress, but the primary focus was on the organizational context and less on the characteristics of the experienced stress.

One consequence of these theoretical roots has been that the predominant research questions have focused more on social and interpersonal factors in the workplace and less on individual variables. A second consequence is that burnout did not attract the attention of researchers doing work on stress and physical health, and thus there has not been the kind of biomedical perspective that is traditionally associated with stress research.

The initial research on burnout was exploratory and relied primarily on qualitative techniques. What emerged from this descriptive work were the three dimensions of the burnout experience. The *exhaustion dimension* was also described as wearing out, loss of energy, depletion, debilitation, and fatigue. The *cynicism dimension* was originally called depersonalization (given the nature of human services occupations), but was also described as negative or inappropriate attitudes toward clients, irritability, loss of idealism, and withdrawal. The *inefficacy dimension* was originally called reduced personal accomplishment and was also described as reduced productivity or capability, low morale, and an inability to cope.

The emergence of this multidimensional model of burnout occurred at the same time as a shift to more quantitative and empirical research. One of the first tasks of this new research phase was the development of standardized measures of the burnout experience. The only measure that assesses all three dimensions is the Maslach Burnout Inventory (MBI), so it has been considered the standard tool for research in this field (see Maslach et al., 1996, for the most recent edition). The original version of the MBI was designed for use with people working in the human services and health care; a slightly modified version was then developed for use by people working in educational settings. More recently, given the increasing interest in burnout within occupations that are not so clearly people oriented, a third, general version of the MBI was developed (the MBI–General Survey, or MBI-GS). The MBI-GS assesses the same three dimensions as the original measure, using slightly revised items, and maintains a consistent factor structure across a variety of occupations.

At first, the multidimensional quality of the burnout construct and its measure posed statistical challenges for researchers who wanted a single score that could be correlated with scores on other variables. With the development of more sophisticated methodology and statistical tools that could manage complex constructs, researchers were able to analyze the interrelationships between the burnout dimensions and other factors, and to develop structural models. As a result, researchers have been able to examine the contribution of many potential influences and consequences simultaneously, separating unique contributors from those that are redundant.

The initial research on burnout was concentrated in the U.S., and then it gradually expanded to other English-speaking countries, such as Canada and Great Britain. With the translations of articles and research measures into other languages, burnout began to be studied in many European countries and in Israel. Currently, burnout research is being conducted in many other countries around the world, with the bulk of the work occurring in postindustrialized nations. Although the psychometric properties of the MBI are similar across cultures, there appear to be national differences in average levels of burnout. For example, Europeans show lower average scores than North Americans (Schaufeli & Enzmann, 1998), and other researchers have found cultural differences in multinational data sets (Golembiewski et al., 1996; Savicki, 2002). However, given that these studies were not designed to test cultural hypotheses and did not use random and representative comparative samples, it is difficult to draw strong conclusions about the cultural implications of the findings.

A recent development in burnout research has been to expand the focus to the positive antithesis of burnout, rather than just focusing on the negative state that it represents. This positive state has been called job engagement, but it has been conceptualized in different ways. One approach has been to define engagement as the opposite of burnout; thus, it is comprised of the same three basic dimensions, but with the positive endpoints of energy, involvement, and efficacy (Leiter & Maslach, 1998). By implication, engagement is assessed by the opposite pattern of scores on the three MBI dimensions. A different approach has defined engagement as a persistent, positive affective–motivational state of fulfillment that is characterized by the three components of vigor, dedication, and absorption. Schaufeli and his colleagues have developed a new measure to assess this positive state, and the preliminary results show that while the scores are negatively correlated with burnout, they are most strongly related to the positive endpoint of efficacy (see Maslach et al., 2001, for a more extensive comparison of these two approaches).

ISSUES IN CONCEPTUALIZING BURNOUT

Throughout the history of burnout research, there have been a number of debates about key theoretical points. Some of these have focused on what burnout is (and is not), and others have tried to deal with how burnout develops and changes over time.

MULTIDIMENSIONAL VS. ONE-DIMENSIONAL CONSTRUCTS

All theoretical perspectives on burnout have included exhaustion as a key defining dimension. The concept of exhaustion captures the basic stress experienced by an individual, as it refers to feelings of being overextended and depleted of one's emotional and physical resources. When people describe themselves or others as experiencing burnout, they are often referring to the experience of exhaustion (e.g., Pick & Leiter, 1991). In the research literature on burnout, exhaustion is the most widely reported and most thoroughly analyzed component of this syndrome. In some one-dimensional theories of burnout, exhaustion has been the sole defining criterion (Freudenberger, 1983; Pines et al., 1981; Shirom, 1989). The strong identification of exhaustion with burnout has led some to argue that the other two aspects of the syndrome are incidental or unnecessary. However, the fact that exhaustion is a necessary criterion for burnout does not mean it is sufficient. If one were to look at burnout out of context and simply focus on the individual exhaustion component, one would lose sight of the phenomenon entirely.

Although exhaustion reflects the stress dimension of burnout, it fails to capture the critical aspects of the relationship people have with their work. Exhaustion is not something that is simply experienced — rather, it prompts actions to distance oneself emotionally and cognitively from one's work, presumably as a way to cope with the work overload. Within the human services, the emotional demands of the work can exhaust a service provider's capacity to be involved with, and responsive to, the needs of service recipients. Cynicism (or depersonalization) is an attempt to put distance between oneself and service recipients by actively ignoring the qualities that make them unique and engaging people. Their demands are more manageable when they are considered impersonal objects of one's work. Outside of the human services, people use cognitive distancing by developing an indifferent or cynical attitude when they are exhausted and discouraged. Distancing is such an immediate reaction to exhaustion that a strong relationship from exhaustion to cynicism is found consistently in burnout research, across a wide range of organizational and occupational settings.

The relationship of inefficacy to the other two aspects of burnout is somewhat more complex. In some instances, it appears to be a function, to some degree, of either exhaustion or cynicism, or a combination of the two (Byrne 1994; Lee & Ashforth 1996). A work situation with chronic, overwhelming demands that contribute to exhaustion or cynicism is likely to erode one's sense of effectiveness. Further, the experience of exhaustion or cynicism interferes with effectiveness; it is difficult to gain a sense of accomplishment when feeling exhausted or when helping people toward whom one is indifferent. However, in other job contexts, inefficacy appears to develop in parallel with the other two burnout aspects, rather than sequentially (Leiter, 1993). Here the lack of efficacy seems to arise more clearly from a lack of relevant resources, while exhaustion and cynicism emerge from the presence of work overload and social conflict. An alternative view is that inefficacy is more strongly related to personality than are the other two burnout dimensions, and this is why it does not show consistent relationships with situational variables (Schaufeli & Enzmann, 1998).

Diagnosis of Burnout as Mental Ill Health

In the early stages of conceptual work on burnout, one of the major questions was whether burnout was a form of mental illness and, if so, what was the type of disorder and its diagnostic criteria. It is possible that this focus on framing burnout as mental illness was a factor in retarding the later recognition of burnout as a stress phenomenon (as noted earlier). The issues surrounding the conceptualization of burnout as a form of ill health continue to this day, and more research is clearly needed.

Early research conducted during the development of the MBI found burnout to be correlated with measures of anxiety and depression. Some argued that burnout was simply a form of depression, but subsequent empirical research established a clear distinction between burnout and depression (Bakker et al., 2000a; Glass & McKnight, 1996; Leiter & Durup, 1994). This research demonstrated that burnout is a problem that is specific to the work context, in contrast to depression, which tends to pervade every domain of a person's life. These findings lent empirical support to earlier claims that burnout is job related and situation specific, as opposed to depression, which is general and context-free (Freudenberger, 1983; Warr, 1987). However, as noted later, individuals who are more depression-prone (as indicated by higher scores on neuroticism) are more vulnerable to burnout.

An analysis of various conceptualizations of burnout noted five common criteria for the burnout phenomenon (Maslach & Schaufeli, 1993). First, there is a predominance of dysphoric symptoms such as mental or emotional exhaustion, fatigue, and depression. Second, the emphasis is on mental and behavioral symptoms more than physical ones. Third, burnout symptoms are work related. Fourth, the symptoms manifest themselves in normal persons who did not suffer from psychopathology before. Fifth, decreased effectiveness and work performance occur because of negative attitudes and behaviors. Most of these elements are represented in the diagnosis for job-related neurasthenia (WHO, 1992), so recent research has been utilizing this diagnosis as the psychiatric equivalent of burnout. A recent study has found that burnout scores on the MBI can distinguish psychiatric outpatients diagnosed with job-related neurasthenia from outpatients diagnosed with other mental disorders, and that the former group shows a less pathological profile than the latter (Schaufeli et al., 2001).

The link between job-related neurasthenia and burnout might support the argument that burnout is itself a form of mental illness. However, a more common assumption has been that burnout causes mental dysfunction — that is, it precipitates negative effects in terms of mental health, such as anxiety, depression, drops in self-esteem, and so forth. Unfortunately, this assumption has not been tested with the necessary longitudinal research. An alternative argument is that people who are mentally healthy are better able to cope with chronic stressors and thus less likely to experience burnout. Although not assessing burnout directly, one study addressed this question by analyzing archival longitudinal data of people who worked in interpersonally demanding jobs (i.e., emotionally demanding "helper" roles or jobs that deal with people in stressful situations). The results showed that people who were psychologically healthier in adolescence and early adulthood were more likely to enter, and remain in, such jobs, and they showed greater involvement and satisfaction with their work (Jenkins & Maslach, 1994). Given this longitudinal data set, this study was better able to establish possible causal relationships than is true for the typical correlational studies.

The Development of Burnout Over Time

There have been various theoretical proposals about how burnout develops and changes over time, in terms of the sequential progression of the three dimensions.

One approach is the phase model, in which the three burnout dimensions are split into high and low categories, yielding eight different patterns, or phases, of burnout (Golembiewski & Munzenrider, 1988). The phase model has hypothesized that cynicism is the early minimum phase of burnout, followed by the addition of inefficacy and finally by exhaustion. An alternative process model has hypothesized that the occurrence of one dimension precipitates the development of subsequent ones. Exhaustion occurs first, which leads to the development of cynicism, which then leads to inefficacy (Leiter & Maslach, 1988). The latter approach has received stronger empirical evidence for the first of these two linkages than for the latter, as mentioned earlier. Much of that research has relied primarily on cross-sectional studies and statistical causal models, but there have been some recent longitudinal studies that have provided empirical support for this process sequence (Bakker et al., 2000b; Leiter & Maslach, 2004; Toppinen-Tanner et al., 2002).

Other theorizing about burnout over time has focused on the causes and effects of burnout, rather than the interrelationships between the three dimensions. Cherniss (1980b) proposed a transactional model of burnout, which has three stages. The first stage is an imbalance between work demands and individual resources (job stressors), the second stage involves an emotional response of exhaustion and anxiety (individual strain), and the third stage involves changes in attitudes and behavior, such as greater cynicism (defensive coping). Several studies have provided empirical support for this transactional model (Burke et al., 1984; Burke & Greenglass, 1989). More recently, a mediation model of burnout has been proposed by Leiter and Maslach (2004), in which burnout mediates the impact of job stressors on individual outcomes. Like the transactional model, the mediation model frames job stressors in terms of person–job imbalances, or mismatches, but identifies six key areas in which these imbalances take place (these areas will be reviewed later in this paper). These stressors affect an individual's level of experienced burnout (which is defined to combine both exhaustion and cynicism, as well as inefficacy), and this level of burnout in turn determines various individual outcomes, such as work behaviors (e.g., performance, absenteeism), social behaviors (e.g., quality of home life), and personal health. Initial empirical support for this mediation model has been provided by both cross-sectional and longitudinal analyses.

CAUSES AND CONSEQUENCES OF BURNOUT

Both the transactional and mediation models of burnout make explicit the causal theorizing that has always been implicit in burnout research: certain factors (both situational and individual) cause people to experience burnout, and once burnout occurs, it causes certain outcomes (both situational and individual). However, these causal assumptions have rarely been able to be tested directly. Most research on burnout has involved cross-sectional designs or studies using statistical causal models. This correlational database has provided support for many of the hypothesized links between burnout and its sources and effects, but it is unable to address the presumed causality of those linkages. The recent increase in longitudinal studies, as mentioned earlier, will begin to provide a better opportunity to test sequential hypotheses, but stronger causal inferences will also require appropriate methodological designs (and these are often difficult to implement in applied settings). One other critical constraint to keep in mind while reviewing the research findings is that many of the variables have been assessed by self-report measures (rather than other indices of behavior or health). Given these caveats, this section will provide an overview of the major research findings on the predictors and outcomes of burnout.

Situational Predictors of Burnout

Over two decades of research on burnout has identified a plethora of organizational risk factors across many occupations in various countries (see Maslach et al., 2001; Schaufeli & Enzmann, 1998). In analyzing this research literature, Maslach and Leiter (1997, 1999) identified six key domains: workload, control, reward, community, fairness, and values. The first two areas are reflected in the demand–control model of job stress (Karasek & Theorell, 1990), and reward refers to the power of reinforcements to shape behavior. Community captures all of the work on social support and interpersonal conflict, while fairness emerges from the literature on equity and social justice. Finally, the area of values picks up the cognitive-emotional power of job goals and expectations.

Workload

A commonly discussed source of burnout is overload: job demands exceeding human limits. People have to do too much in too little time with too few resources. Increased workload has a consistent relationship with burnout, especially with the exhaustion dimension (Cordes & Dougherty, 1993; Maslach et al., 2001; Schaufeli & Enzmann, 1998). Structural models of burnout have shown that exhaustion then mediates the relationship of workload with the other two dimensions of burnout (Lee & Ashforth, 1996; Leiter & Harvie, 1998). This association reflects the relationship of work demands with occupational stress in the stress and coping literature (Cox et al., 1993). Both qualitative and quantitative work overload contribute to exhaustion by depleting the capacity of people to meet the demands of the job. The critical point occurs when people are unable to recover from work demands. That is, acute fatigue resulting from an especially demanding event at work — meeting a deadline or addressing a crisis — need not lead to burnout if people have an opportunity to recover during restful periods at work or at home (Shinn et al., 1984). When this kind of overload is a chronic job condition, not an occasional emergency, there is little opportunity to rest, recover, and restore balance. A sustainable workload, in contrast, provides opportunities to use and refine existing skills as well as to become effective in new areas of activity (Landsbergis, 1988).

Control

The demand–control theory of job stress (Karasek & Theorell, 1990) has made the case for the enabling role of control. This area includes employees' perceived capacity to influence decisions that affect their work, to exercise professional autonomy, and to gain access to the resources necessary to do an effective job. A major control problem occurs when people experience role conflict. Many burnout studies have found that greater role conflict is strongly and positively associated with greater exhaustion (Cordes & Dougherty, 1993; Maslach et al., 1996). Role conflict arises from multiple authorities with conflicting demands or incongruent values, and people in this situation cannot exercise effective control in their job. Role conflict is not simply an indicator of additional work demands, but is emotionally exhausting in itself (e.g., Siefert et al., 1991; Starnaman & Miller, 1992). Studies that examine role conflict usually also consider role ambiguity — the absence of direction in work. Generally, role ambiguity is associated with greater burnout, but the relationship is not nearly as consistent as that of role conflict (Cordes & Dougherty, 1993; Maslach et al., 1996). Ambiguity can enhance some work contexts by providing the freedom to pursue one's values, while conflict directly inhibits a course of action. When people have more control in their work, their actions are more freely chosen — and this can lead to greater satisfaction with the job and more commitment to it. Active participation in organizational decision making has been consistently found to be associated with higher levels of efficacy and lower levels of exhaustion (Cherniss, 1980a; Lee & Ashforth, 1993; Leiter, 1992).

Reward

The research literature on reward addresses the extent to which rewards — monetary, social, and intrinsic — are consistent with expectations. The results of various studies have shown that insufficient reward (whether financial, institutional, or social) increases people's vulnerability to burnout (e.g., Chappell & Novak, 1992; Glicken, 1983; Maslanka, 1996; Siefert et al., 1991). Lack of recognition from service recipients, colleagues, managers, and external stakeholders devalues both the work and the workers and is closely associated with feelings of inefficacy (Cordes & Dougherty, 1993; Maslach et al., 1996). In contrast, consistency in the reward dimension between the person and the job means that there are both material rewards and opportunities for intrinsic satisfaction (Richardsen et al., 1992). Intrinsic rewards (such as pride in doing something of importance and doing it well) can be just as critical as extrinsic rewards, if not more so. What keeps work involving for most people is the pleasure and satisfaction they experience with the day-to-day flow of work that is going well (Leiter, 1992).

Community

Community is the overall quality of social interaction at work, including issues of conflict, mutual support, closeness, and the capacity to work as a team. Burnout research has focused primarily on social support from supervisors, coworkers, and family members (Cordes & Dougherty, 1993; Greenglass et al., 1988, 1994; Maslach et al., 1996). Distinct patterns have been found for informal coworker support and supervisor support (Jackson et al., 1986; Leiter & Maslach, 1988). Supervisor support has been more consistently associated with exhaustion, reflecting the supervisors' impact on staff members' workload. Coworker support is more closely related to accomplishment or efficacy, reflecting the value staff members put on the expert evaluation by their peers. A sense of community has been found to buffer the impact of feelings of inequity at work (Truchot & Deregard, 2001). Regardless of its specific form, social support has been found to be associated with greater engagement (Leiter & Maslach, 1988, Schnorpfeil et al., 2002).

Research on the social context of burnout has also attended to the broader issues associated with a sense of community in an organization (Drory & Shamir, 1988; Farber, 1984; Royal & Rossi, 1996). Research on community orientation (Buunk & Schaufeli, 1993) provides a distinct but consistent perspective. Both of these approaches consider ways in which the overall quality of personal interactions among people in an organization has an impact on the relationships people have with their work. The consistent finding throughout this research is that a lively, attentive, responsive community is incompatible with burnout. People's subjective appraisal of their social context — their sense of community with colleagues or their communal orientation toward their clients or customers — reflects the extent to which the organizational community is consistent with their expectations.

Fairness

Fairness is the extent to which decisions at work are perceived as being fair and equitable. Relevant research on procedural justice (e.g., Lawler, 1968; Tyler, 1990) has shown that people are more concerned with the fairness of the process than with the favorableness of the outcome. People use the quality of the procedures, and their own treatment during the decision-making process, as an index of their place in the community. They will feel alienated from that community if they are subject to unfair, cursory, or disrespectful decision making. In contrast, a fair decision is one in which people have an opportunity to present their arguments and in which they feel treated with respect and politeness. Thus, fairness shares some qualities with community, as well as with reward.

Fairness is central to equity theory (Walster et al., 1973), which posits that perceptions of equity or inequity are based on people's determination of the balance between their inputs (i.e., time, effort, and expertise) and outputs (i.e., rewards and recognition). This core notion of inequity is also reflected in the effort–reward imbalance model (Siegrist, 1996). Research based on these theoretical frameworks has found that a lack of reciprocity, or imbalanced social exchange processes, is predictive of burnout (e.g., Bakker et al., 2000a; Schaufeli et al., 1996). Fairness has also emerged as a critical factor in administrative leadership (e.g., White, 1987). Employees who perceive their supervisors as being both fair and supportive are less susceptible to burnout and are more accepting of major organizational change (Leiter & Harvie, 1997, 1998). It appears that employees value fairness in itself and consider it to be indicative of a genuine concern for the long-term good of the organization's staff, especially during difficult times.

Values

There has not been a lot of research on the impact of values for job stress, but current work suggests that it can play a key role in predicting levels of burnout and engagement (Leiter & Maslach, 2004). Values are the ideals and motivations that originally attracted people to their job, and thus they are the motivating connection between the worker and the workplace, which goes beyond the utilitarian exchange of time for money or advancement. When there is a values conflict on the job, and thus a gap between individual and organizational values, workers will find themselves making a trade-off between work they want to do and work they have to do. In some cases, people might feel constrained by the job to do things that are unethical and not in accord with their own values, or they can be caught between conflicting values of the organization (e.g., high-quality service and cost containment do not always coexist). In other instances, there can be a conflict between personal career aspirations and organizational values, as when people realize that they entered an occupation with mistaken expectations. One resolution of the tension resulting from value conflicts is to bring personal expectations in line with those of the organization (Stevens & O'Neill, 1983); another is to leave the organization in search of more fulfilling career opportunities (Pick & Leiter, 1991). Research has found that a conflict in values is related to all three dimensions of burnout (Leiter & Harvie, 1997).

Integration of the Six Areas

It is not yet clear from the research whether some of these situational factors are more significant than others as predictors of burnout. The six areas are not independent of each other; indeed, problems in one area can be associated with problems in another area. For example, excessive workload often indicates problems in control and autonomy, because much of what people identify as excessive work demands are externally imposed tasks (rather than internally chosen ones). As another example, an organization that has a strong sense of community is likely to treat employees fairly and provide meaningful rewards.

However, recent research on the interrelationships of these six areas suggests that there is a consistent and complex pattern that predicts the level of experienced burnout. Using a new measure to assess person–job incongruities, or imbalances, in these six areas, Leiter and Maslach (2004) found that workload and control each play critical roles (thus replicating the demand–control model) but are not sufficient. Reward, community, and fairness add further power to predict values, which in turn was the critical predictor of the three dimensions of burnout.

Another possibility to consider in future research is whether the weighting of the importance of these six areas can reflect an important individual difference. For example, some people might place a higher weight on rewards than on values, and thus might be more distressed by insufficient rewards than by value conflicts.

Individual Predictors of Burnout

It is interesting to note that the empirical research on risk factors for burnout is far less for personal variables than for situational ones. This can reflect, to some extent, the theoretical orientations of the leading researchers in the field, but the pattern of findings suggests that personal factors play a less critical role as sources of burnout. Although some individual characteristics have been correlated with burnout, these relationships are not as great in size as those for situational factors, which implies that burnout is more of a social phenomenon than an individual one.

Several demographic variables have been studied in relation to burnout, but the studies are relatively few and the findings are not that consistent (see Schaufeli & Enzmann, 1998, for a review). Age is the one variable that shows a more consistent correlation with burnout. Among younger employees the level of burnout is reported to be higher than it is among those aged over 30 or 40 years. Age is confounded with work experience, so burnout appears to be more of a risk earlier in one's career, rather than later. The reasons for such an interpretation have not been studied very thoroughly. However, these findings should be viewed with caution because of the problem of survival bias — i.e., those who burn out early in their careers are likely to quit their jobs, leaving behind the survivors, who consequently exhibit lower levels of burnout. The demographic variable of sex has not been a strong predictor of burnout. The one small but consistent sex difference is that males often score slightly higher on cynicism. There is also a tendency in some studies for women to score slightly higher on exhaustion. These results could be related to gender role stereotypes, but they can also reflect the confounding of sex with occupation (e.g., police officers are more likely to be male, nurses are more likely to be female). With regard to marital status, those who are unmarried seem to be more prone to burnout than those who are married. Singles seem to experience even higher burnout levels than those who are divorced. As for ethnicity, very few studies have assessed this demographic variable, so it is not possible to summarize any empirical trends.

Several personality traits have been studied in an attempt to discover which types of people might be at greater risk for experiencing burnout (see Schaufeli & Enzmann, 1998, for a review). As with demographic variables, there are some suggestive trends but not a large body of consistent empirical findings. Burnout tends to be higher among people who have low self-esteem, an external locus of control, low levels of hardiness, and a type A behavior style. Those who are burned out cope with stressful events in a rather passive, defensive way, whereas active and confronting coping is associated with less burnout. In particular, confronting coping is associated with the dimension of efficacy. More consistent findings have come from research on the big five personality dimensions, which has found that burnout is linked to the dimension of neuroticism (Deary et al., 1996; Hills & Norvell, 1991; Zellars et al., 2000). Neuroticism includes trait anxiety, hostility, depression, self-consciousness, and vulnerability; neurotic individuals are emotionally unstable and prone to psychological distress.

Outcomes of Burnout

Some of the research on burnout has viewed it as an important end state in its own right, particularly when it has been considered to be a form of poor mental health. However, the more common assumption is that the significance of burnout lies in its role as a mediator of other important outcomes. It is presumed that the person experiencing burnout will show a decline in job performance and an increase in job withdrawal (absenteeism, turnover). In addition, given that burnout is a stress phenomenon, the presumption is that it will also have important health outcomes for the individual, and might affect the person's home life as well. All of these outcomes have high costs not only for the individual, but also for the place where he or she works. Despite the importance of such significant outcomes, the research in this area has been relatively sparse.

Burnout has been associated with various forms of negative responses to the job, including job dissatisfaction, low organizational commitment, absenteeism, intention to leave the job, and turnover (see Schaufeli & Enzmann, 1998, for a review). People who are experiencing burnout can have a negative impact on their colleagues, both by causing greater personal conflict and by disrupting job tasks. Thus, burnout can be contagious and perpetuate itself through informal interactions on the job. The hypothesis that burnout leads to poor job performance has not received many empirical tests. However, one study found that nurses experiencing higher levels of burnout were judged by their patients to be providing a lower level of patient care (Leiter et al., 1998), while another study found that burned-out police officers reported more use of violence against civilians (Kop et al., 1999).

Despite all this research evidence, the actual causal linkage between burnout and these negative job outcomes is still a matter of speculation. Does burnout cause people to be dissatisfied with their job? Or does a drop in satisfaction serve as the precursor to burnout? Alternatively, both burnout and job dissatisfaction can be caused by another factor, such as poor working conditions.

Research studies on the connection between work and home life have found that burnout has a negative spillover effect. Workers experiencing burnout were rated by their spouses in more negative ways (Jackson & Maslach, 1982; Zedeck et al., 1988), and they themselves reported that their work has a negative impact on their family and that their marriage is unsatisfactory (Burke & Greenglass, 1989, 2001).

Even though the stress literature provides a clear theoretical basis for a relation between burnout and health, such a relation has not been studied extensively. Of the three burnout dimensions, exhaustion is the closest to an orthodox stress variable, and thus it should be more predictive of stress-related health outcomes than the other two components. Indeed, a consistent finding in burnout research is the correlation between the exhaustion dimension and various physical symptoms of stress: headaches, gastrointestinal disorders, muscle tension, hypertension, cold/flu episodes, and sleep disturbances (e.g., Bhagat et al., 1995; Burke & Deszca, 1986; Golembiewski & Munzenrider, 1988; Hendrix et al., 1995; Jackson & Maslach, 1982; Kahill, 1988). Some research has also found a link between burnout and lifestyle practices that carry health risks, such as smoking and alcohol use (e.g., Burke et al., 1984). In terms of mental health, burnout has been predictive of depression (Greenglass & Burke, 1990; Schonfeld, 1989) and other emotional symptoms.

Despite this link between burnout and stress-related health behaviors, there has not yet been any research on relevant health outcomes, such as the utilization of health care services or the filing of workmen's compensation claims for stress. There has also been no theorizing to suggest that burnout has a connection to the development or progression of specific diseases, and consequently, there is no empirical research on this issue.

CONCLUSION

Significant progress in understanding burnout has been based on the development of new, rather than traditional, theoretical perspectives. What is unique about the burnout syndrome, and what distinguishes it from other types of job stress, is what has been, and needs to be, emphasized in theoretical formulations. Future progress will rest on the further elaboration of all three dimensions of burnout and on their relationship to the six areas of mismatch, or imbalance, between worker and workplace. This theoretical elaboration should generate better hypotheses about the causes and consequences linked to each of these dimensions, and should guide a more informed search for solutions to this important social problem.

REFERENCES

Bakker, A. B., Schaufeli, W. B., Demerouti, E., Janssen, P. M. P., Van der Hulst, R., & Brouwer, J. (2000a). Using equity theory to examine the difference between burnout and depression. *Anxiety, Stress and Coping*, 13, 247–268.

Bakker, A. B., Schaufeli, W. B., Sixma, H. J., Bosveld, W., & VanDierendonck, D. (2000b). Patient demands, lack of reciprocity, and burnout: A five-year longitudinal study among general practitioners. *Journal of Organizational Behavior*, 21, 425–441.

Bhagat, R. S., Allie, S. M., & Ford, Jr., D. L. (1995). Coping with stressful life events: An empirical analysis. In R. Crandall & P. L. Perrewe (Eds.), *Occupational Stress: A Handbook* (pp. 93–112). Washington, DC: Taylor & Francis.

Burke, R. J., & Deszca, E. (1986). Correlates of psychological burnout phases among police officers. *Human Relations*, 39, 487–502.

Burke, R. J., & Greenglass, E. R. (1989). Psychological burnout among men and women in teaching: An examination of the Cherniss model. *Human Relations*, 42, 261–273.

Burke, R. J., & Greenglass, E. R. (2001). Hospital restructuring, work-family conflict and psychological burnout among nursing staff. *Psychology and Health*, 16, 83–94.

Burke, R. J., Shearer, J., & Deszca, G. (1984). Burnout among men and women in police work: An examination of the Cherniss model. *Journal of Health and Human Resources Administration*, 7, 162–188.

Buunk, B. P., & Schaufeli, W. B. (1993). Professional burnout: A perspective from social comparison theory. In W. B. Schaufeli, C. Maslach, & T. Marek (Eds.), *Professional Burnout: Recent Developments in Theory and Research* (pp. 53–69). Washington, DC: Taylor & Francis.

Byrne, B.M. (1994). Burnout: Testing for the validity, replication, and invariance of causal structure across elementary, intermediate, and secondary teachers. *American Educational Research Journal*, 31, 645–673.

Chappell, N. L., & Novak, M. (1992). The role of support in alleviating stress among nursing assistants. *Gerontologist*, 32, 351–359.

Cherniss, C. (1980a). *Professional Burnout in Human Service Organizations*. New York: Praeger.

Cherniss, C. (1980b). *Staff Burnout: Job Stress in the Human Services*. Beverly Hills, CA: Sage.

Cordes C. L., & Dougherty, T. W. (1993). A review and an integration of research on job burnout. *Academy of Management Review*, 18, 621–656.

Cox, T., Kuk, G., & Leiter, M. P. (1993). Burnout, health, work stress, and organizational healthiness. In W. Schaufeli, C. Maslach, & Marek, T. (Eds.), *Professional Burnout: Recent Developments in Theory and Research* (pp. 177–193). Washington, DC: Taylor & Francis.

Deary, I. J., Blenkin, H., Agius, R. M., et al. (1996). Models of job-related stress and personal achievement among consultant doctors. *British Journal of Psychology*, 87, 3–29.

Drory, A., & Shamir, B. (1988). Effects of organizational and life variables on job satisfaction and burnout. *Group and Organization Studies*, 13, 441–455.

Farber, B. A. (1984). Stress and burnout in suburban teachers. *Journal of Educational Research*, 77, 325–331.

Freudenberger, H. J. (1983). Burnout: Contemporary issues, trends, and concerns. In BA Farber (Ed.), *Stress and Burnout in the Human Service Professions* (pp. 23–28). New York: Pergamon.

Glass, D. C., & McKnight, J. D. (1996). Perceived control, depressive symptomatology, and professional burnout: A review of the evidence. *Psychology and Health*, 11, 23–48.

Glicken, M. D. (1983). A counseling approach to employee burnout. *Personnel Journal*, 62, 222–228.

Golembiewski, R. T., Boudreau, R. A., Munzenrider, R. F., & Luo, H. (1996). *Global Burnout: A World-Wide Pandemic Explored by the Phase Model*. Greenwich, CT: JAI Press.

Golembiewski, R. T., & Munzenrider R. (1988). *Phases of Burnout: Developments in Concepts and Applications*. New York: Praeger.

Greenglass, E. R., & Burke, R. J. (1990). Burnout over time. *Journal of Health and Human Resources Administration*, 13, 192–204.

Greenglass, E. R., Fiksenbaum, L., & Burke, R. J. (1994). The relationship between social support and burnout over time in teachers. *Journal of Social Behavior and Personality*, 9, 219–230.

Greenglass, E. R., Pantony, K.-L., & Burke, R. J. (1988). A gender-role perspective on role conflict, work stress and social support. *Journal of Social Behavior and Personality*, 3, 317–328.

Hendrix, W. H., Summers, T. P., Leap, T. L., & Steel, R. P. (1995). Antecedents and organizational effectiveness outcomes of employee stress and health. In R. Crandall & P. L. Perrewe (Eds.), *Occupational Stress: A Handbook* (pp. 73–92). Washington, DC: Taylor & Francis.

Hills, H., & Norvell, N. (1991). An examination of hardiness and neuroticism as potential moderators of stress outcomes. *Behavioral Medicine*, 17, 31–38.

Jackson, S. E., & Maslach, C. (1982). After-effects of job-related stress: Families as victims. *Journal of Occupational Behaviour*, 3, 63–77.

Jackson, S. E., Schwab, R. L., & Schuler, R. S. (1986). Toward an understanding of the burnout phenomenon. *Journal of Applied Psychology*, 7, 630–640.

Jenkins, S. R., & Maslach, C. (1994). Psychological health and involvement in interpersonally demanding occupations: A longitudinal perspective. *Journal of Organizational Behavior*, 15, 101–127.

Kahill, S. (1988). Symptoms of professional burnout: A review of the empirical evidence. *Canadian Psychology*, 29, 284–297.

Kahn, R. L., & Byosiere, P. (1992). Stress in organizations. In M. D. Dunnette & L. M. Hough (Eds.), *Handbook of Industrial and Organizational Psychology*, Vol. 3 (pp. 571–650). Palo Alto, CA: Consulting Psychologists Press.

Karasek, R., and Theorell, T. (1990). *Stress, Productivity, and the Reconstruction of Working Life*. New York: Basic Books.

Kop, N., Euwema, M., & Schaufeli, W. (1999). Burnout, job stress, and violent behaviour among Dutch police officers. *Work and Stress*, 13, 326–340.

Landsbergis, P.A. (1988). Occupational stress among health care workers: A test of the job demands-control model. *Journal of Organizational Behavior*, 9(), 217–239.

Lawler III, E. E. (1968). Equity theory as a predictor of productivity and work quality. *Psychological Bulletin*, 70, 596–610.

Lee, R. T., & Ashforth, B. E. (1993). A longitudinal study of burnout among supervisors and managers: Comparisons between the Leiter and Maslach (1988) and Golembiewski et al. (1986) models. *Organizational Behavior and Human Decision Processes*, 54, 369–398.

Lee, R. T., & Ashforth, B.E. (1996). A meta-analytic examination of the correlates of the three dimensions of job burnout. *Journal of Applied Psychology*, 81, 123–133.

Leiter, M. P. (1992). Burnout as a crisis in professional role structures: Measurement and conceptual issues. *Anxiety, Stress and Coping*, 5, 79–93.

Leiter, M. P. (1993). Burnout as a developmental process: Consideration of models. In W. B. Schaufeli, C. Maslach, & T. Marek (Eds.), *Professional Burnout: Recent Developments in Theory and Research* (pp. 237–250). Washington, DC: Taylor & Francis.

Leiter, M. P., & Durup, J. (1994). The discriminant validity of burnout and depression: A confirmatory factor analytic study. *Anxiety, Stress and Coping*, 7, 357–373.

Leiter, M. P., & Harvie, P. (1997). The correspondence of supervisor and subordinate perspectives on major organizational change. *Journal of Occupational Health Psychology*, 2, 1–10.

Leiter, M. P., & Harvie, P. (1998). Conditions for staff acceptance of organizational change: Burnout as a mediating construct. *Anxiety, Stress and Coping*, 11, 1–25.

Leiter, M. P., Harvie, P., & Frizzell, C. (1998). The correspondence of patient satisfaction and nurse burnout. *Social Science and Medicine*, 47, 1611–1617.

Leiter, M. P., & Maslach, C. (1988). The impact of interpersonal environment on burnout and organizational commitment. *Journal of Organizational Behavior*, 9, 297–308.

Leiter, M. P., & Maslach, C. (1998). Burnout. In H. Friedman (Ed.), *Encyclopedia of Mental Health*. San Diego: Academic Press.

Leiter, M. P., & Maslach, C. (2004). Areas of worklife: A structured approach to organizational predictors of job burnout. In P. Perrewé & D.C. Ganster (Eds.), *Research in Occupational Stress and Well Being*, Vol. 3. Oxford, U.K.: Elsevier Science, Ltd.

Maslach, C. (1982). *Burnout: The Cost of Caring*. Englewood Cliffs, NJ: Prentice Hall.

Maslach, C. (1993). Burnout: A multidimensional perspective. In W. B. Schaufeli, C. Maslach, & T. Marek (Eds.), *Professional Burnout: Recent Developments in Theory and Research* (pp. 19–32). Washington, DC: Taylor & Francis.

Maslach, C., Jackson, S. E., & Leiter, M. P. (1996). *The Maslach Burnout Inventory*, 3rd ed. Palo Alto, CA: Consulting Psychologists Press.

Maslach, C., & Leiter, M. P. (1997). *The Truth about Burnout*. San Francisco: Jossey-Bass.

Maslach, C., & Leiter, M. P. (1999). Burnout and engagement in the workplace: A contextual analysis, *Advances in Motivation and Achievement*, 11, 275–302.

Maslach, C., & Schaufeli, W. B. (1993). Historical and conceptual development of burnout. In W. B. Schaufeli, C. Maslach, & T. Marek (Eds.), *Professional Burnout: Recent Developments in Theory and Research* (pp. 1–16). Washington, DC: Taylor & Francis.

Maslach, D., Schaufeli, W. B., & Leiter, M. P. (2001). Job burnout. *Annual Review of Psychology*, 52, 397–422.

Maslanka, H. (1996). Burnout, social support and AIDS volunteers. *AIDS Care*, 8, 195–206.

Pick, D., & Leiter, M. P. (1991). Nurses' perceptions of the nature and causes of burnout: A comparison of self-reports and standardized measures. *The Canadian Journal of Nursing Research*, 23, 33–48.

Pines, A., Aronson, E., & Kafry, D. (1981). *Burnout: From Tedium to Personal Growth*. New York: Free Press.

Richardsen, A. M., Burke, R. J., & Leiter, M. P. (1992). Occupational demands, psychological burnout, and anxiety among hospital personnel in Norway. *Anxiety, Stress and Coping*, 5, 62–78.

Royal, M. A., & Rossi, R. J. (1996). Individual level correlates of sense of community: Findings from workplace and school. *Journal of Community Psychology*, 24, 395–416.

Sauter, S. L., & Murphy, L. R. (Eds.). (1995). *Organizational Risk Factors for Job Stress*. Washington, DC: American Psychological Association.

Savicki, V. (2002). *Burnout across Thirteen Cultures: Stress and Coping in Child and Youth Care Workers*. Westport, CT: Praeger.

Schaufeli, W. B., Bakker, A. B., Hoogduin, K., Schaap, C., & Kladler, A. (2001). The clinical validity of the Maslach Burnout Inventory and the Burnout Measure. *Psychology and Health*, 16, 565–582.

Schaufeli, W. B., & Enzmann, D. (1998). *The Burnout Companion to Study and Practice: A Critical Analysis*. London: Taylor & Francis.

Schaufeli, W. B., van Dierendonck, D., & van Gorp, K. (1996). Burnout and reciprocity: Towards a dual-level social exchange model. *Work and Stress*, 10, 225–237.

Schnorpfeil, P., Noll, A., Wirtz, P., Schulze, R., Ehlert, U., Frey, K., & Fischer, J.E. (2002). Assessment of exhaustion and related risk factors in employees in the manufacturing industry: A cross-sectional study. *International Archives of Occupational and Environmental Health*, 75, 535–540.

Schonfeld, I. S. (1989). Psychological distress in a sample of teachers. *Journal of Psychology*, 124, 321–338.

Selye, H. (1967). *Stress in Health and Disease*. Boston: Butterworth.

Shinn, M., Rosario, M., Morch, H., & Chestnut, D.E. (1984). Coping with job stress and burnout in the human services. *Journal of Personality and Social Psychology*, 46, 864–876.

Shirom, A. (1989). Burnout in work organizations. In C. L. Cooper & I. T. Robertson (Eds.), *International Review of Industrial and Organizational Psychology* (pp. 25–48). Washington, DC: American Psychological Association.

Siefert, K., Jayaratne, S., Chess, W.A. & Wayne, A. (1991). Job satisfaction, burnout, and turnover in health care social workers. *Health and Social Work*, 16, 193–202.

Siegrist, J. (1996). Adverse health effects of high-effort/low-reward conditions. *Journal of Occupational Health Psychology*, 1, 27–41.

Starnaman, S. M., & Miller, K. I. (1992). A test of a causal model of communication and burnout in the teaching profession. *Communication Education*, 41, 40–53.

Stevens, G. B., & O'Neill, P. (1983). Expectation and burnout in the developmental disabilities field. *American Journal of Community Psychology*, 11, 615–627.

Toppinen-Tanner, S., Kalimo, R., & Mutanen, P. (2002). The process of burnout in white-collar and blue-collar jobs: An eight-year prospective study of exhaustion, *Journal of Organizational Behavior*, 23, 555–570.

Truchot, D., & Deregard, M. (2001). Perceived inequity, communal orientation and burnout: The role of helping models. *Work and Stress*, 15, 347–356.

Tyler, T.R. (1990). *Why People Obey the Law*. New Haven, CT: Yale University Press.

Walster, E., Berscheid, E., & Walster, G. W. (1973). New directions in equity research. *Journal of Personality and Social Psychology*, 25, 151–176.

Warr, P.B. (1987). *Work, Unemployment and Mental Health*. Oxford: Clarendon Press.

White, S.L. (1987). Human resource development: The future through people. *Administration in Mental Health*, 14, 199–208.

World Health Organization (1992). The ICD-10 classification of mental and behavioral disorders, Geneva: WHO.

Zedeck, S., Maslach, C., Mosier, K., & Skitka, L. (1988). Affective response to work and quality of family life: Employee and spouse perspectives. *Journal of Social Behavior and Personality*, 3, 135–157.

Zellars, K.L., Perrewé, P. L., & Hochwarter, W. A. (2000). Burnout in health care: The role of the five factors of personality. *Journal of Applied Social Psychology*, 30, 1570–1598.

9 Organizational Interventions to Alleviate Burnout and Build Engagement with Work

Michael P. Leiter and Christina Maslach

CONTENTS

0-8493-1820-3/05/$0.00+$1.50

Early in the development of the burnout research literature, authors noted three potential levels of intervention: individual treatment, group education, and organizational intervention (Golembiewski & Munzenrider, 1988; Leiter, 1991; Maslach, 1982; Shinn et al., 1984). These levels of intervention are not crisply distinct from one another — an organization can introduce an employee assistance program to provide individual treatment — but they identify three important entry points for the burnout process.

It is reasonable to consider that the individual, the work group, and the organization are all credible points of entry for addressing burnout. This chapter focuses on organizational interventions because they have the greatest potential to affect the lives of a large number of people and to make changes with a potential to endure. This focus on organizational interventions does not imply a view that individual interventions do not make a contribution. There are studies that have demonstrated an impact of interventions designed to alleviate burnout, at least on a short-term basis, using individual insight or enhancement of coping skills (Golembiewski & Munzenrider, 1988; Shinn et al., 1984; van Dierendonck et al., 1998). The emphasis on organizational interventions reflects the authors' perspective on burnout as a phenomenon brought about by incongruence of individuals with the organizations in which they work. It reflects as well a view that the widespread prevalence of burnout with its close correlation with the workplace requires a profound, enduring, and extensive change in the way people work.

OVERVIEW OF INTERVENTION ISSUES

Schaufeli and Enzmann (1998) provide the most thorough consideration of intervention approaches to burnout. They differentiate between approaches that focus on the individual, those that focus on the individual–organizational interface, and those that focus on the organization.

Individual approaches draw from established techniques for gaining insight, learning new skills or perspectives, and reducing negative arousal. For example, some interventions arise from an individual's resolve to live a healthier lifestyle through regular physical exercise (McDonald & Hodgdon, 1991; Ross & Altmaier, 1994). In reviewing research on lifestyle approaches, Schaufeli and Enzmann (1998) note that "physical exercise is perhaps the most powerful antidote to stress" (p. 148). Another widely used approach is relaxation training (Higgins, 1986). In general, these approaches build an individual's resilience to withstand the demands, frustrations, and pressures of the present-day workplace. This resilience is not exclusively relevant to burnout; a stronger, healthier, more informed person is better prepared to address a wide range of life demands at work or in any other domain of life.

Schaufeli and Enzmann's (1998) consideration of the individual–organizational interface includes a range of interventions, training programs, or support systems that assist individuals in addressing the specific demands at work. In these approaches, the workplace remains constant — except for the introduction of these programs. The objective is to assist individual employees in coping with specific work demands. A prime example of a training program is time management courses. These are educational interventions that intend to increase employees' capacity to establish personal objectives, set priorities, and use their time effectively. Other training programs focus on interpersonal skills, balancing work with family, and gaining a realistic understanding of a new job. In addition to educational programs, the individual–organizational interface includes initiatives to establish peer support groups, peer counseling, and career planning advice. Organizations can in various ways encourage and sustain social support networks (Burke & Greenglass, 2000; Hobfoll & Shirom, 2000) alone or in conjunction with other initiatives to address stress or burnout. Organizations can deliver these programs with in-house resources or outsource them. In terms of treatment, organizations can refer employees to psychotherapy or counseling with burnout as the individual's primary complaint.

Organizational approaches to alleviating burnout look to managers as a source of initiative, consistent with their role in stress management programs (Quick et al., 1996). Initially, proposals for organizational interventions focused largely on controlling workload, especially hours of direct client contact for human service providers (Cherniss, 1980; Maslach, 1982). More recently, research has concentrated on broadly based organizational interventions that change other aspects of work life (Cherniss, 1995). Schaufeli and Enzmann's (1998) review includes as organizational interventions corporate wellness programs (Batman, 1994) despite their objective of enhancing individual resilience, because these programs approach the workplace as a whole rather than focus exclusively on individuals experiencing problems. Corporate wellness approaches are encouraged increasingly by government legislation calling for organizations to take proactive steps to address stress and encourage healthy workplaces (de Gier, 1995). These prevention programs can be complemented by corporate employee assistance programs (EAPs) to facilitate employees' access to treatment for established problems (Lee & Gray, 1994).

For practitioners, the thin research findings provide little solid ground for implementing organizational interventions. Kasl and Sexner (1992) stated that there was little data on record that confirmed the impact of organizational interventions on burnout, and there are few signs of progress recently (Shirom, 2003). Few studies have confirmed the impact of burnout workshops on exhaustion (Pines & Aronson, 1983; Schaufeli, 1995; van Dierendonck et al., 1998). This shortfall is not specific to burnout, but appears to characterize the field of stress management as well (Briner & Reynolds, 1999). Making matters more complex, few interventions at any level — individual or organizational — are specific to burnout. That is, physical exercise and relaxation help people address a wide variety of problems, such as tension or cardiovascular health; they are not exclusively related to burnout. Their primary benefit might even be addressing problems other than burnout.

Despite repeated calls over the years for the assessment of organizational interventions to prevent and alleviate burnout, the research literature has little to offer. In light of the current state of affairs, the salient question is not, what does the research have to say about the effectiveness of organizational interventions? The central question is, why are organizational interventions so difficult? That is, in light of the extensive research demonstrating the correspondence of burnout with problematic areas of work life (Maslach & Leiter, 1997; Schaufeli & Enzmann, 1998), what factors inhibit manipulating workplaces to address problems with burnout?

Although the research literature makes a compelling case for organizational approaches, each implementation is somewhat experimental. Without clear, rigorously assessed procedures, each intervention project requires a clear and explicit conceptual base. That is, it is not possible to work from a checklist of proven approaches to organizational intervention, because such a list does not exist. Justifying a specific approach requires a thorough grasp of its foundations: What was the basis of recommending a given approach to alleviating or preventing burnout? The following section considers ideas for developing effective organizationally based interventions.

QUALITIES OF ORGANIZATIONAL INTERVENTIONS

Despite a wealth of research findings consistently pointing toward organizational factors as the primary issues driving burnout, there are no rigorous, long-term research studies that have applied — successfully or not — organizational interventions to address the problem. As noted by Maslach and Goldberg (1998), there are logistic and conceptual issues behind this gap. The experiences of implementing intervention projects provide lessons that are potentially useful to subsequent initiatives. This discussion is guided by the mediation model of burnout (illustrated in Figure 9.1), described fully in the companion chapter in this volume.

- **Flexibility**. The model favors organizational interventions that increase employees' options for finding their preferred resolution within the six areas of work life. This is not a one-size-fits-all approach. Lacking a model of an ideal work setting for everyone, the approach works to facilitate employees' pursuit of the resolution that makes sense to them.
- **Collaboration**. A key to successful interventions is the process through which the interventions were developed. The active involvement of a diverse group of employees in developing, implementing, and assessing an intervention contributes considerably to the intervention's potential to have a lasting impact.
- **Leadership**. It is important that the senior management of an organization explicitly support the initiatives arising from a survey project. This support gives credibility to the process and publicly confirms the organization's values regarding the well-being of employees and their potential to make an enduring contribution to an organization's productivity. On another level, it is critical that the people managing the survey process and each intervention process play an active leadership role in engaging employees in the process, keeping the initiatives on senior management's agenda, and pushing for creative solutions to meaningful problems.
- **Iterative Process**. There is a certain amount of trial and error in an employee finding his preferred level of control or reward or any other area of work life. Ideally, an intervention provides employees with the time and opportunity to explore a new approach to managing an area of work life to find a resolution that works. Not only is there not one size that fits all, but an intervention will not necessarily work on the first try.

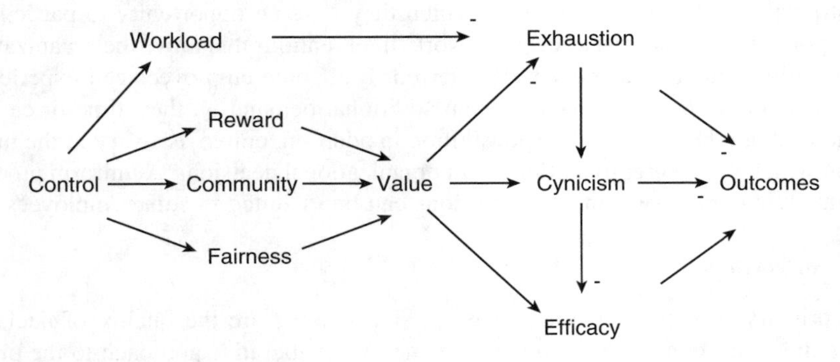

FIGURE 9.1 Mediation model of burnout.

- **Information Flow**. Successful interventions establish an information flow to monitor their success. In the dynamic and sometimes contradictory world of organizations in a turbulent environment, any innovation, especially one that requires ongoing maintenance, must continually justify itself. The availability of valid and reliable instruments for assessing burnout and employees' perceptions of work life is a valuable asset in this regard. Accompanying these measures with relevant data regarding the performance of individuals or organizational units extends their persuasiveness considerably.

FLEXIBILITY

The research is clear that a one-size-fits-all solution for burnout is not available. There is too much complexity on both sides of the equation. Work settings are too complex in their structures, missions, management processes, and demands. People not only vary widely in their career aspirations, abilities, and resilience, but these qualities change markedly over the span of a person's working life. Any broadly successful approach an organization takes to preventing burnout and building engagement will be sufficiently flexible to accommodate a diverse range of solutions.

The definitive benefit of increasing flexibility in organizational life is that it opens possibilities for individual employees to find resolutions in their work life that work for them. Maslach and Leiter (1997) depicted the driving force in burnout to be chronic mismatches of individual aspirations and inclinations with the structures and processes in their work environments. Rigidly constrained work environments that prescribe limited patterns of workload, decision-making involvement, reward systems, etc., will provide fewer options. A rigidly structured work environment places the burden on employees to develop the skills, attitudes, and resilience necessary to experience energy, involvement, and effectiveness within the work environment as it is. To the extent that a mismatch persists, the employees have the responsibility to address it.

Some interventions might hit the mark with most people, providing that the intervention is guided by sound general ideas about people in general or at least about those people who are employees of the organization in question. For example, most people prefer work settings in which they have an opportunity to participate in important decisions that affect their work. Interventions that move the organization in that direction are generally well received. But, some employees can experience a greater role in decision making as an additional demand on their time or can be anxious about the additional responsibility. In addition, employees vary in the manner in which they prefer to participate in organizational decisions. A uniform process for involving employees in such decisions can be ill suited to some employees.

Collaboration

The primary benefits of participative decision making are the quality of decision and employees' commitment to the outcome. A collaborative approach to the problem solving and decision making that make up an organizational intervention calls upon the expertise resident among the participants. These people know the work and, to the extent that they are committed to the organization's core mission, wish to do that work well.

A unilateral approach to designing or implementing organizational interventions takes a major risk of neglecting expertise and a further risk of introducing a program that will not be fully implemented. While individuals from management, human resource units, or external consulting firms can bring essential expertise to an intervention, the local knowledge of frontline or supervisory employees makes a vital contribution to the organization's capacity to use that expertise.

Leadership

Organizational interventions call for proactive leadership. Left to their own momentum, organizations tend to continue in their present directions. To produce a distinctly different work environment requires a concerted effort. A major intervention requires an individual or group to take the initiative to introduce an intervention process, to maintain concerted efforts toward implementing that change, to assess the impact of the intervention, and to decide upon modifications of the intervention as it unfolds.

Iterative Process

Intervention is an iterative process in which a work group tests ideas, adapting the intervention plan in light of experience. This approach requires participants to keep an open mind. It also requires a reliable flow of information about the initial impact of any intervention plan. An essential contribution of workplace audits, such as the Checkup Survey (Leiter & Maslach, 2000), is their capacity to establish and maintain such an information flow.

Information Flow

Maslach and Goldberg (1998) noted that interventions are often lacking in reliable, valid indicators of the intervention's impact, especially the persistence of impact over time. Even with studies that include the Maslach Burnout Inventory (MBI) (Maslach et al., 1996) as a measure of burnout per se, there are inadequate measures of other relevant concepts. There is little consensus on the critical elements of work life to measure; the reliable, valid measures of these states; or the amount of change necessary to effect a meaningful impact on burnout.

Leiter and Maslach (2000, 2004) proposed a measure, the Areas of Worklife Scale (AWS), to provide consistency in the assessment of organizational environments. The scale comprises 29 items that provide six subscales pertaining to the areas of work life that research over the previous two decades has identified as the primary correlates of burnout: workload, control, reward, community, fairness, and values. The items are worded generally to encompass a wide range of occupational situations and professional roles. A central objective of the scale development was to establish a multidimensional perspective on work environments that was relevant to employees throughout a large, complex organization. One of the primary development settings for this measure was a large teaching hospital that encompassed physicians, nurses, occupational therapists, cafeteria workers, custodians, accountants, security personnel, and a plethora of other occupational groups of various supervisory statuses and with work experience ranging from trainee positions to senior mentors. Rather than delve into the specific workplace challenges of these diverse occupational groups, the AWS assesses the respondents' perspectives on the extent to which the work environment is consistent with their aspirations and expectations. By focusing on the relationships of people with their work environments, the AWS foregoes defining an ideal work environment. The scale design assumes that people bring distinct expectations, aspirations, talents, and vulnerabilities to a workplace. As well, work environments are not uniform throughout a complex, spatially dispersed organization, but contain subcultures, working groups, or management levels with distinct challenges and opportunities pertaining to the six key areas of work life. The interaction of these unique personal qualities with the distinct qualities of the setting in which work occurs is the focal point of the AWS. The objective is not to identify the extent to which an entire organization departs from an ideal, but to identify consistent themes in the gaps employees experience between their proclivities for a work setting and the context in which they work.

Logistic Challenges to Implementing Burnout Interventions

In addition to these conceptual and measurement issues, organizational intervention projects face major logistical challenges. Organizations attempting to address burnout often face major crises that have implications for their capacity to make long-term commitments. The consultative process that is at the heart of effective organizational interventions to prevent or alleviate burnout is both technically and politically challenging to implement. Another logistic challenge is establishing an organizational unit or function to assess the impact of interventions on the energy, involvement, and efficacy of participants as well as on the organization's performance. These challenges are considerable, bringing about the premature demise of more long-term intervention studies.

In summary, there is an inherent dilemma in the design and implementation of major interventions between the leadership necessary to initiate the project and the stability needed to see it to completion. The initial commitment to the project requires a visionary, courageous, and dedicated senior management team. It requires more than an ordinary amount of ability and leadership. The contradiction is that visionary leaders are vulnerable, especially in the public service sector, in which they can be seen as a liability by governments attempting to pursue ambitious agendas with modest resources. Initiatives to enhance the quality of work life often come about during major transitions in the life of an organization. These are times of opportunity to bring about meaningful changes through implementing new ways of work. They are also times of vulnerability in which an organization's change can be encompassed in larger-scale transitions. These events have a profound and lasting impact on the people working in these organizations and on their clientele.

CONSULTATIVE PROCESSES

A consultative process is demanding. It adds new dimensions to employees' jobs. It might well increase workload in the short run, a factor that could aggravate burnout rather than alleviate it. Consultative processes introduce uncertainty into the process. When working with a group to develop a creative solution, adapted to the specific challenges and resources of the work group, it is often difficult to predict where things are going to go. The process can produce interventions that exceed management's initial concept of the initiative or that encompass a range of issues broader than burnout per se.

Active participation in the design, implementation, and evaluation of interventions contributes to their effectiveness. It increases participants' commitment to the intervention and draws upon a wide range of relevant expertise. But it does not come easy; often it requires effective leadership at various levels of the organization and considerable expertise on group problem solving, decision making, and conflict resolution.

TRACKING INTERVENTIONS

A third logistic challenge in this research is the difficulty in establishing a systematic approach to assessing the impact of interventions. Burnout is a pervasive problem with diverse links to myriad aspects of the organizational work environment. The approach outlined in Leiter and Maslach (2000) emphasizes the need for a thorough initial assessment of a work setting to determine the specific mix of matches, mismatches, and strains evident in an organization at a specific time. Although some aspects of the six areas of work life assessed in the Areas of Worklife Scale will have close relationships with the energy, involvement, and efficacy that people bring to their work, a current survey is necessary to determine those areas of work life that are pertinent at a given time.

With a diverse range of interventions custom-made by organizational units, an organization faces a serious challenge in evaluation. As work units develop unique solutions to address their primary challenges, the organization lacks a unified goal for interventions. It might be difficult to bring together a complete list of the organization's initiatives. It is certainly difficult to determine in an overall way whether it is attaining its objectives. Addressing this challenge requires an organizational commitment to assessing a broad range of relevant factors over time.

GOALS OF INTERVENTION

The primary long-term goal of the organizational interventions considered here is to alleviate or prevent burnout. A complementary goal is to build engagement with work. Although these two goals overlap to a large extent, they have distinct qualities. Building engagement with work is a more all-encompassing goal in that an organization can prevent burnout without necessarily building engagement, but can only build engagement in a work context that prevents or alleviates burnout. That is, one can prevent burnout, bringing an organization to a neutral point of a somewhat safe and perhaps bland existence. Engagement with work is never bland and safe; it is a lively relationship with work that is incompatible with burnout and with a neutral perspective on work life.

The most direct approach to burnout interventions is to define the goals of intervention in terms of the three aspects of burnout. The strength of this perspective is that it keeps the focus on the explicit target of concern: the levels of exhaustion, cynicism, or inefficacy that provided the occasion for designing the intervention in the first place. It also has the advantage of including a means of assessing progress through the quantified scores on the MBI–General Survey (MBI-GS). In this way the approach keeps things simple by focusing on the core issue and defining progress in a reliable, valid, quantifiable way.

This straightforward approach is not always readily available. Although one can reliably measure employees' levels of energy, involvement, and efficacy, the means for directly affecting these psychological states might not be apparent. An indirect approach implicit in the mediation model is to reduce burnout by enhancing the areas of work life that influence employees' relationships with their work. While the overall goal remains to reduce indicators of burnout among staff members, the immediate points of focus are the areas of work life that contribute to these psychological states. The rationale for focusing on areas of work life is that they are the direct responsibility of management; the psychological states of employees are not. Management has the capacity and the responsibility for developing the best possible areas of work life. Management has more constrained authority regarding employees' psychological states.

Measuring the downstream consequences of preventing burnout is a major challenge for organizations that lack systematic procedures for assessing their overall performance. The mediation model depicts burnout as an intermediate psychological state between the nature of the workplace and important organizational or personal outcomes. Although reducing burnout can be considered a sufficient goal in itself, major interventions, especially those that fundamentally change the way that work is done within an organization, often require a more thoroughgoing justification in terms of the organization's core mission. With this approach, the objective is not reducing or preventing burnout, but enhancing qualities of organizational performance that are affected by employees' energy, involvement, and efficacy. Evaluating the relationship between burnout and organizational performance requires valid measures of all aspects of the equation.

Aspects of Burnout

In quantifiable terms, alleviating burnout is equivalent to bringing the overall scores on the three aspects of burnout, as measured by the MBI (Maslach et al., 1996), close to the established norms for a specific occupational group. Occupational norms provide a credible reference point for determining the alleviation of burnout. They imply that the average level of exhaustion, cynicism, and professional efficacy for an occupation is indicative of a manageable and sustainable work life. Although one might aspire to alleviate burnout to such an extent that the overall average for the work setting is noticeably lower than that of the occupational group, this goal goes beyond alleviating burnout, strictly speaking, and moves into the territory of building engagement.

Energy

The energy dimension plays a pivotal role in alleviating burnout. In the mediation model it is evident that exhaustion not only is a problem in itself, but aggravates cynicism and inefficacy. The mechanisms through which exhaustion affects the other two aspects of burnout have not been rigorously tested. Maslach and Leiter (1997) have proposed that a critical element is the contribution of physical, emotional, and creative energy to a subjective sense of well-being. Even a temporary lapse of energy can be discouraging. Prolonged, chronic exhaustion as assessed by the MBI profoundly undermines optimism, the capacity to become engaged in work, and confidence in one's abilities.

Three general approaches to enhancing the subjective experience of energy are (1) to prompt excitement or enthusiasm, (2) to provide opportunities for rest and revitalization, and (3) to design work in a manner that helps employees sustain their energy. Organizations seek to prompt excitement and enthusiasm through various means, including inspirational speakers or retreats, charismatic leaders, and revitalizing their organizational mission. Despite considerable anecdotal evidence of a short-term lift in spirits from inspirational speakers or charismatic leaders, the enduring impact of these approaches is uncertain. As Collins (2001) demonstrates in his consideration of companies that maintain impressive performance over the long term, low-profile leaders with modest personal styles build more effective teams than do their more flamboyant, charismatic counterparts. Revitalizing the organizational mission has a potential for enduring influence if it provides the impetus for strategic planning that affects the day-to-day life of employees. Without the translation into new patterns of work or cooperation among employees, a revised mission plan in itself is likely to share with inspirational speakers and charismatic leaders the limitation of a short-term impact on employees' energy levels.

The workplace has a limited capacity to facilitate rest and revitalization of employees. Although doing so is very much to the organization's advantage, its capacity to influence the process is restricted in that much of rest and revitalization occurs away from work. Often, being away from work in itself is a critical part of the process. The primary points of intervention for the organization are (1) reviewing and changing values that encourage employees in exhausting work patterns; (2) anticipating and scheduling for demanding episodes of work to keep overtime commitments at a reasonable, sustainable level; and (3) developing family-friendly policies that help employees sustain personal lives that support their capacity to be effective, creative contributors over the long run.

Involvement and Efficacy

The line from exhaustion to cynicism in the mediation model suggests one approach to reducing cynicism is through reducing exhaustion. This approach would lead to considering the full range of strategies considered in the previous section. The other source of influence on cynicism and efficacy is from values, suggesting that a greater congruence of personal and organizational values could be effective in reducing cynicism and enhancing efficacy.

Directly influencing employees' involvement in their work presents special challenges. Cynicism reduces employees' openness to external influence, as it brings a tendency to be dismissive toward the thoughts and feelings of other people, be they service recipients, colleagues, or supervisors. The greatest challenge for management interventions is that employees often direct cynical thoughts toward the organization's management. Cynicism would tend to diminish the impact of motivational speakers or efforts to revitalize the organizational mission through an inclusive process.

In light of the skepticism inherent in cynicism, an enduring enhancement of employees' involvement in their work requires meaningful changes in their work situation. It is insufficient for an organization to profess congruence with employees' values. Employees attend more closely to their day-to-day working conditions as an indicator of organizational values than to statements by management. Similarly, although the model proposes that a greater congruence of values enhances efficacy, that congruity becomes credible only when it is reinforced by the nature of the work environment. From this perspective, it is important to look behind values per se to other areas of work life that provide the basis of value congruence in the mediation model.

Areas of Work Life

The mediation model identifies an indirect route of influencing the three aspects of burnout through improving employees' evaluation of six areas of work life. These six areas encompass the factors that research has identified as the primary predictors of exhaustion, cynicism, and efficacy. Their integral role in organizational environments puts them firmly within the authority and responsibility of management. Although management cannot always identify the optimal solution to an incongruence between organizational design and employee expectations, it clearly has a responsibility to address problems within that environment.

The Areas of Worklife Scale (Leiter and Maslach, 2000) provides a means of assessing the immediate impact of interventions to enhance the quality of the work environment. Although the long-term objective of the intervention is generally to change the three aspects of burnout as assessed by the MBI, it is critical to determine the extent to which employees experience these interventions as having a meaningful impact on the work environment. Without this confirmation, the means through which an intervention has an impact would remain unclear, even if the intervention was successful. In a more practical sense, it is likely that the impact on burnout of an intervention to change an area of work life would only be evident after an extended period.

The primary challenge in changing areas of work life is resistance to change. Significant organizational change is rarely welcomed universally among employees. Generally, any silver lining is going to have a cloud for someone in the organization. Successful intervention planning includes a serious consideration of who is going to lose as well as who is going to benefit from a given change in the way the organization operates. While the goal might be to establish win–win changes to the benefit of everyone, it is a major challenge to develop and implement such a scheme flawlessly. It is even more of a challenge to convince everyone along the way that the change is undoubtedly to everyone's benefit. Employees often doubt the potential benefit of a major change until the benefit has been proven through an implementation that was successful despite their best efforts to the contrary.

And frontline employees are not the only source of resistance to change. Management has established the organizational structures and procedures currently in place. Usually, they established things for a good reason from the organization's strategic perspective. Even when convinced that the strategic perspective has given inadequate consideration to supporting employees' engagement in work and alleviating pressures toward burnout, management might hesitate to change the way it does business. In the short term, interventions that enhance the quality of work life might be in direct conflict with structures and procedures that protect the organization's bottom line. A negative impact on the bottom line can occur much more quickly than the time frame required for the impact of a more effective workforce to enhance organizational performance.

This time frame emphasizes the importance of two critical elements of organizational interventions. First, successful interventions require a serious commitment from employees and from management within a time frame that is appropriate to the objectives of change. If the intervention requires changing the organization's core values and procedures, that impact requires a long time. Second, ongoing assessment with valid and reliable measures is essential to obtain markers of meaningful progress prior to the impact on the ultimate measures of employee burnout or organizational performance.

Workload

Workload is an obvious target for interventions designed to alleviate or prevent burnout. There are a variety of ways in which workload aggravates the experience of exhaustion. The most obvious is the amount of work that must be completed in a limited time, but the type of work is an additional factor, as is the employees' mastery of the work. Recognizing the potential impact of overwhelming work demands on employees' energy levels does not require advanced scientific insight. It is obvious that reducing workload would be a good way to reduce exhaustion and assure that employees maintain sufficient energy to maintain involvement in their work and to perform more effectively. And reducing workload in itself can often be straightforward. It could necessitate reducing the required caseload, shortening working hours, or loosening deadlines so that employees have more time to do what needs to be done. Addressing workload mismatches while maintaining organizational productivity requires a clear, strategic view of the organization's work.

- **Eliminating Low-Priority Tasks**. Organizations working in volatile environments constantly adapt and innovate to keep up to date. In some organizations, the addition of new tasks and procedures is driven primarily by management. In other organizations, innovation is driven primarily by employees. Employees' initiatives occur often in organizations that employ professionals — such as health care, research, or education settings — as the employees are motivated to keep their skills and work experience current. A new service, technology, or activity can appear so attractive that employees cheerfully accept the new responsibilities at first.

  Organizations often find it much more difficult to eliminate old tasks than to add new tasks. Management often assumes that employees will somehow fit the new tasks into their day, while employees often assume that management will allocate additional resources to address the additional work. When neither occurs and the initial excitement associated with the innovation fades, employees find themselves overwhelmed by excessive workload, some of which is a result of their own initiative. A thorough strategic assessment of workload can prioritize tasks to identify activities whose importance has been supplanted by the new initiatives. Ideally, this assessment occurs prior to introducing an initiative, but often it is not prompted until employees experience exhaustion.
- **Finding New Ways to Do Things**. Organizations settle into ways of doing things that perpetuate themselves despite obvious inefficiencies. An additional advantage to an inclusive survey project is the opportunity to encourage employees to reflect on how work is done and to propose new ways of doing the work. An explicit process through a task force on reviewing work procedures to improve their effectiveness can be beneficial in its direct results, but also in promoting a value of improved effectiveness through the workforce.
- **Teamwork**. Teamwork is often a means of improving quality at the expense of additional time and effort necessary to attend to coordinating and reviewing shared activity. It can also be a means of sharing workload more effectively. Individuals within a multidisciplinary work setting might be carrying excessive responsibility because of unique credentials or expertise. A review of the working procedures of the group can identify more effective ways for them to operate as a team, sharing some qualities

of what might be developing as a bottleneck in the work process with other members of the team.

Control

Control is sometimes a contradictory area of work life in that people might seek more control only to find that the price in terms of additional responsibilities is more than they bargained for. In any case, it is a point that requires a careful negotiation of perspectives between management and employees. From some perspectives, control or power is a zero-sum game in which a gain by one person or group appears to be at the expense of another. Making shared control mutually enhancing is a tough challenge requiring the active participation of those affected by the shift in control.

- **Building Frontline Decision Making**. An effective approach to building congruence between organizational decision and the aspirations of employees is providing clear direction on the specific points on which a collaborative process is expected. Frontline supervisors benefit from policies that take a clear position on their range of decision-making authority and the expectations on employee participation. Such policies reduce uncertainty regarding situations that call for strong action on the part of supervisors and those that require consensus building.
- **Supervisor Training**. Frontline supervisors can accept readily the rationale for including employees in decisions that affect the quality of employees' work life. They might also lack the expertise and perspective necessary to put intentions into action. While there are many generic programs in team building available, it is important for the training to be localized to an organization's specific situation. Relevant issues include communication strategies to provide supervisors with operating rules to guide their approach to sharing information from upper management. Too often, supervisors keep information to themselves that would be more effectively shared with employees. In this situation, management is disseminating information through the supervisory structure, but the information is not reaching the intended audience. A second issue is leading the decision-making process within a work group. There is a delicate balance between moving quickly through the agenda of a busy work group and assuring a thorough discussion of the matter at hand. Without appropriately inclusive procedures, employees can feel left out of decisions despite their attendance at meetings in which the decisions are made. Developing the capacity for inclusive leadership in frontline supervisors, and supporting this approach by modeling it throughout the organization's management structure, is a basis for a meaningful enhancement of the control area of work life.

Reward

The focus of the reward subscale of the AWS is recognition by colleagues and management. While financial rewards are certainly relevant to employees' feelings and actions about their workplace, those concerns appear to be distinct from perspectives on recognition or intrinsic reward. The relevance of financial rewards to burnout is unclear, but research has identified consistent correlations of nonfinancial rewards with burnout (Leiter & Maslach, 2000).

- **Increasing the Relevance of Recognition Events**. Major recognition events within organizations can miss their mark. In some organizations the events are poorly attended; in others, employees attend with a fairly skeptical attitude. In organizations with both kinds of problems, the primary intervention is to launch a process through which employees feel the process is their own. In some organizations this involves a consultative process that generates extensive discussions on reward and recognition across the various departments and subgroups in the organization. In others, there is little discussion, but the process of planning and staging the events is delegated to individuals and groups that serve as important opinion leaders in the organization. As employees become more involved in the process of recognition and reward, the events' impacts grow.
- **Management and Supervisor Training**. A second source of interventions to enhance the reward area of work life is training managers and frontline supervisors in providing recognition and support to employees in the course of their day-to-day work. These training programs are more effective when accompanied by revising managers' performance evaluation process to give greater weight to evidence of providing recognition to subordinates.

Community

Enhancing the community area of work life encompasses a wide variety of interventions to enhance the quality of social relationships among employees. The specific target of the intervention varies across organizations, focusing on coworker relationships in one setting and supervisor–subordinate relationships in another. The overall goals of these interventions are enhancing the supportive quality of social interactions, reducing conflict, and building a greater capacity for teamwork appropriate to the work to be done.

- **Mediation Processes**. Organizations with enduring conflict among employees have contracted with external professionals to provide mediation services. Although the actual mediation processes are reactive — responding to persistent problems — and limited to specific settings, the organization's initiative in establishing the process provides a signal to employees that management is taking the concerns associated with enduring conflict, bullying, or harassment seriously.
- **Team Building**. Organizations are accessing a variety of approaches to team building to enhance the capacity of employees to work together more effectively. A key element of these approaches is enhancing the capacity of coworkers to provide mutual support and to rely on one another for

integrating their work on complex tasks. The AWS provides a means of assessing the short-term impact of such interventions by assessing their impact on employees' perceptions of community at work.

Fairness

Enhancing employees' perception of an organization's capacity to treat them with respect and fairness is a powerful source of intervention. These interventions are usually going against the tide of employees' perceptions, as the AWS consistently shows the greatest mismatches to be in the workload and fairness areas of work life (Leiter & Maslach, 2002). These two areas are generally in the mismatch range (below the neutral 3.00 rating on the assessment scale).

- **Equity**. Senior managers are often surprised to read the written comments associated with a survey to discover the extent to which employees attribute frustrations in their careers or tense interaction with other employees to discrimination. With the limited information available to employees in the complex world of organizations, people tend to call upon personal explanations of events that have a personal impact. Without a comprehensive perspective on an open process for selecting among various employees for a promotion or reward, employees attribute their lack of success to personal animosity rather than to personal shortcomings. The feelings and perceptions resulting from personal frustrations of this sort at work have the potential to undermine relationships with work, aggravating the burnout process. Organizations have found the most effective way of addressing these concerns to be establishing a formal process to address allegations or suspicions of discrimination, harassment, or other forms of adverse treatment from managers or coworkers.

Values

The values area of work life integrates employees' perception of the other areas of work life in the model. It is the point in the model at which employees build a coherent view of how the workplace fits together in regard to the aspirations and expectations that they bring to their jobs and careers.

- **Reviewing Core Values**. The most direct approach to addressing a mismatch of organizational and personal values is a value clarification process. The process becomes elaborate in large organizations as it is built upon a thorough consultative process. A core group leads a reiterative process comprising successive waves of discussions and questionnaires throughout the organizational hierarchy from senior management and the board of directors to the frontline units. It encompasses the organization's range of occupational groups, departments, and sites. The process focuses primarily on distilling a set of core values shared throughout the organization, but can also note subcultures within a large organization that have distinct perspectives on the issue pertaining to their work, history, or location.

- **New Employee Orientation**. Organizations become most aware of their values — at least their espoused values — when they orient new employees. The process of introducing new employees to the organization requires explicit consideration of value issues that are rarely discussed in the day-to-day life of many organizations. For some organizations, the key intervention is to incorporate a defined discussion of organizational values into the orientation process that might otherwise be dominated by the logistics of the job with little consideration for the organization's mission, vision, and values. Organizations that already include this focus in their orientation have taken a more strategic approach to involving existing employees into the values element of the orientation process. Rather than relying on managers or trainers to clarify the core values, the orientation process brings existing employees into the process. Doing so increases the salience of the core values for the existing employees and brings an additional element of credibility to the discussion.

Overall, the six areas of work life provide specific focal points for organizational interventions to enhance employees' capacities to develop more constructive and fulfilling relationships with their work. The immediate impact of the kinds of interventions discussed here is to change the processes and structures through which organizations conduct their work. The longer-term impact is focused on the cognitive and emotional states of energy, involvement, and efficacy that underlie burnout.

CONCLUSION

Preventing and alleviating burnout is a major challenge that is only beginning to be assessed by rigorous research models. The field at present faces considerable challenges in regard to conceptual frameworks, measurement, and logistics. At present, the biggest challenge is the logistics. Research in recent years, built primarily on cross-sectional research supplemented by a few key longitudinal studies, has developed conceptual models that make sense and that are supported by the data that are available. Although researchers continue to explore alternative measures of burnout, the MBI in its various forms is so clearly dominant in the field that it can be accepted as the definitive indicator of changes in burnout over time. The logistic challenges are the serious challenge for researchers who need to build productive, ongoing relationships with organizations as a basis for working with these organizations through assessment, planning, implementation, and evaluation phases of large-scale projects. They need to work with organizations to identify and sometimes develop afresh measures of key organizational outcomes that can be readily associated with questionnaire surveys of employees' levels of burnout and perceptions of work areas. The challenge is considerable, but the benefits in terms of enhancing the quality of work life and furthering knowledge of the relationships people develop with their work are enormous.

REFERENCES

Batman, D. C. (1994). Development of a corporate wellness programme: Nestle UK Ltd. In D. L. Cooper & S. Williams (Eds.), *Creating Healthy Work Organizations* (pp. 25–48). Chichester, U.K.: John Wiley.

Briner, R. B., & Reynolds, S. (1999). The costs, benefits, and limitations of organizational level stress interventions. *Journal of Organizational Behavior*, 20, 647–664.

Burke, R. J., & Greenglass, E. (2000). A longitudinal study of teacher burnout and perceived self-efficacy in classroom management. *Teaching and Teacher Education*, 16, 239–253.

Cherniss, C. (1980). *Professional Burnout in Human Service Organizations*. New York: Praeger.

Cherniss, C. (1995). *Beyond Burnout: Helping Teachers, Nurses, Therapists, and Lawyers Recover from Stress and Disillusionment*. New York: Routledge.

Collins, J. (2001). *Good to Great: Why Some Companies Make the Leap and Others Don't*. New York: Harper Business.

de Gier, E. (1995). Occupational welfare in the European Community: Past, present, and future. In L. W. Murphy, J. J. Hurrell, S. L. Sauter, and G P. Keita (Eds.), *Job Stress Interventions* (pp. 405–416). Washington, DC: American Psychological Association.

Golembiewski R. T., & Munzenrider R. (1988). *Phases of Burnout: Developments in Concepts and Applications*. New York: Praeger.

Higgins, N. C. (1986). Occupational stress and working women: The effectiveness of two stress reduction programs. *Journal of Vocational Behavior*, 29, 66–78.

Hobfoll, S. E., & Shirom, A. (2000). Conservation of resources theory: Applications to stress and management in the workplace. In R. T. Golembiewski (Ed.), *Handbook of Organizational Behavior*, 2nd rev. ed. (pp. 57–81). New York: Dekker.

Kasl, S. V., & Sexner, S. (1992). Health promotion at the worksite. In S. Maes, H. Leventhal, & M. Johnston (Eds.), *International Review of Health Psychology* (pp. 111–142). Chichester, U.K.: John Wiley.

Lee, C., & Gray, J. A. (1994). The role of employee assistance programmes. In C. L. Cooper and S. Williams (Eds.), *Creating Healthy Work Organizations* (pp. 215–242). Chichester, U.K.: John Wiley.

Leiter, M. P. (1991). Coping patterns as predictors of burnout: The function of control and escapist coping patterns. *Journal of Organizational Behaviour*, 12, 123–144.

Leiter, M. P., & Maslach, C. (2000). *Preventing Burnout and Building Engagement: A Complete Program for Organizational Renewal*. San Francisco: Jossey Bass.

Leiter, M.P., & Maslach, C. (2002). *Areas of Worklife Manual*, Technical Report. Centre for Organizational Research & Development, Acadia University, Wolfville, Nova Scotia, Canada.

Leiter, M.P., & Maslach, C. (2004). Areas of worklife: A structured approach to organizational predictors of job burnout. In P. Perrewé & D. C. Ganster (Eds.), *Research in Occupational Stress and Well Being*, Vol. 3. *Emotional and Physiological Processes and Positive Intervention*: 91–34, Oxford, U.K., JAI Press/Elsevier.

Maslach, C. 1982. *Burnout: The Cost of Caring*. Englewood Cliffs, NJ: Prentice Hall.

Maslach, C., & Goldberg, J. (1998). Prevention of burnout: New perspectives. *Applied and Preventative Psychology*, 7, 63–74.

Maslach, C., Jackson, S. E., & Leiter, M. P. (1996). *Maslach Burnout Inventory Manual*, 3rd ed. Palo Alto, CA: Consulting Psychologists Press.

Maslach, C., & Leiter, M. P. (1997). *The Truth about Burnout*. San Francisco: Jossey Bass.

Maslach, D., Schaufeli, W. B., & Leiter, M. P. (2001). Job burnout. *Annual Review of Psychology*, 52, 397–422.

McDonald, D. G., & Hodgdon, J. A. (1991). *Psychological Effect of Aerobic Fitness Training: Research and Theory.* New York: Springer.

Pines, A., & Aronson, E. (1983). Combating burnout. *Children and Youth Services Review*, 5, 263–275.

Quick, J. C., Paulus, P. B., Whittengton, J. L., Lary, T. S., & Newlson, D. L. (1996). Management development, well-being, and health. In M. J. Schabracq, J. A. M. Winnubst, and C. L. Cooper (Eds.), *Handbook of Work and Health Psychology* (pp. 369–388). Colchester, U.K.: John Wiley.

Ross, R. R., & Altmaier, E. M. (1994). *Interventions in Occupational Stress*. London: Sage.

Schaufeli, W. B. (1995). The evaluation of a burnout workshop for community nurses. *Journal of Health and Human Services Administration*, 18, 11–31.

Schaufeli, W. B., & Enzmann, D. (1998). *The Burnout Companion to Study and Practice: A Critical Analysis*. London: Taylor & Francis.

Shinn, M., Rosario, M., Morch, H., & Chestnut, D. E. (1984). Coping with job stress and burnout in the human services. *Journal of Personality and Social Psychology*, 46, 864–876.

Shirom, A. (2003). Job-related burnout: A review. In J. C. Quick & L. E. Tetrick (Eds.), *Handbook of Occupational Health Psychology.* Washington, DC: APA.

van Dierendonck, D., Schaufeli, W. B., & Buunk, B. P. (1998). The evaluation of an individual burnout intervention program: The role of inequity and social support. *Journal of Applied Psychology*, 83, 392–407.

10 Hardy Personality, Stress, and Health

Terry A. Beehr and Nathan A. Bowling

CONTENTS

Hardiness is the ability to endure hardship; in relation to stress, it is the ability to endure otherwise stressful situations without suffering illness. In the stress literature, and relevant to this section (personality) of the present book, hardiness is a personality construct. A hardy personality is expected to affect health, because by definition, hardy individuals suffer relatively little ill health when exposed to stressors. It should

0-8493-1820-3/05/$0.00+$1.50

be noted that this definition defines hardiness in part by its effects, as dictionary definitions of the word *hardiness* do.

Stress processes involve the presence of an environmental event or condition that produces negative health consequences. Unfortunately, much confusion surrounds the terminology used in stress research. Following the suggestions of Jex et al. (1992), among others, we label aspects of one's environment that negatively impact health as *stressors* and the negative health consequences experienced as the result of stressors as *strains*. The term *stress* is used to refer to the general field of study or practice, rather than to a specific variable. It seems likely that there is an immediate, common, psychological or physical stress response that occurs after the stressor but before health consequences occur. The trouble is that there is no broad agreement on what this response is (e.g., secretion of adrenaline or noradrenaline, secretion of cortisol, experience of emotions, or cognitive appraisal), and it is beyond the scope of this chapter to address the issue; therefore, we offer a black-box definition of stress leading to illness, with unidentified intermediate processes.

As is discussed in this section of the book, personality plays an important role in the experience of stressors and strains. The current chapter reviews the role of hardiness as a set of personality characteristics that can lead to reduced strain (Kobasa, 1979). We first define hardiness and then review research on the potential effects of personality on stressors and strains. In doing this, we examine the possibilities that personality is both an antecedent and consequence of stressors and strains, that it moderates the relationships between stressors and strains, and that some of its effects might be related to coping efforts.

DEFINING THE HARDY PERSONALITY

Hardiness was introduced by Kobasa (1979) as a personality variable that buffers or moderates the stressor–strain relationship. She described hardy individuals as believing that they have control over the events in their lives, as being committed to their life activities, and as viewing change as positive and challenging, rather than as negative and threatening. These three facets of hardiness are labeled control, commitment, and challenge, respectively. This seems to imply that hardiness might be a set of personality characteristics rather than a single one. In fact, Kobasa measured it with more than one personality measure. In the development of the concept by Kobasa and colleagues, the personality dimensions common to many studies were measured by existing scales of alienation from self and work, security, internal locus of control, powerlessness, and sometimes cognitive structure (e.g., Kobasa, 1979; Kobasa et al., 1981, 1982a, 1982b, 1983, 1985; Kobasa & Puccetti, 1983), although Semmer (2003) observed that some recent studies have developed specific hardiness scales instead of relying on existing multiple personality scales. It should be noted that internal locus of control has been consistently included as one part of hardiness in research on hardiness and stress. Readers interested in hardiness should note that there is another chapter in this book specifically on locus of control.

Critics of hardiness research have questioned the original three-dimensional structure of the construct. Funk and Houston (1987), for example, found that measures of control, commitment, and challenge loaded onto two rather than three factors, with the control subscales splitting between the two factors. Others have noted inconsistency in the literature concerning whether hardiness should be treated as one or three constructs (Hull et al., 1987). Consistent with the notion that hardiness is multidimensional, Hull et al. presented evidence that the three facets of hardiness are differentially associated with health outcomes. Specifically, commitment and control have generally been found to have their hypothesized effects on health, whereas challenge has not. This might be attributable to the low internal consistency reliability of challenge measures (alpha = .40), which could attenuate any relationships with those measures.

Logically, if the hardiness domain is the set of personality characteristics that protect people from the negative effects of stress, then other personality characteristics fitting this criterion might also be considered part of the domain, whether or not they are included in Kobasa's (1979) three-part conceptualization of hardiness. Based on a review of research, these personality characteristics include type A, negative affectivity (NA), positive affectivity (PA), some characteristics of the five-factor model, self-esteem and self-efficacy, sense of humor, and religiosity. Although we recognize the importance of type A behavior in stress research, we do not discuss this personality characteristic here because it is thoroughly examined in other chapters of this book.

EFFECTS OF PERSONALITY ON STRESSORS AND STRAINS

There are several potential effects of personality on stressors and strains that have been considered by researchers. First, personality characteristics might have a main effect on stressors. That is, personality might predict the extent to which one tends to (1) be exposed to stressful situations, for instance, by selection or self-selection; (2) to perceive situations as stressful; or (3) even to create one's own stressors by the way one behaves. Second, personality might have main effects on strains. Some personality traits, in other words, might influence the development (or the report) of negative mental and physical health consequences. The first of these two effects implies that the relationship between personality and strains is mediated by stressors, as personality factors would influence the experience of stressors which, in turn, would influence the development of strain. Personality might also moderate the relationship between stressors and strains. This occurs when the strength of the relationship between stressors and strains varies across individuals with different personalities. As an example, Kobasa (1979) predicted and found that the relationships between stressors and strains were weaker for hardy than for nonhardy individuals.

Spector et al. (2000) outlined these effects of personality on the stress process while discussing negative affectivity as a personality characteristic, and these effects are just as relevant for hardiness. A difference, of course, is that NA is posited to have deleterious effects and hardiness is expected to have favorable effects.

In addition to the effects of personality on stress identified by Spector et al., personality also could influence stressors and strains by influencing the actions people take regarding stress, actions that can broadly be considered coping. Coping with stress is a very broad concept, so much so that it sometimes can be difficult to identify what behaviors are *not* coping (Beehr & McGrath, 1996). Obtaining social support is a good example. Personality could influence the amount of social support one receives, which in turn impacts one's experiences of stressors and strains. Zellars and Perrewe (2001), for example, found that extraversion, agreeableness, and neuroticism influenced the amount and content of emotional social support that one receives at work. Presumably, people with some types of personality were more likely to act in a way that led to their receipt of social support, and these actions can be considered coping behaviors. It has been argued that the coping concept is very broad and can be invoked for behaviors that are intended or not intended to deal with stress; for behaviors that occur before, during, or after the appearance of a stressors or strain; and for traits themselves (Beehr & McGrath, 1996).

Personality also could influence whether individuals use other effective or ineffective stress coping strategies. Kobasa (1979), for example, suggests that some of the health benefits of the control facet of hardiness occur because individuals who feel in control of their lives have a more diverse repertoire of coping strategies and are more persistent in their coping efforts than are individuals who do not feel in control of their lives. It makes perfect sense that people who believe they can control their situations will make stronger efforts at problem solving, which has been linked with positive outcomes.

IMPACT OF HARDINESS

Since Kobasa (1979) first proposed the concept of hardiness, a growing number of studies have supported the importance of the personality characteristic in stress and health research. A recent meta-analysis, for example, found that hardiness was among the personality variables that were most predictive of subjective well-being (DeNeve & Cooper, 1998). In this section, we review research on the relationships between hardiness, as traditionally defined, and stress variables. We pay special attention to the underlying mechanisms by which hardiness influences stressors and strains.

EFFECTS OF HARDINESS ON STRESS AND HEALTH

As suggested above, personality characteristics such as hardiness can affect health and stress variables in multiple ways. Evidence for these effects is discussed here.

Hardiness and Hyposensitivity to Stressors: The Moderating Effect

Observing that a select number of individuals suffer relatively few health consequences as a result of exposure to stressors, Kobasa (1979) proposed that hardiness would act as a buffer of the stressor–strain relationship. In that initial study, business executives were asked to complete measures of negative life events, illness, and hardiness. Results indicated that participants who did not become ill after exposure to high levels of stressors scored higher on each of the three facets of hardiness (i.e., control, commitment, and challenge) than did participants who did become ill after exposure to high levels of stressors.

A longitudinal study by Kobasa et al. (1982a) found that hardiness moderated the relationship between negative life events and physical and mental health among business executives. The presence of negative life events had a less negative effect on the health of hardy than of nonhardy participants. Hardiness likewise acted as a buffer against undesirable life change in a sample of women (Rhodewalt & Zone, 1989). Specifically, the presence of undesirable life change had stronger relationships with depression and illness for nonhardy than for hardy participants. In a sample of female undergraduates, Ganellen and Blaney (1984) found that commitment (measured via an alienation-from-self scale), but not control and challenge, acted as a buffer of the relationship between life change and depression.

Sinclair and Tetrick (2000), however, found only weak support for buffering effects. Specifically, they found that only negatively worded hardiness items moderated the role stressor–anxiety relationship (they had also conducted moderator analyses with depression as a strain), and these moderating effects, although statistically significant, were relatively weak. Moreover, many studies have failed to support the buffering effect of hardiness. King et al. (1998), for example, examined the effects of hardiness in 1,632 veterans who were exposed to war-related stressors. Results indicated that hardiness did not moderate the relationship between war-related stressors and posttraumatic stress disorder (PTSD). Similarly, using a sample of college students, Roth et al. (1989) found that hardiness did not moderate the relationship between negative life events and physical illness. In a sample of university secretaries, hardiness did not buffer the relationship between negative life events and illness (Schmied & Lawler, 1986). Both cross-sectional and longitudinal analyses found that hardiness did not moderate the relationships between negative life events and strains (physical illness and depression) in a sample of undergraduates (Funk & Houston, 1987). In sum, the notion that hardiness acts as a buffer of the deleterious effects of stressors has received at best only mixed support. The general lack of evidence for the buffering effect of hardiness was noted in the early years of hardiness research by other authors (Funk & Houston, 1987; Hull et al., 1987).

Hardiness, Perception of Stressors, and Self-Selection of Stressors

Spector et al. (2000) suggest that personality is important in stress research because it could potentially influence one's subjective judgment concerning the presence of stressors. Hardiness is likely to impact one's perception of stressors for many reasons. People who are high in internal control, for example, are likely to perceive a negative situation as less threatening (i.e., less of a stressor), because they believe that they are able to modify and improve the situation. Likewise, those high in commitment are less likely to view a negative situation as a stressor, because they have a sense of direction in their lives. Finally, people who are high in challenge are likely to judge a negative situation not as a stressor, but as an opportunity to grow and succeed.

Kobasa and Puccetti (1983), for example, found that hardiness correlated –.18 with reports of stressful life events among business executives. Hardiness was also negatively associated with the frequency ($r = -.39$) and severity ($r = -.36$) of negative life events reported in a group of university secretaries (Schmied & Lawler, 1986).

In another study, nonhardy women judged a greater number of recent life events as undesirable and uncontrollable than did hardy women (Rhodewalt & Zone, 1989), even though there were no significant differences between hardy and nonhardy participants in the appraisal of desirable life events. Epstein and Katz (1992) found that a global measure of hardiness ($r = -.21$) and a commitment subscale ($r = -.20$) were negatively associated with undergraduates' reports of total stressors (the sum of externally produced and self-produced stressors). Global hardiness and each of its facets, however, were not significantly related to externally produced stressors alone. Data collected from a sample of military personnel found that each of the facets of hardiness was negatively associated with the extent to which participants perceived military training as threatening (Florian et al., 1995). Specifically, perceptions of threat correlated –.44 with commitment, –.39 with control, and –.20 with challenge. Finally, Rhodewalt and Agustsdottir (1984) found that although hardiness did not influence the extent to which college students reported the occurrence of any given negative life event, hardy participants were more likely than nonhardy participants to perceive life events as controllable and desirable.

Thus, across a wide variety of types of people and situations, hardiness and its elements tend to be negatively related to self-described stressful situations. The extent to which this means hardy people are less exposed to stressful situations (e.g., because they are treated with more respect, trusted with more challenging tasks, etc.), have selected themselves into less stressful situations, or have actively created less stressful situations (e.g., by proactive, preventive coping) vs. simply perceived ordinary situations as more stressful is uncertain. It could be argued that studies measuring differences in the occurrence of somewhat objective events, such as the Kobasa and Pucetti (1983) study, lend more support to the former explanation. The Florian et al. (1995) and Rhodewalt and Agutsdottir (1984) studies are examples that can lend themselves to the latter explanation, however, because hardiness was related to differential reports of stressfulness of similar situations. If one looks closely at the studies, it can be seen that while this might be a generally valid interpretation, the evidence is not overwhelming for either conclusion. The military training experience (e.g., the way everyone was treated) is not exactly the same for every person, for example, and there have been arguments about the degree of objectivity of life stressful events scales (e.g., Spector et al., 2000).

Hardiness and Creation of Stressors

Hardiness might provide health benefits by influencing the extent to which individuals actively engage in behaviors that produce stressors. Unfortunately, we are aware of little research that examines this possibility. One way to test this hypothesis is to examine the relationship between hardiness and the extent to which one reports the presence of stressors that are under his or her control. In one study already described above, data collected from a sample of undergraduates indicated that a global measure of hardiness correlated –.21 with self-produced stressors (e.g., contracted a venereal disease; Epstein & Katz, 1992). Self-produced stressors were also predicted by commitment ($r = -.21$) and control ($r = -.16$). Another way to test whether hardiness impacts the self-creation of stressors would be to examine whether specific stressor-producing behaviors mediate the relationship between hardiness and strains. Hardiness, for example, might result in one being less overworked via effects on procrastination behavior. The roles of such mediators of the hardiness–stressor relationship, however, have largely been overlooked by researchers.

Hardiness and the Receipt of Social Support

Another possibility, mentioned earlier, is that hardiness provides health benefits via its effects on social support. Ganellen and Blaney (1984), for example, found that the commitment and challenge dimensions of hardiness were positively associated with the amount of social support received in a sample of undergraduate students (r values ranged from .35 to .42). In a sample of business executives, Kobasa and Puccetti (1983) found that hardiness was positively associated with the amount of social support provided from one's boss ($r = .29$). The relationship between hardiness and social support provided by one's family, however, was nonsignificant. King et al. (1998) hypothesized and found that hardiness was positively related with the receipt of social support. Commitment, however, was unrelated to social support in a sample of attorneys (Kobasa, 1982).

There are several reasons why hardiness might be related to social support. Hardy individuals might be more willing to seek out or accept social support, or they might be more attractive targets for the providers of social support than their nonhardy counterparts (Kobasa, 1979). Florian et al. (1995), for example, found that challenge ($r = .22$), but not the other facets of hardiness, was associated with seeking support. Another possibility is that hardy individuals tend to provide others with social support and that these others reciprocate by providing social support in return. For the most part, however, these possibilities are untested.

Hardiness and Coping Strategies

Efforts to obtain social support can be considered a coping strategy, but there are many other coping strategies that might be affected by hardiness. Kobasa (1982), for example, found that commitment influenced mental and physical health in a sample of lawyers via a negative relationship with regressive coping (e.g., denying or escaping the stressor). Using data collected from a sample of Israeli soldiers, Florian et al. (1995) found that commitment predicted the use of emotion-focused coping ($r = -.38$) and distancing coping ($r = -.21$); that control predicted problem-focused coping ($r = .25$), emotion-focused coping ($r = -.26$), and distancing coping ($r = -.14$); and that challenge predicted problem-focused coping ($r = .15$), emotion-focused coping ($r = -.27$), and distancing coping ($r = -.17$). Mediation analysis indicated that commitment contributed to mental health via effects on emotion-focused coping and that control contributed to mental health via effects on problem-focused coping. Rhodewalt and Zone (1989), using a more qualitative methodological approach, asked female participants to indicate which of a series of events they had experienced in the last 12 months and to indicate how easily they coped with events that they judged as undesirable. Nonhardy women reported more difficulty coping with the negative events than did hardy women.

Direct Effects of Hardiness on Strains

A final possibility is that hardiness has direct effects on strains. Hull et al. (1987), for example, suggest that lack of commitment and lack of control are stressful in their own right. Research has generally supported the direct negative effects of hardiness on health (Funk & Houston, 1987), especially for commitment and control (Hull et al., 1987). Kobasa and Puccetti (1983), for example, found that hardiness was negatively correlated with a measure of physical and mental health (r = .30). In cross-sectional analyses, Florian et al. (1995) found that the facets of hardiness were each related to mental health in a sample of Israeli soldiers cross-sectionally, but not longitudinally. Specifically, commitment (r = .44) and control (r = .38) were positively associated with well-being, while commitment (r = –.55), control (r = –.44), and challenge (r = –.24) were negatively associated with distress. Longitudinal data from that study, however, failed to support a link between hardiness and strains, throwing doubt on the true meaning of the cross-sectional results. Data collected from a sample of undergraduates indicated that a global measure of hardiness correlated –.22 with emotional strains, such as depression and anxiety, and correlated .26 with satisfaction with health (Epstein & Katz, 1992). Likewise, commitment correlated –.27 with emotional strains and .25 with health satisfaction, and control correlated –.19 with emotional strains and .26 with health satisfaction. Although not statistically significant, global hardiness, as well as commitment and control, were generally associated with a number of physical and behavioral strains in the expected (negative) direction. In another study, hardiness correlated .25 with life satisfaction (Rhodewalt & Zone, 1989). Schmied and Lawler (1986), however, found that hardiness was unrelated to the frequency of illness reported by a sample of female secretaries. In cross-sectional analyses, Funk and Houston (1987) found that although hardiness predicted both physical health problems and depression in an undergraduate sample; these relationships disappeared after controlling for maladjustment, suggesting that hardiness can, to a considerable degree, measure adjustment. In longitudinal analyses, hardiness predicted depression, even after controlling for maladjustment. However, hardiness at T1 was unrelated to physical health at T2. Overall, there seems to be a clear relationship between hardiness and strain cross-sectionally, but the effects are greatly diminished or even disappear when longitudinal data are examined. This throws doubt on the strength of the effect for hardiness on health.

The Effects of Stressors and Health on Hardiness

Above we discussed the potential effect that personality might have on stressors and strains. Another possibility is that stressors and strains affect personality. Spector et al. (2000), for example, suggested that trait negative affectivity might be affected by exposure to work-related stressors. Several of the cross-sectional studies reviewed above could be interpreted as supporting the argument that stressors and strains cause personality. Using a cross-sectional design, Kobasa and Puccetti (1983), for example, found that hardiness was negatively associated with stressors and strains. One interpretation of these findings, which we have considered above, is that hardiness was the cause of stressors and strains. It is also possible, however, that stressors and strains caused hardiness.

Likewise, Kobasa (1979) first identified groups of executives who had experienced either high stressors with little strain or high stressors with high strain. Three months later she administered hardiness measures to these two groups and found that the low-strain group scored higher on the hardiness measures than did the high-strain group. Kobasa interpreted these results as showing that hardiness moderates the relationship between stressors and strains. It is also possible, however, that individuals in the high-strain group scored low on hardiness because they already were experiencing poor health. Finally, Florian et al. (1995) found that when measured simultaneously, hardiness was associated with strains. However, the fact that T1 hardiness was unrelated to T2 strains suggests that hardiness might not cause strains after all. What, then, would explain the cross-sectional relationship between hardiness and strains? One possibility is that strains caused people to be less hardy.

Assuming that one cannot feasibly manipulate hardiness in an experimental design or strongly manipulate stress (for ethical reasons), the most rigorous test of whether stressors and strains impact hardiness or vice versa would involve a longitudinal design. Stressors, strains, and hardiness would be assessed at multiple times. Analyses showing that stressors and strains measured at earlier times are related to hardiness at later times while controlling for initial scores on hardiness would provide strong support for the prediction that personality is an outcome of stressors and strains. Many administrations of the measure could be used to examine whether any effects on hardiness are temporary or permanent. Unfortunately, no research that we are aware of has taken this approach. Because it is assumed that hardiness is relatively stable across time, most longitudinal studies have assessed hardiness only during the earliest measurement period (e.g., Florian et al., 1995). Such designs do not allow tests of the possibility that stressors and strains cause hardiness.

CRITICISMS OF HARDINESS RESEARCH

Several criticisms have been levied against hardiness research. Rather than measuring hardiness directly, many studies use negative indicators of hardiness (Funk & Houston, 1987). A measure of alienation, for example, is often used to assess commitment, or powerlessness is used to assess control. Unfortunately, it is unclear that these negative indicators are actually valid reverse-coded measures of the facets of hardiness. Indeed, Funk and Houston (1987) suggest that these negative indicators are actually measures of maladjustment or psychopathology, and Sinclair and Tetrick (2000) found empirical overlap between the negative items and neuroticism. Semmer (2003) noted that recently developed hardiness scales often omit alienation. In fact, data Funk and Houston collected from a sample of undergraduates suggest that several of the scales used to assess hardiness correlated moderately with measures of maladjustment. In some cases, the correlation between hardiness and maladjustment was nearly as strong as the correlation between two measures of maladjustment. This is strikingly parallel to a controversial issue in stress research regarding negative affectivity, perhaps at the extreme when very similar items are to be found in both negative affectivity and psychological strain measures. If a negative affectivity scale includes items such as scared, nervous, distressed, upset, jittery, and afraid, it is no surprise that it would correlate with measures of psychological strain or distress, such as depression or anxiety — in principle, the main difference is that one scale asks how one feels recently, and the other asks how one feels in general. Negative affectivity, a personality construct, and psychological strain measures sometimes look almost interchangeable. Sinclair and Tetrick (2000) noted that hardiness measures typically included mostly negatively worded items, and their studies suggested that the negatively worded items in hardiness might have some redundancy with neuroticism.

Funk and Houston (1987) also noted that in many cases, items used to assess hardiness have little resemblance to the construct as defined by Kobasa (1982). For example, the item "Public supported medical care is the right of everyone" is included in a scale commonly used to assess the challenge dimension of hardiness. It is difficult to argue for even the face validity of this item as a measure of internal control, commitment, or challenge.

Finally, they criticize the use of analysis of variance (ANOVA), which is common in much of the research on hardiness (Funk & Houston, 1987). As one example of the use of ANOVA, Kobasa (1979) identified a group of high-stressor/high-strain and a group of high-stressor/low-strain executives and examined (using *t*-tests) group differences in hardiness measures as tests of the buffering effect of hardiness. Funk and Houston (1987), however, found strikingly different results when using regression rather than ANOVA for the retrospective analyses. When using data obtained with continuous measures, collapsing the data into a small number of categories introduces error into the measures. A common practice in this research is to divide the sample at the median, which reassigns the scores of the highest-scoring person and the person barely above the median to the same value; the best estimate of each person's value, however, is his or her original score, and thus the data are likely to be made less accurate using this method. In addition, converting continuous scores into categories is likely to attenuate relationships between variables by reducing variance.

EXPANDING THE HARDINESS CONSTRUCT

The limited number of traits that are traditionally considered to define hardiness might be too few; other personality traits might act in the same way, and it would be logical to consider them as indicators of hardiness as well. Although hardiness is often conceived as a specific, small set of personal characteristics, at its core, the hardiness concept and the definition of the English word, hardiness simply indicates that some people possess characteristics that enable them to endure otherwise stressful conditions while experiencing less strain than would be expected — hardiness is a moderator of the stressor–strain relationship. The favorite category of personal characteristics in hardiness seems to be personality rather than, say, abilities or physical characteristics; hardiness seems to be a conglomerate of personality or personality-like characteristics that have this moderating effect. When such concepts are developed, it is common for researchers to add and subtract elements as research shows them to be more or less viable as moderators. Thus, consistent with the theme of hardiness, any personality characteristic that empirically moderates the relationship between stressors and strains could be considered to make the person hardy. Over time, researchers have examined many personality characteristics as potential moderators of the relationship between stressors and strains, including negative and positive affectivity, self-esteem and self-efficacy, and, of course, any of the characteristics in the five-factor model of personality.

Negative Affectivity

Negative affectivity is a personal trait epitomized by the tendency to experience negative emotions (Watson & Clark, 1984), and Semmer (2003) argue that the traditional concept of hardiness is more cognitive or belief oriented, while negative affectivity is more emotional. There is an obvious link between negative affectivity and psychological strain, because psychological strain *is* the experience of negative emotions (due to current environmental stressors). It is thought to be measured by a number of negative personality measures, including anxiety, depression, and neuroticism scales. In fact, it appears that the primary difference between negative affectivity and psychological strain is their duration or the extent to which the emotion is a stable trait or a temporary state. NA is highly likely, therefore, to be correlated with psychological strain, and a recent meta-analysis (Thoresen et al., 2003) found that the average cross-study correlation between NA and emotional exhaustion (a psychological strain that is part of burnout and that resembles NA) was .43 (.52 corrected). Given the resemblance between NA and psychological strain, that is to be expected, but a main concern here is whether NA can also moderate the relationships between stressors and strains (psychological or otherwise).

There has been a great deal of research on negative affectivity and stress, much of it in the context of work-related stress. Often, NA has been used as a control variable; i.e., researchers examine the potential effects of stressors on strains while controlling for NA. This is done because NA is often considered a nuisance variable that influences both stressors and strains. A relationship between stressors and strains usually remains even while controlling NA (e.g., Adler et al., 2000; Jeurissen & Nyklicek, 2001; Spector et al., 2000), and it is noteworthy that even the idea of controlling NA in stress studies is not without controversy, especially in the occupational stress research domain (e.g., see Judge et al., 2000; Payne, 2000; Spector et al., 2000).

Research results regarding NA's moderating effects are inconsistent, with some research finding stressor–strain relations moderated (e.g., Cassar & Tattersall, 1998; Moyle, 1995; Parkes, 1990) and some not (e.g., Houkes et al., 2003; Mak & Mueller, 2000; Walker et al., 2001; Zellars et al., 1999). To some extent, therefore, having (low) negative affectivity might be considered part of being hardy.

Positive Affectivity

Positive affectivity is the extent to which one is pleasantly aroused, excited, and activated across a wide range of situations (Watson et al., 1988). If negative affectivity might moderate the stressor–strain relationship, what about positive affectivity? Very little research has been conducted on this issue, and so the results should be considered more tentative. A large portion of the studies of PA also included NA as a variable. The Thoresen et al. (2003) meta-analysis found an average correlation of –.26 (–.32 corrected) between PA and emotional exhaustion, although only eleven studies of this relationship were found. As with negative affectivity, some research uses PA as a control variable, usually finding that the stressor–strain relationships remain after controlling for PA (e.g., Jeurissen & Nyklicek, 2001), but our main concern is again the potential moderating effects of PA. More studies, however, seem to have failed to find a moderating effect of PA than to have found one, (e.g., Iverson et al., 1998; Mak & Mueller, 2000).

The Five-Factor Model of Personality

If the five-factor or big-five model covers all personality factors, as is often purported (e.g., McCrae & Costa, 1987), then positive and negative affectivity must be covered by its five factors. Negative affectivity is widely considered to be the factor of neuroticism, and PA might be part of extraversion (Watson et al., 1988). Some studies examined relationships of personality with either stressors or strains, but few studies have examined personality specific to elements of the five-factor model as potential moderators of the stressor–strain relationship. One study found that two of the five personality characteristics moderated this relationship: neuroticism and extraversion (Hudiburg et al., 1999). To the extent that these overlap with NA and PA, this finding might be redundant with the results for negative and positive affectivity. Overall, the big-five personality factors have not been used explicitly very often in studies searching for personality moderators of the stressor–strain relationship, with the exception of factors that might substitute for NA and PA.

Self-esteem and Self-efficacy

Self-esteem and self-efficacy are cognitive beliefs people have about their capabilities. Whereas self-esteem consists of general positive beliefs about one's self, self-efficacy is more specifically one's belief that he or she is capable of performing well in general or in some specific domain, task, or activity (Bandura, 1982) — perhaps in the workplace or in some even more specific domain such as conducting a meeting in which one must engage in public speaking. Logically, this fits with the traditional hardiness dimension, control. To the extent that these beliefs are stable and represent action tendencies, they might act like, or even be, personality characteristics. There has been some suggestion that they, especially self-efficacy in task-relevant situations such as the workplace, should be studied as potential moderators of the relationships between stressors and strains (e.g., Hastings & Bham, 2003). Its moderating effect might occur through its influence on coping efforts (Bandura, 1982); if one has high self-efficacy, coping efforts should be more likely to be seen as worthwhile and to be attempted.

Research has sometimes supported the moderating effects of self-efficacy on the stressor–strain relationship. Jex and colleagues (Jex & Bliese, 1999; Jex et al., 2001) found this effect in studies of military personnel, although its two-way interaction with stressors depended upon a three-way interaction involving use of specific coping styles in one study (Jex et al., 2001). They also found the effect among university employees (although only collective efficacy and not individual self-efficacy had moderating effects; Jex & Gudanowski, 1992). Salanova et al. (2002) also found something more complex than the simple two-way interaction. They found a three-way interaction of job demand (a stressor), control, and a relatively specific measure of computer self-efficacy (but not their more general measure of self-efficacy) predicting information technology employees' burnout. In addition, a Japanese study (Matsui & Onglatco, 1992) found that the direction of the moderating effect of self-efficacy might even be "backward" depending on the nature of the stressor. That is, high self-efficacy might strengthen the relationship between some stressors and strains. Apparently, any moderating effects of self-efficacy on stressor–strain relationships might be quite complex.

It should be noted that while self-efficacy might resemble a personality trait, it also might lack some trait-like qualities. It can be less stable than most personality traits, assuming it can more easily be altered by experience. Indeed, a longitudinal stress study by Holman and Wall (2002) investigated self-efficacy as a dependent variable, implying that it is not stable (even though they did not find its predictors). How does one come to believe that he or she is good at math — perhaps by previous successful experiences with math? On the other hand, to some extent, it might be easier to alter one's efficacy beliefs in most domains upward than downward. That is, once people believe they can ride a bicycle, their efficacy beliefs probably do not revert all the way to being certain that they *cannot* ride one. In this way, efficacy beliefs in many domains might be more stable downward than upward.

Sense of Humor

Stress researchers have long been interested in the role of sense of humor. In a recent review article, however, Martin (2001) suggested that the effects of sense of humor on health are at best weak and that sense of humor has not been consistently found to moderate the relationship between stressors and physical strains. There is some evidence that sense of humor might even have negative effects on physical health. In a longitudinal study of 1178 participants that spanned seven decades, Friedman et al. (1993) unexpectedly found that cheerfulness/humor was negatively associated with longevity.

Some research, however, does suggest that sense of humor has benefits for psychological health. Sense of humor buffered or moderated the effects of negative life event stressors on depression in a sample of college students (Nezu et al., 1988). However, sense of humor did not moderate the relationship between negative life events and anxiety. Using data from three student samples, Martin and Lefcourt (1983) found that sense of humor moderated the relationship between negative life events and negative mood.

Some authors have argued that sense of humor can benefit one's health by attracting social support (Martin, 2001; Nezu et al., 1988). However, we tested this hypothesis in a sample of high school employees and found that sense of humor was unrelated to the amount of social support received from others at work (Bowling et al., 2004).

Religiosity

Religiosity, or the extent to which people consider religion to be an important part of their lives, also has been hypothesized to protect individuals from the harmful effects of stressors. Whether religiosity is a personality trait is open to question; the idea has seldom been addressed. It might be a belief system, for example, rather than a personality trait. Important conceptual similarities might sometimes exist, however, between religiosity and the commitment facet of hardiness. Whereas commitment concerns the extent to which an individual is connected to various aspects of one's life, such as self, work, family, and friends (Kobasa, 1979), religiosity is more specific in that it involves an engagement with one's spiritual life. Thus, religiosity could be thought of as a specific aspect of commitment.

A few studies investigated whether religiosity moderates the relationship between stressors and strains. One way this might work is that stressors could result in more strains for nonreligious individuals than for religious individuals, because those who are high in religiosity believe that they have access to the resources of a higher power when confronted with stressors. A longitudinal study by Hettler and Cohen (1998) found that religiosity moderated the relationship between negative life events and depression for members of liberal Protestant congregations, but not for members of conservative Protestant congregations. Park et al. (1990) found that religiosity moderated the relationship between negative life events and depression for Protestants but not for Catholics. Among Protestants, the regression slope for the relationship between negative life events and depression was stronger for low-religiosity individuals than for high-religiosity individuals. The relationship between uncontrollable life events and depression was actually negative for high-religiosity Protestants. Data collected from older Japanese adults also support the buffering hypothesis of religiosity (Krause et al., 2002). Experiencing the death of a loved one was less likely to result in hypertension for participants who believed in an afterlife. In a sample of African-American youths, religious involvement moderated the relationship between stressful life events and psychological symptoms for females but not for males (Grant et al., 2000). Krause and Van Tran (1989), however, found that religious involvement did not moderate the relationships of negative life events with self-esteem and personal control in a sample of older African-Americans.

In summary, although hardiness is traditionally considered to be composed of a limited number of personality traits (perhaps as few as three), it is logical to consider any personality trait moderating the stressor–strain relationship to be an element of the hardiness concept. Here, positive and negative affectivity, elements of the five-factor model, self-esteem and self-efficacy, sense of humor, and religiosity are considered. In addition, readers are referred to other chapters in this book for thorough discussions of types A and B and internal locus of control.

SUMMARY AND CONCLUSIONS

Hardiness is by definition the ability to withstand stressors without being seriously harmed by them. The early research by Kobasa and colleagues (e.g., Kobasa, 1979, 1982; Kobasa et al., 1982b; Kobasa & Pucetti, 1983) tended to focus on moderating effects that hardiness has on the relationships between stressors and strains, and this is in some ways the most interesting effect from a stress standpoint. Hardiness also might help people by having a main effect on their health, however, and this appears probable. Indeed, the research discussed here provides more support for the main effects of hardiness than for moderating effects. As suggested above, these main effects might occur via a number of mechanisms. Future research should clarify these processes.

Some well-known cognitive approaches to stress emphasize appraisal and coping (e.g., Folkman et al., 1979; Lazarus & Launier, 1978), and hardiness seems to be related to these two activities of stressed people. In primary appraisal, people can interpret elements of their environments as *challenge* vs. threat, for example, and challenge is traditionally a part of hardiness. In secondary appraisal of potentially stressful situations, people can judge that they have the resources to cope with or handle the situation, which is similar to believing in their own internal *control*, another element of hardiness. Future research might investigate the overlap and interplay of hardiness and cognitive theories of stress.

We have also argued that personality characteristics other than those specifically identified in Kobasa's (1979) conceptualization of hardiness could potentially protect individuals from the ill effects of stressors. Because of this, the time might have come to redefine the concept of hardiness operationally. There is good reason, for example, to believe that researchers should rethink whether challenge should be included as an aspect of hardiness (Hull et al., 1987). Advances might also be made by improving the measures and research designs used in hardiness studies (Funk & Houston, 1987). As illustrated by Florian et al. (1995), future research should utilize longitudinal designs.

One interesting avenue of research would involve examining Kobasa's (1979) concept of hardiness in conjunction with other personality characteristics addressed in this chapter. For example, factor analysis could be used to examine whether other personality characteristics should be included as facets of hardiness. Kobasa et al. (1983) made a start in this area by showing that the elements of hardiness they measured were empirically distinct from type A characteristics. Similarly, future research might also consider whether hardiness predicts stressors and strains after controlling for other personality characteristics.

It also should be noted that many of the early studies by Kobasa and colleagues apparently were conducted on white male managers working in the same utility company (e.g., Kobasa, 1979; Kobasa et al., 1981, 1982a, 1982b, 1983, 1985; Kobasa & Puccetti, 1983). Many times these appeared to be the same set of people, although in some studies they were a subset of these people; furthermore, new data were collected from some of the people to examine longitudinal issues in some of the studies. We conclude from this observation, however, that the early results on hardiness, stress, and health should be considered less robust than one might have expected, given the number of studies reported. Fortunately, more studies have now been reported on very different and, as a set, more diverse samples.

Finally, researchers should consider hardiness within the context of the bandwidth fidelity debate (Ones & Viswesvaran, 1996). If hardiness is regarded as a broad heterogeneous personality trait, as Kobasa (1979) described it, then it could be expected to better predict broadly defined outcomes than more narrow ones. For example, hardiness could be expected to be a better predictor of the number of stressors encountered in life in general than in a specific aspect of one's life, such as work or marriage.

ACKNOWLEDGMENTS

Michael O'Driscoll and Norbert Semmer provided helpful feedback on an earlier draft of this chapter.

REFERENCES

Bandura, A. (1982). Self-efficacy mechanism in human agency. *American Psychologist*, 37, 122–147.

Beehr, T.A., & McGrath, J.E. (1996). The methodology of research on coping: Conceptual, strategic, and operational-level issues. In M. Zeidner & N.S. Endler (Eds.), *Handbook of Coping: Theory, Research, Applications* , (pp. 65–82). New York: John Wiley & Sons.

Bowling, N.A., Beehr, T.A., Johnson, A.L., Semmer, N.K., Hendricks, E.A., & Webster, H.A., (in press). Explaining antecedents of workplace social support: reciprocity or attractiveness?

Cassar, V., & Tattersall, A. (1998). Occupational stress and negative affectivity in Maltese nurses: Testing moderating influences. *Work and Stress*, 12, 85–94.

DeNeve, K., & Cooper, H. (1998). The happy personality: A meta-analysis of 137 personality traits and subjective well-being. *Psychological Bulletin*, 124, 197–229.

Epstein, S., & Katz, L. (1992). Coping ability, stress, productive load, and symptoms. *Journal of Personality and Social Psychology*, 62, 813–825.

Florian, V., Mikulincer, M., & Taubman, O. (1995). Does hardiness contribute to mental health during a stressful real-life situation? The roles of appraisal and coping. *Journal of Personality and Social Psychology*, 68, 687–695.

Folkman, S., Schaefer, C., & Lazarus, R.S. (1979). Cognitive processes as mediators of stress and coping. In V. Hamilton & D. M. Warburton (Eds.), *Human Stress and Cognition: An Information Processing Approach* (pp. 265–298). New York: Wiley.

Friedman, H.S., Tucker, J.S., Tomlinson-Keasey, C., Schwartz, J.E., Wingard, D.L., & Criqui, M.H. (1993). Does childhood personality predict longevity? *Journal of Personality and Social Psychology*, 65, 176–185.

Funk, S.C., & Houston, B.K. (1987). A critical analysis of the Hardiness Scale's validity and utility. *Journal of Personality and Social Psychology*, 53, 572–578.

Ganellen, R.J., & Blaney, P.H. (1984). Hardiness and social support as moderators of the effects of life stress. *Journal of Personality and Social Psychology*, 47, 156–163.

Hastings, R.P., & Bham, M.S. (2003). The relationship between student behaviour patterns and teacher burnout. *School Psychology International*, 24, 115–127.

Hettler, T.R., & Cohen, L.H. (1998). Intrinsic religiousness as a stress-moderator for adult Protestant churchgoers. *Journal of Community Psychology* , 26, 597–609.

Holman, D.J., & Wall, T.D. (2002). Work characteristics, learning-related outcomes, and strain: A test of competing direct effects, mediated, and moderated models. *Journal of Occupational Health Psychology*, 7, 283–301.

Hudiburg, R.A., Pashaj, I., & Wolfe, R. (1999). Preliminary investigation of computer stress and the Big Five personality factors. *Psychological Reports*, 85, 473–480.

Hull, J.G., Van Treuren, R.R., & Virnelli, S. (1987). Hardiness and health: A critique and alternative approach. *Journal of Personality and Social Psychology*, 53, 518–530.

Iverson, R.C., Olekalns, M., & Erwin, P.J. (1998). Affectivity, organizational stressors, and absenteeism: A causal model of burnout and its consequences. *Journal of Vocational Behavior*, 52, 1–23.

Jeurissen, T., & Nyklicek, I. (2001). Testing the vitamin model of stress in Dutch health care workers. *Work & Stress*, 15, 254–264.

Jex, S.M., Beehr, T.A., & Roberts, C.K. (1992). The meaning of occupational stress items to survey respondents. *Journal of Applied Psychology*, 77, 623–628.

Jex, S.M., Bliese, P.D., Buzzell, S., & Primeau, J. (2001). The impact of self-efficacy in stressor-strain relations: Coping style as an explanatory mechanism. *Journal of Applied Psychology*, 86, 401–409.

Judge, T. A, Erez, A., Thoresen, C. J. (2000). Why negative affectivity (and self-deception) should be included in job stress research: Bathing the baby with the bathwater. *Journal of Organizational Behavior*, 21, 101–111.

King, L.A., King, D.W., Fairbank, J.A., Keane, T.M., & Adams, G.A. (1998). Resilience-recovery factors in post-traumatic stress disorder among female and male Vietnam veterans: Hardiness, postwar social support, and additional stressful life events. *Journal of Personality and Social Psychology*, 74, 420–434.

Kobasa, S.C. (1979). Stressful life events, personality and health: An inquiry into hardiness. *Journal of Personality and Social Psychology*, 37, 1–11.

Kobasa, S.C. (1982). Commitment and coping in stress resistance among lawyers. *Journal of Personality and Social Psychology*, 42, 707–717.

Kobasa, S.C., Maddi, S.R., & Courington, S. (1981). Personality and constitution as mediators in the stress-illness relationship. *Journal of Health and Social Behavior*, 22, 368–378.

Kobasa, S.C., Maddi, S.R., & Kahn S. (1982a). Hardiness and health: A prospective study. *Journal of Personality and Social Psychology*, 42, 168–177.

Kobasa, S.C., Maddi, S.R., & Puccetti, M.C. (1982b). Personality and exercise as buffers in the stress-illness relationship. *Journal of Behavioral Medicine*, 5, 391–404.

Kobasa, S.C., Maddi, S.R., Puccetti, M.C., & Zola, M.A. (1985). Effectiveness of hardiness, exercise, and social support as resources against illness. *Journal of Psychosomatic Research*, 29, 525–533.

Kobasa, S.C., Maddi, S.R., & Zola, M.A. (1983). Type A and hardiness. *Journal of Behavioral Medicine*, 6, 41–51.

Kobasa, S.C.O., & Puccetti, M.C. (1983). Personality and social resources in stress resistance. *Journal of Personality and Social Psychology*, 45, 839–850.

Krause, N., Liang, J., Shaw, G.A., Sugisawa, H., Kim, H., & Sugihara, Y. (2002). Religion, death of a loved one, and hypertension among older adults in Japan. *Journals of Gerontology*, 57, S96–S107.

Krause, N., & Van Tran, T. (1989). Stress and religious involvement among older Blacks. *Journals of Gerontology*, 4, S4–S13.

Lazarus, R.S., & Launier, R. (1978). Stress-related transactions between person and environment. In L.A. Pervin & M. Lewis (Eds.), *Perspectives in Interactional Psychology* (pp. 287–327). New York: Plenum.

McCrae, R. R., & Costa, P. T. (1987). Validation of the five-factor model of personality across instruments and observers. *Journal of Personality and Social Psychology*, 52, 81–90.

Mak, A.S., & Mueller, J. (2000). Job insecurity, coping resources and personality dispositions in occupational strain. *Work and Stress*, 14, 312–328.

Martin, R.A. (2001). Humor, laughter, and physical health: Methodological issues and research findings. *Psychological Bulletin*, 127, 504–519.

Martin, R.A., & Lefcourt, H.M. (1983). Sense of humor as a moderator of the relation between stressors and moods. *Journal of Personality and Social Psychology*, 45, 1313–1324.

Matsui, T., & Onglatco, M.L. (1992). Career self-efficacy as a moderator of the relation between occupational stress and strain. *Journal of Vocational Behavior*, 41, 79–88.

Moyle, P. (1995). The role of negative affectivity in the stress process: Tests of alternative models. *Journal of Organizational Behavior*, 16, 647–668.

Nezu, A.M., Nezu, C.M., & Blissett, S.E. (1988). Sense of humor as a moderator of the relation between stressful events and psychological distress: A prospective analysis. *Journal of Personality and Social Psychology*, 54, 520–525.

Ones, D.S., & Viswesvaran, C. (1996). Bandwidth-fidelity dilemma in personality measurement for personnel selection. *Journal of Organizational Behavior*, 17, 609–626.

Park, C., Cohen, L.H., & Herb, L. (1990). Intrinsic religiousness and religious coping as life stress moderators for Catholics versus Protestants. *Journal of Personality and Social Psychology*, 59, 562–574.

Parkes, K.R. (1990). Coping, negative affectivity, and the work environment: Additive and interactive predictors of mental health. *Journal of Applied Psychology*, 75, 399–409.

Payne, R.L. (2000). Comments on "Why negative affectivity should not be controlled in job stress research: Don't throw the baby out with the bathwater." *Journal of Organizational Behavior*, 21, 97–99.

Rhodewalt, F., & Agustsdottier, S. (1984). On the relationship of hardiness to the type A behavior pattern: Perception of life events versus coping with life events. *Journal of Research in Personality*, 18, 212–223.

Rhodewalt, F., & Zone, J.B. (1989). Appraisal of life change, depression, and illness in hardy and nonhardy women. *Journal of Personality and Social Psychology*, 56, 81–88.

Roth, D.L., Wiebe, D.J., Fillingim, R.B., & Shay, K.A. (1989). Life events, fitness, hardiness, and health: A simultaneous analysis of proposed stress-resistance effects. *Journal of Personality and Social Psychology*, 57, 136–142.

Salanova, M., Peiro, J.M., & Schaufeli, W.B. (2002). Self-efficacy specificity and burnout among information technology workers: An extension of the job demand-control model. *European Journal of Work and Organizational Psychology* , 11, 1–25.

Schmied, L.A., & Lawler, K.A. (1986). Hardiness, type A behavior, and the stress-illness relation in working women. *Journal of Personality and Social Psychology*, 51, 1218–1223.

Semmer, N.K. (2003). Individual differences, work stress and health. In M.J. Schabracq, J.A.M. Winnubst, & C.L. Cooper (Eds.), *The Handbook of Work and Health Psychology*, 2nd ed. (pp. 83–120). New York: John Wiley & Sons.

Sinclair, R.R., & Tetrick, L.E. (2000). Implications for item wording for hardiness, structure, relationship with neuroticism, and stress buffering. *Journal of Research in Personality*, 34, 1–25.

Spector, P.E., Zapf, D., Chen, P.Y., & Frese, M. (2000). Why negative affectivity should not be controlled in job stress research: Don't throw out the baby with the bath water. *Journal of Organizational Behavior*, 21, 79–95.

Thoresen, C.J., Kaplan, S.A., Barsky, A.P., & Warren, C.R. (2003). The Affective Underpinnings of Job Perceptions and Attitudes: A Meta-Analytic Review and Integration. Paper presented at the annual meeting of the Society for Industrial and Organizational Psychology, Orlando FL, April.

Watson, D., & Clark, L.A. (1984). Negative affectivity: The disposition to experience aversive emotional states. *Psychological Bulletin*, 96, 465–490.

Watson, D., Clark, L.A., & Tellegen, A. (1988). Development and validation of brief measures of positive and negative affect: The PANAS scales. *Journal of Personality and Social Psychology*, 54, 1063–1070.

Zellars, K.L., & Perrewé, P.L. (2001). Affective personality and the content of emotional social support: Coping in organizations. *Journal of Applied Psychology*, 86, 459–467.

Zellars, K.L., Perrewé, P.L., & Hochwater, W. A. (1999). Mitigating burnout among high-NA employees in health care: What can organizations do? *Journal of Applied Social Psychology*, 29, 2250–2271.

11 Stress, Culture, and Personality

Pittu Laungani

CONTENTS

INTRODUCTION

Let us visualize a scenario. It is a warm, beautiful summer afternoon. The sun shines out of a clear, cloudless blue sky. Shading our eyes against the bright sunlight, we look up as the distant sound of a light aircraft reaches our ears. The plane flying at a height of about 8,000 ft whizzes past, does a wide sweep, and returns. Just then, the steel doors open, and a man dressed in his flying gear, goggles, helmet, and a parachute tucked behind him dives into space. Arms and legs spread-eagled, he performs a few free-fall aerobatics. Our mouths agape, we watch, mesmerized. A couple of heart-stopping minutes later, he pulls the parachute cord and it blows open, and shimmering in the sunlight, he drifts sensuously in the air and lands a few minutes later with just a slight thud in the open field — to the thunderous applause of the large crowd that has gathered to see this remarkable feat.

To most of the people on terra firma, the feat seems enthralling, stressful, and even terrifying beyond words — a paradox of conflicting emotions. Not for all the Klondike diamonds would many onlookers have consented to emulate the parachutist. The very idea, to say the least, seems unimaginable. Some, however, might have felt envious and even wished they had the courage to take a plunge. A few with a feeling of supercilious righteousness might have looked upon the entire show as a sham, a pathetic attempt at self-aggrandizement. And among those few, a minuscule

0-8493-1820-3/05/$0.00+$1.50

minority — collectors of macabre memorabilia — might have felt acutely disappointed at seeing the parachutist landing safely on the field.

Although I have chosen an extreme example, it is clear that there are variations in our perceptions and evaluations of the event. A situation, an event, an episode that is stressful to one person might be a thrill to another, disappointing to a third, and a matter of indifference to a fourth. We do not all perceive a situation in an identical manner, nor do we all react to it in an identical fashion. Our perceptions are often subjective, the subjectivity based on our own underlying intuitive, theoretical, experiential, and empirical assumptions. Pursuing this line of reasoning further, it is reasonable to argue that past learning experiences, one's familiarity with stressful events, one's own culturally accepted norms and values, and one's personality factors have a major role to play in one's perception and evaluation of events, and the subsequent label one assigns to one's observations of the events — a field of great interest to phenomenologists and philosophers.

The major aim of this chapter is to undertake a careful analysis of the three constructs that form the title of this chapter: *stress*, *culture*, and *personality.* It is hoped that such an analysis will lead to a clearer understanding of the complex issues surrounding this important area of human stress.

NATURE OF STRESS: WESTERN PERSPECTIVES

The point that often escapes many people, even occasionally some academics, working in this area is that stress is *not* a material entity. It is not part of one's DNA structure, which can be subjected to a systematic biochemical analysis. To reify the concept is to misunderstand it. Yet one never ceases to hear statements such as "I have a lot of stress in me," "I am a very stressed person," "I am a worrier," and so on. If stress is not a material entity, what is stress? How does one define it?

There are as many definitions of stress as there are people whose opinions are solicited. Like the term *intelligence*, the term *stress*, too, is a ubiquitous concept that carries within it diverse shades of meaning. Euphemism aside, this suggests a lack of consensus regarding its meaning.

Hans Selye (1950, 1956, 1974, 1980) was one of the earliest researchers in the area. He formulated the general adaptation syndrome (GAS), which is a general physiological response when the human or animal organism experiences threat. Although Selye's model served as an initial guide to research, it soon outgrew its usefulness. Since then, skillful definitions have been offered. Their focus has been on (1) stimulus factors, viz., stress is seen as a negative force impinging upon an individual; (2) response factors, viz., an individual's emotional, behavioral, or physiological response to external or internal environmental events; and (3) an interactive process, viz., an individual's perceptual and cognitive appraisal of the individual's internal and external environments. Lazarus and Folkman (1984), in proposing an interactive view, go on to add that individuals can engage in a process of *primary appraisal* when confronted with a new or a changing situation, and *secondary appraisal* when assessing their coping abilities required to meet the challenge or the possible harm of the potential event.

Mason (1975), on the other hand, suggests that the term stress has been examined in at least four different ways:

1. It is a stimulus or external force acting on the organism.
2. It is a response or a set of physiological changes acting upon the individual.
3. It is an interaction between an external force and the resistance opposed to it, as in biology.
4. It is a comprehensive phenomenon encompassing all three.

It is clear that the differences in definitions reflect different theoretical perspectives of professionals from different disciplines. The diverse perspectives impose a severe strain on any meaningful comparative investigations. But this has not prevented the area of stress management from becoming big business. In the last 50 years, however, research into stress has mushroomed into a booming, buzzing, business enterprise of gargantuan proportions. According to Sauter (1992), about 600,000 workers in the U.S. tend to be seriously affected by stress and other psychological disorders. This costs around $5.5 billion in annual payments to the affected individuals and their families. And when one takes other hidden costs into account, such as reduced productivity, absenteeism, etc., the figure rises. Wright and Smye (1996) have estimated that the overall cost to business and industry in terms of burnout and depression among employees in the U.S. varies between $150 billion and $180 billion a year. It is estimated that in Britain, up to or over 5 million people experience stress ranging from severe to very severe, and the cost of dealing with this problem runs £3.7 billion a year.

Given the colossal sums of money involved, it is hardly surprising that stress and its management should become a gigantic industry. However, what is unique and remarkable about the stress industry is that it lacks an identifiable monolithic corporate image such as one might attribute to Microsoft or Esso. The *stress industry* solicits the services of multinational insurance companies, legal and paralegal firms, management consultants, medical practitioners, psychiatrists, psychologists, psychotherapists, social workers, and a host of counselors of known and unknown theoretical persuasions. An industry that promises substantial rewards, an industry that does not have the means or any statutory powers to look too closely into the credentials of its practitioners, also attracts, as is only to be expected, a large number of fakes, fraudsters, and charlatans. The entire industry comes into service to help the poor, helpless, inadequate victims, some of whom, without sounding unduly cynical, are often the beneficiaries of their stress-related disorders, when gigantic claims are settled in their favor. Thus, everyone gets a share, and everyone is happy, before another posttraumatic stress disorder (PTSD) occurs or is invented. Sadly, the good that genuine and concerned academics, research workers, and management consultants of impeccable qualifications and integrity do does not always get its due recognition and is "oft interred with their bones."

In this scramble, the process gets murkier and muddier. This, among other things, prompted Cooper (1983) to suggest in a firm but polite manner that what is lacking in the field of stress is an integrative framework that would explain the majority of the research findings in a logical, integrative theoretical perspective. Cooper's comments become even more relevant when one moves away from Western conceptualizations of stress to non-Western ones.

NATURE OF STRESS: NON-WESTERN PERSPECTIVES

It is worth noting in this context that the word *stress* itself is not easily understood in non-Western countries, such as India, Pakistan, and other South Asian countries, including Sri Lanka, Malaysia, and Indonesia, and consequently does not share similar sets of meanings associated with the term in the West. As an example of cultural differences, let us consider the issue from an Indian perspective.

For instance, there is no equivalent word for stress in the languages of India; its meaning has to be gleaned from a variety of social, philosophical, psychophysical, and somatic indices. Ramachandra Rao (1983) has highlighted two Indian concepts, *klesha* and *dukha,* which, according to him, correspond reasonably closely to Western concepts of stress. These concepts have been derived from the Indian indigenous systems known as *Samkhya Yoga* and *Ayurveda.* The word *klesha* refers to the stressor aspect, and the word *dukha* refers to the range of sorrowful experiences that individuals go through in the course of their interactions with the world around them. However, when the word *klesha* is translated into common parlance, it refers to life's unavoidable and inevitable vicissitudes, and *dukha* refers to sorrow or unhappiness. Sorrow, within the framework of the Indian philosophical tradition known as *Advaita Vedanta*, formulated by Sankara, is a fundamental part of the human condition (Radhakrishnan, 1923/1989; Sharma, 2000; Zimmer, 1951/1989). Such a notion of sorrow also forms an integral part of Buddhist philosophy. In Vedantic philosophy, the external world in which we live, although seemingly real and permanent, is ever changing. It lacks permanence. It is illusory. It is referred to as *maya.* At an abstract philosophical level the term *stress* does not arouse the same concerns among Indians as it does among Westerners. It is clear, therefore, that the two Indian words *klesha* and *dukha* do not really convey the same meaning of stress, as it is understood in the West. In addition to Ramchandra Rao's conceptual model of stress, Palsane et al. (1986) have also presented a model of stress based on ancient Indian treatises. Stress in Indian thinking is also conceptualized in holistic terms. It affects individuals both at their inner spiritual and metaphysical level and at their behavioral level.

For instance, the day-to-day religious and secular behaviors of Hindus make sense when seen within the context of pollution and purification. Hindus view pollution and purification largely in *spiritual terms* and not in terms of hygiene (Filippi, 1996; Flood, 1996; Fuller, 1992). The nonperformance of daily purification rites and rituals often leads to acute stress. The status of a person in India is determined by his or her position on the caste hierarchy and by the degree of contact with the polluting agent. Proximity to a polluting agent can constitute a permanent pollution. This would mean that certain occupations are permanently polluting. Such a form of pollution is *collective* — the entire family remains polluted. It is also *hereditary.*

Pollution can be temporary but mild, temporary but severe, or permanent. One is in a state of mild impurity upon waking up in the morning, prior to performing one's morning ablutions, when one has eaten food, and when one has not prayed.

Mild states of pollution are easily overcome by appropriate actions, such as baths, prayers, wearing clean, washed clothes, and engaging in appropriate cleansing and purification rituals. Severe pollution occurs when high-caste Hindus come into physical or social contact with persons of the lowest caste, or when they eat meat (particularly beef), or when the strict rules governing commensality are abrogated. Commensality is concerned with hospitality, with extending and receiving hospitality. It carries a special religious meaning within Hindu culture. There are strict taboos of ritual purity associated with offering and receiving food and water, and great care has to be taken in terms of who one offers food to and whom one receives food from. To offer food to an outsider results in breaking the taboos of ritual purity.

No high-caste Hindu is expected to accept (or offer) cooked food or water from a low-caste Hindu. Nor is it appropriate for a low-caste Hindu to receive cooked food or water from a high-caste Hindu. This feature applies not only to intercaste encounters, but also to within-caste encounters. A person of higher grading within a given subcaste can neither offer nor receive cooked food from a person of lower grading from the same subcaste. A Brahmin engaged in temple duties will not accept hospitality from a Brahmin involved in funeral rites. The temple Brahmin is seen as being ritually superior to the former. The privileges of superiority are fiercely protected. To overcome this form of pollution, it is necessary for the polluted individual (in some instances the entire family can get polluted) to perform a series of appropriate propitiation rites, rituals, and religious ceremonies under the guidance of his family priest. Any breakdown in the performance of ritualistic duties related to purification leads to severe stress both for the individual concerned and, in many instances, for the entire family. The stresses experienced under such conditions can be extremely damaging for the individual, the family, and, in some cases, for their progeny. Such concerns are devoid of any meaning within Western cultures. It is clear that cultures vary in terms of their own value systems, which have a significant bearing on the religious beliefs, the kinship patterns, and the social arrangements of the people of that culture.

Non-Western cultures, it should be emphasized, are communalistic, or collectivist, societies (Laungani, 1996, 2001a, 2001b, 2003, in press). And this very important factor needs to be given its due consideration when attempting to appraise the nature of stress in such societies. Although an individual might experience stress in a given situation, it can in many situations — a few of which have been outlined above — transmit itself to the rest of the members of the family. To ignore the impact of one's experience of stress on the members of the family, and in certain instances on one's entire subcommunity, would betray either indifference to or ignorance of cultural nuances, beliefs, values, and variations.

In addition to the differential religious and value-laden beliefs that contribute to stress within and between cultures, attention also needs to be paid to the influence of geographic, climatic, economic, political, and social factors on stress. For at a day-to-day behavioral level too, common sense confirms the observation that stress varies from one cultural group to another. For those living in the Sahara Desert, the perceptions of stressors will be significantly different from those for persons living on the fringes of the Arctic Circle. The ecology of each culture produces it own unique sets of stressors.

Given the vast differences in the manner in which stress is conceptualized and perceived both within and between cultures, it becomes a daunting task to find acceptable ways by which the intensity and severity of stress can be measured across cultures.

MEASUREMENT OF STRESS: METHODOLOGICAL ISSUES

In keeping with the natural science paradigm, there is a belief shared by many behavioral scientists that anything that varies in any quantity can be measured. And since stress, or rather its experience, varies within and between groups of individuals, it can be measured. Like physiological and neurological measures, such as body temperature, pulse rates, blood pressure, heartbeats, cardiac rhythms, oxygen levels, cortical arousal, etc., there is a belief that psychological measures, such as cognitive arousal, levels of anxiety, depression, introversion–extraversion, neuroticism, intelligence, creativity, anger, aggression, attitudes, beliefs, values, and a host of other psychological attributes, can also be measured with significant degrees of accuracy. And of course stress.

Several strategies of great ingenuity have been employed by research workers in this area to measure stress: self-reports, life change, physiological measures of arousal, biochemical markers, heart rate, and blood pressure, to name but a few. However, from among the variety of measurement strategies that have been adopted over the years, the construction of psychological tests and questionnaires has been the most important. Great thought, time, and ingenuity has gone into the construction and validation of stress tests. The major tests in the field of stress and personality are too well known to merit a detailed exposure. Suffice it to say that within the field of personality and stress, most test users are familiar with the ones designed by Aaron Beck, Adorno, Raymond Cattell, Cary Cooper, Hans Eysenck, Herman Rorschach, Julian Rotter, and Charles Spielberger, not to mention the psychodynamic tests, such as the Rorschach and the ATIC Apperception Test (TAT), of which there are quite a few. But despite the efforts, extending over several decades, that have gone into the design and construction of psychological instruments, there remain a few unresolved problems, which merit a brief discussion.

PSYCHOMETRIC MEASURES: PHILOSOPHICAL CONSIDERATIONS

A psychological test is defined as an objective and standardized measure of a sample of behavior (Janda, 1998). It measures behavior at an overt level — in other words, day-to-day behavior. It is not concerned with inner levels of one's existence. This is because inner levels or metaphysical concerns do not form part of mainstream Western psychology (Janda, 1998).

The fact that one's overt behavior is often motivated and driven by one's inner (metaphysical) considerations does not enter into the equation of test construction. In their adherence to the positivistic model of science, psychologists have discarded the study of the inner person. Sigmund Koch (1961, 1971) laments this loss and points out that he would "prefer a defective understanding of something of value over a safely defended description of something trite" (quoted by Robinson, 2001, p. 420). To fully appreciate the value of psychometric tests in general, including those designed to measure stress, it would therefore be necessary to have a degree of consensus concerning one's overall view of humanity, one's concept of what a human being is, and what it means to be human. In other words, it would be essential to take the inner person — the metaphysical and the spiritual — and the outer or observable person as a whole and not separate them, as appears to be the case with many psychologists involved in test construction. The two, the inner and outer — as William James had explained many years ago, the "I" and the "Me" — are inextricably related. One cannot separate one's inner world from one's outer world just as one cannot separate shadow from substance.

Were William James alive today he would point out that despite the great advances made in psychological tests over the years, what most psychological tests measure are the external statements endorsed by persons responding to a psychological test, — in other words, the outer person. Although many of the tests imply the nebulous existence of an inner person, the manner in which the questions are framed and the responses recorded, scored, analyzed, and interpreted makes the inner person seem but a headpiece filled with straw. After all, the standard definition of a psychological test is that it measures a sample of behavior (Murphy & Davidshofer, 1998).

Like history repeating itself, it is refreshing to note that the metaphysical concepts jettisoned by psychologists in the 1930s, 1940s, and 1950s are beginning to reappear through the backdoor, as it were, in the flourishing field of cognitive neuroscience. In other words, psychology appears to be turning full circle.

It should also be made clear that scientific research does not occur in a social and cultural vacuum. The dominant values prevailing in a culture have a bearing not only on the kind of research that is undertaken, the problems that are investigated, and the manner in which the research is undertaken, but also on the appropriateness of the research enterprise. The investigator is part of the historical and social context in which he or she works. Contemporary research in psychology therefore needs to be understood from within the framework of the dominant values prevalent in Western societies, such as individualism, secularism, environmentalism, liberalism, capitalism, humanism, Darwinism, the recognition and defense of human rights, the rule of law, political correctness, etc. All these dominant values define and establish limits as to what shall (or shall not) be investigated on whom, how, when, and under what conditions.

For instance, the construction of an intelligence test needs to be seen within the context of the dominant values of the culture in which the test has been constructed. Not even the much publicized Raven's Progressive Matrices — a nonverbal test of intelligence — is entirely culture-free. The universal usage of an instrument can only be justified when it can be demonstrated that the instrument is not culture specific but has universal applicability and that what is being measured is a universal quality or attribute, and that, given certain considerations, one would be able to predict differences (directional, or one-tailed) in performances within and between different cultural groups. The clinical thermometer serves as a good example. It has universal applicability. Regardless of where, when, how, and who constructed the clinical thermometer, it is clear that temperature in humans and animals is a universal attribute, which, given certain acceptable margins of errors, is measurable. For a psychological test to have any meaning, its uses and purposes need to be understood very clearly by the person taking the test. In addition to these assumptions, there is also the underlying assumption that the respondent has some understanding of the rationale underlying a psychological test and what is expected of the respondent in that situation. In other words, the respondent needs to have been socialized into *a culture of testing*.

A psychological test is not constructed in a social and cultural vacuum; it reflects the underlying values of the culture in which it constructed, and in that sense, it is a cultural product. To use such a test meaningfully in another culture, which in several fundamental ways can be completely different from the culture in which the test was originally constructed, can turn out to be a fruitless exercise for the simple reason that like is not being compared with like.

In America, testing is an integral part of school education and children are socialized into a culture of testing from an early age. George Miller (1970), in assessing the impact of testing in American schools, points out that in 1969 alone, over 250 million standardized tests of ability were given to American school children.

Psychological testing in non-Western cultures, on the other hand, is a rare phenomenon. It is only in a handful of large metropolitan cities that some form of psychological tests — such as those measuring stress, anger, and personality — organizational tests, and other occupational tests are offered. Irony aside, it would be amusing to observe how psychological tests would be administered to children and adults from the villages and other rural areas of India, which comprise over 75% of the total Indian population, which at present hovers around the 1.1 billion mark.

Psychometric Measures: Practical Considerations

Despite the vast array of extremely sophisticated techniques that have been employed in the construction of psychological tests, psychometric measures often create a variety of practical problems. It is not the aim of this chapter to consider the major problems related to test construction and validation. For a comprehensive and critical exposition of the problems, refer to Kline (2000). Here we shall concern ourselves largely with two issues:

1. Levels of measurement
2. Cross-cultural issues

Levels of Measurement

Several decades ago, Stevens (1951) described four levels of measurement in scientific research. They are the nominal, ordinal, interval, and ratio levels of measurement. The numbers used in the nominal scale are classificatory, such as when males might be assigned a score of 1, females a score of 2, and so on. The numbers have no other meaning and serve no other function. The ordinal scale is a crude measure that can move from high to low or vice versa, such as house numbers or judging beauty contests. An interval scale, on the other hand, moves in a graduated way, the distance separating one interval from another being assumed to be equal. The clinical thermometer conforms to the interval scale of measurement. Although the clinical thermometer has within it a calibrated zero degree, the zero is an arbitrary zero and does not conform to reality — in other words, water does not necessarily freeze at 0°C, nor does it boil at 100°C. It is certainly more powerful than the other two scales. It is, however, the ratio scale that is seen as being the most powerful level of measurement. The distinguishing feature of the ratio scale is that it has an absolute zero, which conforms to reality. The other three scales, including the interval scale, do not possess this desired attribute.

The significant weakness underlying psychometric measures is that none of the thousands of psychological tests constructed over the 150 years, right from the time of Francis Galton to the present, conforms to the ratio scale measurement. Barring a few exceptions, virtually all the psychological tests that have been constructed so far conform to the ordinal scale of measurement. All that the tests reveal is that the scores range from low to high or vice versa. This sad fact tends to test the very credibility of psychological tests from a scientific point of view (Kline, 2000).

Cross-Cultural Issues

Psychological tests, like cheap wine, have been known not to travel easily across cultures. The difficulties — seen and unseen, known and unknown, anticipated and unanticipated — stand as formidably in their way as the climate, terrain, and local natives might have stood in the way of intrepid travelers of the past. Just as the travelers and the adventurers stumbled along, occasionally scoring a hit, so do the cross-cultural psychologists, endeavoring to surmount the obstacles that stand in their way.

Let us list some of the obstacles that are likely to be experienced by psychologists in (1) the process of designing and translating the test and thereby making it relevant to the culture, (2) administering the test, and (3) explaining the findings in ways that are rational, meaningful, and relevant to the cultural group on whom the tests are used. In addition to the ethical issues underlying the field of testing, there are, at the very least, three major problems that psychologists involved in designing *culture-free tests* have to contend with:

1. Emic-etic dilemmas
2. Considerations of conceptual, metric, and functional equivalence
3. Translation of tests

Emic-Etic Dilemmas

The term *emic* refers to a culture-specific construct and *etic* to a universal construct. For instance, the construct "shame" might be seen as a culture-specific, or emic, construct and "guilt" (in the spiritual sense of the term) might be perceived as an etic construct.

Let us take the notion of "paranoid delusional states" to explain the emic-etic dilemma. Notwithstanding a few disputations concerning the precise symptoms comprising the disorder, there is within Western psychiatry and clinical psychology a fair degree of consensus in terms of markers or parameters that one might use to define, identify, and measure a paranoid delusional state. In other words, there exists a mutually shared meaning among different professionals as to what constitutes paranoid delusional states; they tend to be construed as forms of mental aberrations, serious psychological disturbances, with the patient (or client) lacking awareness into his or her mental state. It is then assumed rightly or wrongly that such paranoid delusional states are universal and are to be found all over the world — thereby proposing an etic formulation of the mental disorder.

Such, of course, might not be the case in non-Western cultures. In several non-Western countries, including India, Pakistan, Bangladesh, Haiti, Sierra Leone, Central America, Sri Lanka, Malaysia, Indonesia, Thailand, the Philippines, and others, it is not uncommon for many healers to display the very behaviors characterized by Western psychiatry as being aberrant, and the person concerned in need of psychiatric treatment (Al-Issa, 1995; Hughes, 1985; Kakar, 1982; Kleiman, 1977; Paniagua, 1994; Roland, 1988, 1991; Torrey, 1986) argues that cross-cultural psychologists often *impose* psychiatric categories of their own culture on other cultures. In so doing, they ignore or disregard indigenous constructions and classifications of distress and disorders, thereby forcing an etic formulation on problems that are essentially culture specific, or emic. From this it follows that a test constructed in Western countries purporting to measure a universal construct would fail when used in non-Western cultures, where the construct is defined, construed, and evaluated differently. For a test designed in one culture to be used meaningfully in another culture, it would need to satisfy a variety of criteria; for a start, the constructs to be measured would without doubt need to be universal — applicable to people all over the world — e.g., intelligence, motivation, anger, aggression, etc. In other words, it must satisfy the criteria of being seen as an etic construct.

Considerations of Equivalence

One would need to know too if the concept shares a similar if not an identical meaning in other cultures. Are the concepts conceptually equivalent? To paraphrase Gertrude Stein, does a rose by any other name smell as sweet? Does the word *stress* convey the same meaning as the Sanskrit word *klesha*, or the Hindi word *dukha*? The next problem that a researcher would need to resolve is the one related to empirical equivalence. Does the person from another culture have an understanding of what the test measures and how it measures what it purports to measure? As was stated earlier, people from non-Western cultures lack familiarity with psychological tests; neither the questions nor the scoring system nor indeed the rationale underlying the test may make any sense to them. Hence, there is no guarantee that the subjects would have a clear understanding of what the scores or values assigned to each question would mean. Finally, it would be important to determine if the test served the same function when used in other cultures.

Psychologists involved in cross-cultural testing are no doubt aware of the pitfalls involved in this form of research, and many of them, working with local psychologists and anthropologists, have designed sophisticated ways of combating the obstacles that stand in their way. Yet problems remain.

We have argued that the role of culture in understanding stress is of undeniable importance. We have seen that not only each culture construes stress differently, but that the importance placed on stress varies from culture to culture. In Western countries, stress appears to have reached epidemic proportions and has become an endemic part of Western society. But in non-Western cultures, stress, sorrow, and pain are seen as part of the human condition and hence unavoidable.

Translation of Tests

Can a test designed in one culture be translated and used successfully in another culture? This question has never been satisfactorily answered. It is not just the terminology and wordings of the questions, or the design and scoring systems used, nor indeed the format of the test and the time — fixed or flexible — allocated for its completion, but more importantly, it is the assumptions underlying the tests that create a bewildering set of problems. Words when translated from one language to another often lose their intended meaning. Let us take a simple sentence to illustrate the difficulty: "John eats well." This simple sentence even in English is open to three distinct interpretations:

1. John has a sophisticated style of eating.
2. John chews and masticates his food before swallowing and thus eats well.
3. John is wealthy and therefore eats well.

Which of the three meanings did the researcher have in mind? And how far does the intended meaning coincide with the answers offered by the person taking the test? Words exercise their own tyrannies. Let me quote a more relevant example to illustrate the point emphatically.

Several years ago, Professor Hans Eysenck and I were involved in a cross-cultural research study in India, which involved administering the Eysenck Personality Questionnaire (EPQ) to a large sample (n = 800+) of English-speaking undergraduate students from Bombay University (Laungani, 1985). The questionnaire was administered in English. One of the questions on the scale was concerned with finding out if the subject had ever been cheeky to his or her parents as a child and caused consternation. The subjects taking the test could not understand the word *cheeky.* We searched around but could find no other English word that would convey the meaning of the term *cheeky* to Indian students. Eventually, after great deliberation, the question was eliminated from our data analysis. However, with the use of complicated factor analytic techniques, we were able to obtain stable factor structures, which were in keeping with the theoretical formulations posited by Eysenck.

It needs to be stressed that even within a single culture, a test designed, say in English, to be used on English-speaking subjects can occasionally lead to unforeseen errors. But when the tests are translated into other languages without due attention being paid to the use of metaphors or colloquialisms and similes, or to which might form part of the original test, it becomes difficult to demonstrate conceptual equivalence between the original test and its translated version.

Below, the relationship between personality and stress is examined.

Personality and Stress

Let us start with a few seemingly innocuous questions. How is personality related to stress? Is stress an integral part of human personality? Are certain people more predisposed by virtue of their personalities to experience stress and distress? If so, what are the predisposing factors that increase the probability of stress? Do situations of severe and continuous stress lead to personality changes? Is there a causal or an interactive relationship between stress and personality?

As stated at the beginning of the chapter, a situation that would turn one individual into a state of trembling jelly would have not the slightest effect on another's sense of calm and equanimity. Although one individual would be thrilled at flying through rain, thunder, and lightning, another fellow passenger would be kissing a rosary and muttering a million and one Hail Mary's. What brings about such differences in reactions? Why is one scared out of his or her wits when the other gloats over the same experience? These questions seem simple enough, but as is often the case, the simplest questions seem the most difficult ones to find valid answers to. For all these questions we would need to presuppose that we have a fairly clear idea as to what constitutes human personality and that there is a chorus of consensus among psychologists, psychiatrists, therapists, and others working in the area concerning the nature of human personality. That, sadly, is not the case.

When one refers to the term *personality*, one soon realizes that within psychology there is no one generally accepted theory of personality. There are scores of personality theories, each with its own sets of assumptions, methodologies and investigative strategies, research protocols, adherents, and, of course, fierce critics. Each theory of personality, as we know, reflects its conceptual model. For instance, the "grand" theories of personality such as the ones propounded by Freud, Adler, and Jung and other post-Freudians not only offer an insight into human personality, but also provide a unique worldview of the human psyche. The conceptual frameworks of such idiographic theories, on the other hand, are vastly different from the scientifically formulated theories. Then, of course, there are theories that are concerned with self-growth, self-development, and self-actualization, e.g., those of the humanist psychologists, including Maslow, Rogers, and others.

The major theories of personality can be classified into four interrelated categories. They are:

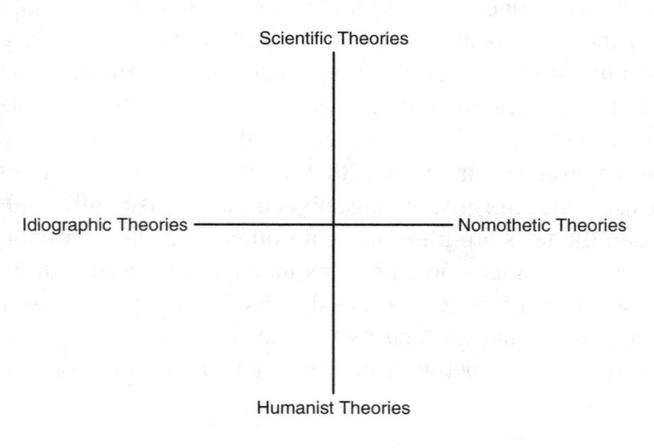

Most, if not all, the theories can be represented along the above two *dimensions* and *between* the four quadrants. The vertical axis expresses the range of personality theories, ranging from the scientific to the humanist. The horizontal axis represents theories ranging from the idiographic end to the nomothetic (or psychometric). It needs to be made clear that the four categories are by no means independent; they are correlated. Theoretically it would be possible to locate their specific positions within each quadrant. At the top end of the vertical axis would be listed a variety of theories purporting to be scientific, e.g., the personality theories of Beck, Eysenck, Cattell, Guilford, Myers-Briggs, and others. Such theories are concerned with establishing a scientific (biological and neurophysiological) basis of human personality through experimentation to establish a firm relationship between biological and neurological processes and human personality. The use of psychometric instruments forms part of their research armory. At the bottom end of the vertical axis are to be found the humanist theories promoted by Erik Erikson, George Kelly, Abraham Maslow, Rollo May, Carl Rogers, and others. Such theories have paid less attention to psychometric measurement and have instead focused their attention on counseling and therapy (individual or group) to enable the client(s) the means in which to grow and develop their full human potential, realizing the spiritual side of their personality. The horizontal axis represents at one end the major pioneering idiographic formulations of Freud, Adler, Jung, Rank, and others. Such theories were unconcerned with the measurement of personality traits, but subsequently, later theorists working within the conceptual framework provided by Freud and the post-Freudians constructed tests such as the Rorschach and the TAT to measure individual deep-rooted (unconscious) personality characteristics. The other end of the horizontal axis represents the attempts by psychologists to design valid psychometric instruments that would enable them to measure any significant features of human personality in which they are interested.

From the multiple theories of personality — some of which are extremely comprehensive, and others quite specific — it becomes difficult to decide which personality theory would best explain the relationship between stress and personality. There was a growing belief within psychology and psychiatry that there were a variety of psychosocial factors that had a negative impact on an individual's physical and mental health. Stress came to be seen as a major risk factor for ill health such as coronary heart disease, cancer, depression, hypertension, loss of self-esteem, prolonged absenteeism from work, a feeling of learned helplessness, pessimism, and inability to cope with stressful life events, such as death of spouse, divorce, unemployment, and imprisonment, to mention a few.

Psychologists and psychiatrists over the years adopted a more pragmatic approach to the problem. As mentioned earlier, it was estimated that about 600,000 workers in the U.S. tend to be seriously affected by stress and other psychological disorders. This costs around $5.5 billion in annual payments to the affected individuals and their families. As a result, psychologists and psychiatrists set out to investigate the major risk factors and other personality variables that mediated the stress–illness relationship. They also designed positive coping strategies (effective management of stress) that would be successful in alleviating stress. Let us briefly consider the major risk factors that mediate between stress and ill health and the coping strategies used.

Risk Factors

Major Life Events — The assumptions that major life events could lead to psychosomatic and psychiatric disorders were first investigated by psychiatrists in the 1960s. Major life events range from the death of a spouse to being unemployed, in debt, in prison, etc. Holmes and Rahe (1967) developed the *Social Readjustment Rating Scale.* It was a self-report scale of critical life events. The subjects had to respond to the scale by indicating all the life events they had experienced in a given period. It was assumed that the severity of the life experiences had a deleterious effect on the individual's physical and mental health. The scale was easy to administer. To assess the predictive validity of the scale, prospective and retrospective studies were carried out. The results of such studies were less promising than had been anticipated initially (Goldberg & Comstock, 1976; Rabkin & Struening, 1976; Theorell et al., 1975). The scale, as some critics have argued, is contaminated by references to specific psychological and physical conditions of illness, thus confounding the findings (Schroeder & Costa, 1984). The earlier positive results obtained by Holmes and Rahe could not be replicated, casting some doubts on the usefulness of the scale.

Locus of Control — The idea underlying the concept *locus of control* was first developed by Julian Rotter (1954, 1966). It grew out of social learning theory. Behavior, Rotter suggests, occurs as a function of expectations about reinforcements in a given situation. He proposed that there were two dimensions of locus of control, which he called the external and the internal locus of control. Persons with a dominant internal locus of control tend to believe that reinforcements are a result of their own behavior. They are capable of influencing the consequences of their behaviors by planning, by rational appraisal, by accepting responsibility for their own actions, and by avoidance of actions that are likely to result in negative consequences to their health, work, social and familial relations, and other day-to-day behaviors. Such persons are less likely to experience severe stress because they take appropriate steps to avoid such negative consequences. In other words, what Rotter is saying is that people who are rational tend to behave rationally, make attempts to maximize their positive reinforcements, and succeed in making an impact on their own environment (Taylor, 1991).

Persons with external control, on the other hand, believe that the consequences of their actions are under the control of external agents: chance, luck, significant people in their lives, coincidence, and so on. They do not often take responsibility for their own actions and the consequences of their actions. Thus, stress, ill health, and minor and major misfortunes might be "explained away" in terms of external factors and even mysterious forces. Rotter's theory, when shorn off its academic jargon, sounds like a eulogy to rationalism, a theme explored, discussed, and articulated by virtually all rationalist philosophers, from Plato and Descartes to Spinoza and Kant (Cottingham, 1984). While there is some confirmatory evidence concerning internal control and preventive health, the scale itself is plagued by serious measurement problems.

At a cross-cultural level, the assumptions underlying the locus-of-control theory run into even more problems. In Eastern cultures, including India, Pakistan, Sri Lanka, Bangladesh, Malaysia, Indonesia, and others, religious beliefs, rituals, and practices play a vital role in one's daily life. To a large extent, life events are construed as being ordained. One prays for succor, for help, for divine intervention in the solution of one's problems related to health, material well-being, the marriage of one's children, happiness, etc., making it difficult at times to disentangle an internal locus-of-control (rationalist) model from an external locus-of-control (religious) model of behavior. The two, like the proverbial Siamese twins, are inextricably enjoined. Events, both positive and negative, that occur are often seen as being the result of mysterious cosmic forces. In fact, in subscribing to an external locus-of-control model, the person concerned is able to explain away and even accept the vicissitudes of life without becoming unduly stressed.

Type A and Type B Behaviors — The ideas underlying type A and type B behaviors owe their origin to two physicians, Friedman and Rosenman, who formulated this concept in 1974. The major thrust of this form of research was to examine the lifestyles of persons to identify persons who possessed type A behavior syndrome and those who possessed type B behavior syndrome. Type A behavior syndrome was considered to be a serious risk factor for coronary heart disease (Cooper et al., 1981; Dembroski et al., 1988). Type A and type B behaviors were measured by means of a questionnaire or through a structured interview, asking people how they responded to situations that made them impatient, aggressive, hostile, etc. The pattern of responses to the self-report questionnaires enabled them to formulate the type A and type B personality syndromes.

People who are classified as having a type A personality tend to be unceasing workers, fiercely competitive, impatient, aggressive, and hostile. Overconscious of time, they endeavor to achieve far more than they are physically able. They have a compelling need to control events and are upset when frustrated in their efforts. Type A persons are often "combat ready" (Myers, 1995). Researchers have found a variety of physiological and psychological differences between the two types. Type A people sleep less, smoke more, consume more drinks, are more likely to meet with accidents, have higher levels of cholesterol, expose themselves to risks, display patterns of risky eating, engage in strenuous exercises, and often create deficient support systems (Cohen & Mathews, 1987). In popular parlance, type A persons work hard, play hard, and experience a variety of health-related problems compared to type B persons.

Type B people, on the other hand, are relaxed and fairly easygoing. They do not feel rushed and are relatively unconcerned about creating unrealistic deadlines, let alone trying to meet them.

Several studies have also established a link between type A personality and stress-related illnesses, such as coronary heart disease (CHD) (Dembroski & Costa, 1988; Lazarus & Folkman, 1984; Rosenman, 1978). However, the much publicized concept of type A personality predisposing a person to die of CHD has been questioned by Eysenck (1995). He argues that "this 'type' has no real existence. The parts of it that predict CHD are anger, hostility, and aggression, linked with heart disease long before Type A saw the light" (Eysenck, 1995, p. 4).

Since the type A personality syndrome is a serious risk factor to health, concerted attempts have been made in recent years to modify such potentially harmful behaviors. A variety of techniques, such as progressive relaxation, physical exercise, meditation, breathing exercises, counseling, avoidance of situations that are stressful or likely to lead to stress, anger control, identifying stressors and learning to avoid them, and short-term and long-term lifestyle changes, are used with varying degrees of success.

Learned Helplessness — Martin Seligman (1975), in keeping with the behaviorist paradigm, proposed the theory of learned helplessness. He is of the opinion that stress produces feelings of helplessness. Seligman's theory rests on three interlocking factors: (1) when a predicted outcome in the environment is beyond one's control, (2) the cessation of those responses that do not produce the desired reinforcements, and (3) the generalized cognitive belief that no voluntary action can control the outcome. He suggests that the theory of learned helplessness is also a theory of achievement. When repeated attempts to achieve the desired reinforcements fail, one begins to see oneself as helpless. He claims that people who acquire this feeling of helplessness easily tend to achieve less — in school, sports, work, and physical health, and "people who are pessimists and experience helplessness will get sicker and perhaps die earlier than optimists" (Seligman, 1975, p. xxxi).

Learned helplessness creates three deficits: (1) motivational, when a person in a state of helplessness makes no effort to change the outcome; (2) helpless persons fail to learn new responses; and (3) helplessness leads to feelings of depression (Seligman et al., 1974).

Seligman's theory, as stated above, springs from a behaviorist paradigm. It is not as unique as it appears to sound at first sight. When one turns away from a behaviorist paradigm and examines the construct from a cognitive social-psychological perspective, one can trace its similarity to the idea of the "self-fulfilling prophecy," which was promoted by Gordon Allport and several other social psychologists in the 1950s. It was argued that "expectations often determine outcomes." If one expects to fail, one often does, and one often succeeds when one expects to succeed. Rosenthal and Jacobson's (1968) classic study on schoolchildren — and their fluctuating scores on intelligence tests — demonstrated the validity of the notion of the self-fulfilling prophecy. The author can testify to the notion of the self-fulfilling prophecy by his personal experience in the intensive care unit into which he was admitted when he became suddenly and critically ill 15 years ago (Laungani, 1992). There was an unvoiced but obvious expectation among the medical staff that he would not survive the critical illness. But his personal expectations ran counter to theirs. There were no *behavioral* strategies that he could resort to because of being totally paralyzed. There was, however, the firm, unshakeable expectation of pulling through, which might have played a vital role in the author's recovery.

SUMMING UP

We have seen that stress varies from individual to individual and from one occasion to another. It also varies across cultures. The variation extends along the familial, social, religious, ecological, environmental, political, and economic parameters, all of which, singly or jointly, contribute to the experience of stress within a particular culture. The prevalent values in a given culture have an influence in terms of what is construed as stress. For a Brahmin priest to touch the statues of the gods in his prayer room at home *before* having bathed and carried out his morning ablutions is to desecrate the statues — an act considered to be extremely stressful and sinful. Few orthodox high-caste Hindus would invite an untouchable into their home, for this would lead to the spiritual pollution of the home, causing untold stress and guilt upon the entire family. There are several such culturally unique constructions of stress around the world. Each culture also promotes its own unique culture-specific techniques for handling and alleviating stress.

However, unresolved stress in any culture tends to predispose an individual to a variety of physical and psychological disorders, including coronary heart disease, high blood pressure, diabetes, anxiety, depression, and several other psychosomatic conditions. Although no unequivocal causal claims can be established between stress and personality, one cannot rule out such a relationship. Whether stress affects and alters human personality at individual and even national levels, as has been proposed by Lynn (1971) in his international studies, or whether certain personality factors predispose an individual to stress is an issue that has not been successfully resolved. Among the personality factors that have been investigated in considerable depth are those related to major life events, locus of control, type A and type B behaviors, and learned helplessness, which were briefly discussed above.

One would not be far off the mark to assert that stress, at least in Western countries, has transformed itself into a fast-spreading "fashionable" illness, which appears to be reaching epidemic proportions. Sadly, in addition to the genuine experts working in the area, a gigantic industry of smooth-talking, ill-trained pseudoexperts has evolved to help the distressed to cope with their individualized problems.

REFERENCES

Al-Issa, I. (1995). Culture and mental illness in international perspective. In I. Al-Issa (Ed.), *Handbook of Culture and Mental Illness: An International Perspective* (pp. 3–49). Madison, CT: International Universities Press.

Cohen, S., & Mathews, K. A. (1987). Social support, type A behaviour, and coronary artery disease. *Psychosomatic Medicine*, 49, 325–330.

Cooper, C. L. (1983). *Stress Research: Issues for the Eighties*. New York: John Wiley.

Cooper, T., Detre, T., & Weiss, S. M. (1981). Coronary-prone behaviour and coronary heart disease: A critical review. *Circulation*, 63, 1199–1215.

Cottingham, J. (1984). *Rationalism*. London: Paladin.

Dembroski, T. M., & Costa, P. T. (1988). Assessment of coronary-prone behaviour: A current overview. *Annals of Behavioural Medicine*, 10, 60–63.

Eysenck, H. J. (1995). The causal role of stress and personality in the aetiology of cancer and coronary heart disease. In C. Spielberger, I. Sarason, J. Brebner, E. Greenglass, P. Laungani, & A. M. O'Roark (Eds.), *Stress and Emotion: Anxiety, Anger, and Curiosity*, Vol. 15 (pp. 3–12). Washington, DC: Taylor & Francis.

Filippi, G. G. (1996). *Mrtyu: Concept of Death in Indian Traditions*. New Delhi: D. K. Printworld (P) Ltd.

Flood, G. (1996). *An Introduction to Hinduism*. Cambridge: Cambridge University Press.

Friedman, M., & Rosenman, R. H. (1974). *Type A Behaviour and Your Heart*. New York: Knopf.

Fuller, C. J. (1992). *The Camphor Fame: Popular Hinduism and Society in India*. Princeton, NJ: Princeton University Press.

Goldberg, E. L., & Comstock, G. W. (1976). Life events and subsequent illness. *American Journal of Epidemiology*, 104, 146–158.

Holmes, T. H., & Rahe, R. H. (1967). The social readjustment rating scale. *Journal of Psychosomatic Research*, 11, 213–218.

Hughes, C. C. (1985). Culture-bound or construct-bound? In R. C. Simmons & C. C. Hughes (Eds.), *The Culture-Bound Syndromes* (pp. 3–24). Boston: D. Reidel.

Janda, L. H. (1998). *Psychological Testing: Theory and Applications*. Needham Heights, MA: Allyn & Bacon.

Kakar, S. (1982). *Shamans, Mystics, and Doctors*. London: Mandala Books.

Kleiman, A. (1977). Depression, somatization and the "new cross-cultural psychiatry." *Social Science and Medicine*, 11, 3–9.

Kline, P. (2000). *Handbook of Psychological Testing*, 2nd ed. London: Routledge.

Koch, S. (1961). Psychological science versus the science-humanism antimony: Intimations of a significant science of man, *American Psychologist*, 16, 629–639.

Koch, S. (1971). Reflections on psychology. *Social Research*, 38, 669–709.

Laungani, P. (1985). *National Differences in Personality: India and England*, Vol. 6, *Personality and Individual Differences*, No. (in press).

Laungani, P. (1992). *It Shouldn't Happen to a Patient: A Survivor's Guide to a Life-Threatening Illness*. London: Whiting & Birch Ltd.

Laungani, P. (1996). Cross-cultural investigations of stress: Conceptual and methodological considerations. *International Journal of Stress Management*, 3, 26–35.

Laungani, P. (2001a). The influence of culture on stress: India and England. In L. L. Adler & U. P. Gielen (Eds.), *Cross-Cultural Topics in Psychology*, 2nd ed. (pp. 149–170). Westport, CT: Praeger.

Laungani, P. (2001b). Culture, cognition, and trauma: Cross-cultural evaluations. In J. F. Schumaker and T. Ward (Eds.), *Cultural Cognition and Psychopathology* (pp. 119–144). Westport, CT: Praeger.

Laungani, P. (2003). Familial stress and obsessive compulsive disorder: A cross-cultural case study. *International Journal of Health Promotion and Education*, 41, 108–116.

Laungani, P. (In press). The experience and management of stress in a life-threatening illness. In D. Spielberger & I. Sarason, (Eds.), *Stress and Emotion*, Vol. 17. Washington, DC: Taylor & Francis.

Lazarus, R.S., & Folkman, S. (1984). *Stress, Appraisal, and Coping*. New York: Springer.

Lynn, R. (1971). *Personality and National Character*. London: Pergammon Press.

Mason, J. W. (1975). A historical view of stress field. *Journal of Human Stress*, March, 6–12.

Miller, G. A. (1970). Assessment of psychotechnology. *American Psychologist*, 25, 11, 991–1001.

Murphy, K. R., & Davidshofer, C. O. (1998). *Psychological Testing: Principles and Applications*, 4th ed. Englewood Cliffs, NJ: Prentice Hall.

Myers, D. G. (1995). *Psychology*, 4th ed. New York: Worth Publishers.

Palsane, M. N., Bhavsar, S. N., Goswami, R. P., & Evans, G. W. (1986). The concept of stress in Indian tradition. *Journal of Indian Psychology*, 5, 1–12.

Paniagua, F. A. (1994). *Assessing and Treating Culturally Diverse Clients*. Thousand Oaks, CA: Sage.

Rabkin, J. G., & Struening, E. L. (1976). Life events, stress, and illness. *Science*, 194, 1013–1020.

Radhakrishnan, S. (1923/1989). *Indian Philosophy*, Vol. 2, centenary ed. Delhi: Oxford University Press.

Ramachandra Rao, S. K. (1983). The conception of stress in Indian thought: The theoretical aspects of stress in Samkhya and Yoga systems. *NIMHANS Journal*, 1, 115–121.

Robinson, D. N. (2001). Sigmund Koch: Philosophically speaking. *American Psychologist*, 56, 420–424.

Roland, A. (1988). *In Search of Self in India and Japan: Toward a Cross-Cultural Psychology.* Princeton, NJ: Princeton University Press.

Roland, A. (1991). Psychoanalysis in India and Japan. Toward a comparative psychoanalysis. *American Journal of Psychoanalysis*, 51, 1–10.

Rosenman, R. H. (1978). The interview method of assessment of the coronary-prone behaviour pattern. In T. Dembroski, S. Weiss, J. Shields, S. Hayes, & M. Feinleib (Eds.), *Coronary-Prone Behaviour.* New York: Springer.

Rosenthal, R., & Jacobson, L. (1968). *Pygmalion in the Classroom*. New York: Holt, Rinehart & Winston.

Rotter, J. B. (1954). *Social Learning and Clinical Psychology.* Englewood Cliffs, NJ: Prentice Hall.

Rotter, J. B. (1966). Generalized expectancies for internal versus external control of reinforcement. *Psychological Monographs*, 80 (whole no. 609, 1).

Sauter, S. L. (1992). Introduction to the NIOSH proposed national strategy. In G. P. Keita & S. L. Sauter (Eds.), *Work and Well-Being: An Agenda for the 1990s* (pp. 11–16). Washington, DC: American Psychological Association.

Schroeder, D. H., & Costa, Jr., P. Y. (1984). Influence of life event stress on physical illness. Substantive effects or methodological flaws? *Journal of Personality and Social Psychology*, 46, 853–863.

Seligman, M. E. P. (1975). *Helplessness: On Depression, Development and Death.* New York: W. H. Freeman and Company.

Seligman, M. E. P., Klein, D. C., & Miller, W. (1974). Depression. In H. Leitenberg (Ed.), *Handbook of Behaviour Therapy.* Englewood Cliffs, NJ: Prentice Hall.

Selye, H. (1950). *Stress*. Montreal: Acat.

Selye, H. (1956). *The Stress of Life*. New York: McGraw-Hill.

Selye, H. (1974). *Stress without Distress*. New York: Lippincott.

Selye, H. (1980). The stress concept today. In I. L. Kutash & L. B. Schlesinger (Eds.), *Handbook of Stress and Anxiety* (pp. 127–129). San Francisco: Josey-Bass.

Sharma, A. (2000). *Classical Hindu Thought: An Introduction*. Delhi: Oxford University Press.

Stevens, S. S. (1951). Mathematical measurement and psychophysics. In Stevens, S. S. (Ed.), *Handbook of Experimental Psychology.* New York, Wiley.

Taylor, S. E. (1991). *Health Psychology*, 2nd ed. New York: McGraw-Hill.

Theorell, T., Lind, E., & Floderus, B. (1975). The relationship of disturbing life changes and emotions to the early development of myocardial infarction and other serious illnesses. *International Journal of Epidemiology*, 4, 281–293.

Torrey, E. (1986). *Witchdoctors and Psychiatrists: The Common Roots of Psychotherapy and Its Future*. New York: Harper & Row.

Wright, L. A., & Smye, M. D. (1996). *Corporate Abuse: How Lean and Mean Robs People and Profits*. New York: Macmillan.

Zimmer, H. (1951/1989). *Philosophies of India: Bollinger Series XXVI*. Princeton, NJ: Princeton University Press.

12 Social Support and Heart Disease

John G. Bruhn

CONTENTS

INTRODUCTION

In an editorial in a well-known medical journal a physician stated that there were few scientifically sound studies that established the relationship between mental state and disease, and therefore, he concluded, to believe that disease is a direct reflection of mental state is largely folklore.[1] More recently, a cardiologist said that he and his colleagues felt uncomfortable with research in the heart–mind area. Despite research findings that depression was a risk factor, he said that he, and those he knew, did not attempt to prevent or treat depression in patients who had experienced a myocardial infarction or who had coronary bypass surgery. He explained that what we know about the heart–mind linkage is not sufficiently *proven* and not generalizable enough to be accepted in the cardiology community.[2]

Science demands that the scientific method be rigorous and that results be replicable before proof can be claimed. Nonetheless, skeptics will always question and challenge what has been proven. How much proof and what kind is needed is an open-ended debate that is fueled in part by scientists' adherence to fashion in research and in part by the comfort of what is considered sufficient proof in one's discipline. Interdisciplinary research or the use of qualitative methods, or indeed any research in the sciences of human behavior, is a target for skeptics and critics from the "hard" sciences who consider only quantifiable proof scientific and valid. Krantz and

0-8493-1820-3/05/$0.00+$1.50

McCeney[3] concluded, in their focused review of carefully designed studies of the involvement of social and behavioral factors in myocardial infarction and coronary bypass surgery, that it was likely that some members in the biomedical community would resist acknowledging the heart–mind relationship regardless of the evidence.

THE EVIDENCE: WHAT KIND AND HOW MUCH?

The scientific evidence linking mental state and disease, and mental state to the morbidity and mortality from myocardial infarction in particular, is substantial but not definitive. Wolf[4] pointed out that changes in the social environment or in the state of the individual have long been known to produce psychological adaptations in the human organism that, when exaggerated, insufficient, or inappropriate, actually *constitute* the manifestations of disease. Perhaps the most common example of the link between mental state and one's psychological state is the anxiety and slightly elevated blood pressure of a normotensive patient at a routine visit to his doctor's office, and how relaxation, reassuring communication, and the human touch can normalize the reading in minutes.[5] Or, more dramatically, how the decline and death of patients in a coronary care unit reflects itself in the changing electrocardiograms of observant neighboring patients. Or, how an episode of angina pectoris can be precipitated in a patient in the coronary care unit by a visiting contentious spouse.[6] These examples are not folklore. The positive and negative relationships between a person's environment, mental state, and bodily reactions are well enough established that many health care professionals put the principles underlying the relationship into practice by teaching patients to become aware of and alter their attitudes and behavior, so that they can reduce their risks for disease, enhance their recovery and longevity from illness, and minimize recurrences.

The problem is not the lack of evidence but gathering the *right kind* of evidence that will convince skeptics and critics.[7] This is a big challenge. It is not always meaningful to study individuals in artificial environments such as laboratory simulations to control variables. Furthermore, not all aspects of human behavior are easily quantifiable. It is also not meaningful to average aspects of human behavior into mean scores or compare individual traits to a range of "normal" values as if all individuals shared the same beliefs and values. In addition, human behavior is a moving target, as people act differently at different times in different environments, in different social settings, and with different people. Because of the interrelationships of human behavior, there is the potential of not being able to clearly differentiate cause from effect, and the variability of human behavior makes it difficult to precisely replicate even the most rigorous study designs.[8] Nonetheless, an attempt to learn about the human organism by separating it from its social cosmos would be senseless and unscientific.

Indeed, it is the complexity and variability of human behavior that causes social and behavioral scientists to differ among themselves as to the definition and appropriate measurement of the same phenomena. Heitzmann and Kaplan,[9] in reviewing the psychometric properties of 23 methods for measuring social support, concluded that the problem of accurately measuring social support appears to be as unique as the subjects being studied. Winemiller and colleagues[10] reviewed 262 empirically based articles about social support published between 1980 and 1987. They found that many social support researchers utilized standardized instruments, but failed to consider the complex, multidimensional nature of social support. Most instruments were objective and assessed support received from close, nuclear relationships, such as those with family, spouse, and friends. This means that our perspective of social support generally excludes an individual's support network; focuses on the social support received rather than on its interactive nature; excludes consideration of cultural and environmental sources of support; and tends to look at an individual's perceptions of available support without concomitant consideration of the support the individual has used and is likely to use in certain circumstances. Furthermore, researchers have not usually taken into consideration the different needs for social support, and the availability and accessibility of supportive resources, at different points in the life cycle.[11,12,]

It will be impossible to gather the *right kind* of evidence as discussed earlier unless we operationalize the concept of social support so that its dynamic nature can be tapped. Mendes de Leon[8] questioned whether *every* aspect of our social relationships is supposed to be supportive and have health benefits. Every source of social support might not be available and accessible all the time, and even persons who have strong support systems available might not use them and, therefore, do not benefit from them. Too much support can be just as deleterious as too little or none at all. The loose network ties of the homeless might be as salubrious as the tight network ties of a homogenous religious community. It depends on who is evaluating social support. As Coyne and De Longis[13] have said, social support is best regarded as a "personal experience," rather than a set of objective circumstances or even a set of interactional processes.

Social support is intimately tied to a person's adaptive repertoire and the situations that cue certain responses. Therefore, to answer the question of *how much* evidence we need to convince scientists that social support (and its absence) impacts health, we will need to collect data from different types of populations, in different cultures and social situations, at different intervals, and during different life experiences.[14] Social support is a process; therefore, the right kind of data cannot be measured only at one point in time. Coyne and De Longis[13] stated that social support is one rung in a ladder in learning about the role of social relationships in adaptation. They noted that we need to learn more about how people find, build, maintain, and end relationships; how they are constrained by their personal characteristics, their circumstances, and the pool of people available; and the benefits and costs that they incur. Existing research methods need to be supplemented with in-depth interview studies and daily diary assessments of stress and support as they unfold over time.[13] And perhaps the most challenging, since social support is a multifaceted concept, is the need for an interdisciplinary approach to studying it.[15]

THE MECHANISM(S): ENVIRONMENTAL STIMULI AND NEUROLOGICAL PATHWAYS

In a literature search from 1978 to early 1999, focusing on prospective studies, Tennant[16] concluded that while life events stress and poor social supports are risk factors for coronary heart disease (CHD) and CHD mortality, the exact mechanism by which stress and social support impact heart disease is not known, although disturbance in mood, especially depression, appears to be the most likely intervening variable. In another review of prospective studies of the role of psychosocial stress and social support in coronary heart disease, Greenwood and his colleagues[17] concluded that social support and stress both had an influence on coronary heart disease — social support more so than stress. Both had a stronger influence on CHD mortality than on initial incidence. The quality of social support was more important than the size of the social network. These authors emphasized the need for interventions to reduce stress and increase social support among normal healthy subjects, subjects at risk for CHD, and patients with CHD to gain insights into the mechanisms by which stress and support work.

When we attempt to measure the amount of social support present in an individual's life by using a Social Network Index[18] based on different types of social connections, we are assessing the quantitative aspects of an individual's personal networks. We can compile a quantifiable index of the presence of social support, but the index does not tell us *how* social support works. Just because there are *sources* of social support available to an individual does not tell us how these sources are *perceived* (some sources of social support might be perceived as generic and others idiosyncratic), and just because there are available sources of social support does not mean that they are accessible and used when they are needed. All of this is to say an individual's environment is a complex network of relationships between people, places, and things. We are continuously confronted with events that arise from the environment, from our brains, and from responses to events. The brain might respond to a stimulus depending on whether it was sensed, perceived, and attended to. However, the brain remembers the characteristics of each event. The brain acts like a social sponge retaining its evaluation of the characteristics of prior events and thereby assisting us in responding in environmentally appropriate ways to new ones.[19] When environmental stimuli or events are transmitted to the brain, they are encapsulated in emotions. Damasio[20] pointed out that emotions provide a natural means for the brain and mind to evaluate the environment within and around the individual and respond accordingly and adaptively. Emotions include an appraisal of the degree of threat to the individual and the extent to which social support has helped counter a prior event or can help counter a new event. The triggering and executing of emotions is a complicated chain of events that involves the brain's memory and evaluation of social situations, including social support. Social support is a mediating variable that links environmental stimuli with neural mechanisms to assist individuals in appraising and coping with events (see Figure 12.1).

Wegner[21] noted that events seldom occur only once in real life; rather there is a sequence of events that create interaction and feedback. He saw real-life tasks and events as creating a "circle of influence" that sets off a chain of events. Observing people's reactions to related events over time usually yields some reliable insights about their behavior. For these reasons, information gathered either from real life or the laboratory alone greatly limits and distorts our learning about the process that links the environment to the brain. The author proposes that potential gains could be realized from richer input stimuli, such as cultural context and social stimuli.

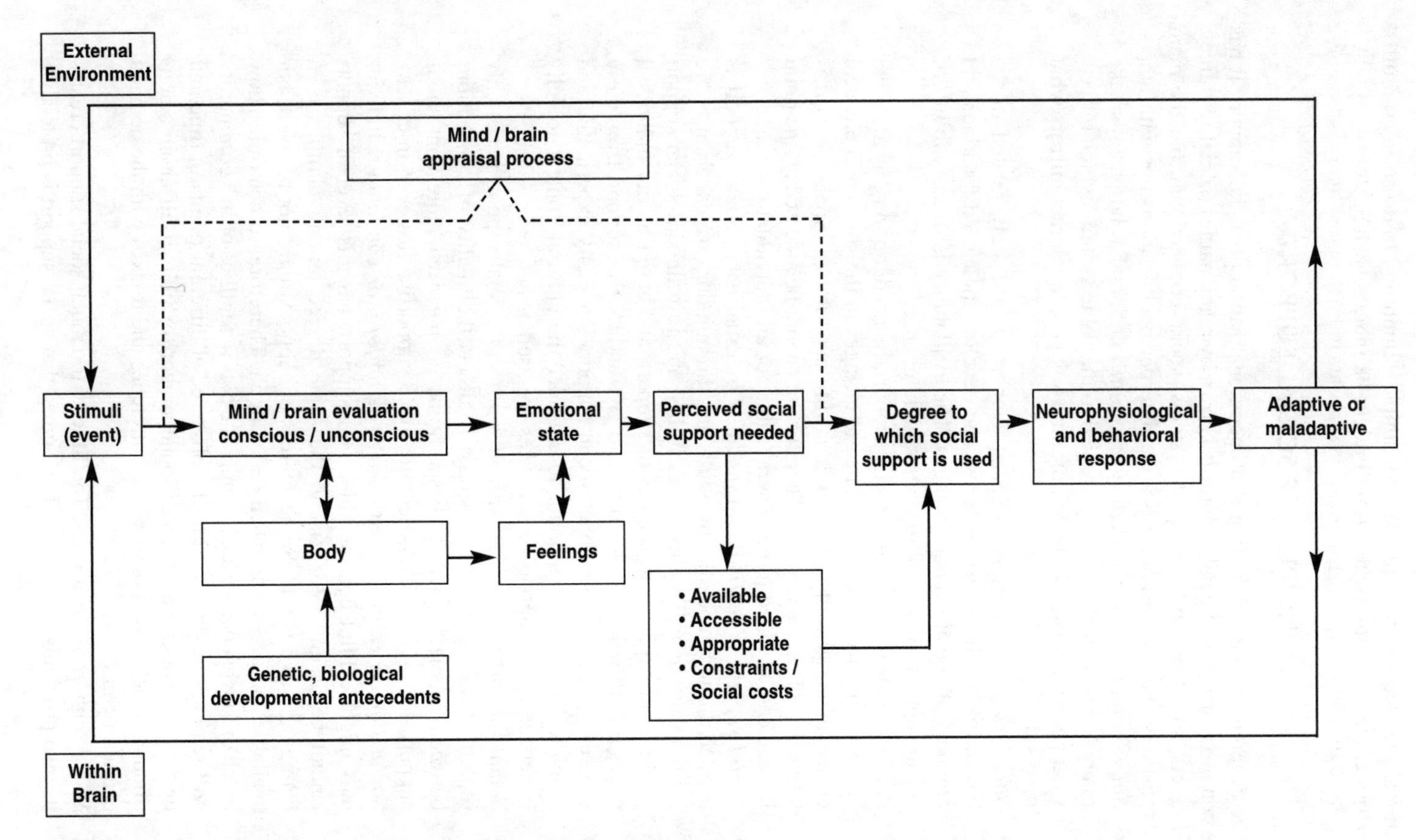

FIGURE 12.1 Social support as a part of the mind–brain appraisal process.

Traditional practice has been to use very simple stimuli and to do so in controlled laboratory contexts. Using richer stimuli might be more revealing.

PRINCIPLES OF SOCIAL SUPPORT

Despite differences in the definition and operationalization of social support, it has some common attributes. Social support is known by many names (social resources, social assets, social networks, support systems, social connections), but the main characteristic is that social support is about interpersonal relationships with others.

- *Social support is embedded in all cultures.* Social relationships take many forms in a culture; they are tied to the value system, which reflects what people consider to be important. How people interact mirrors what they value.
- *Social support is dynamic.* Social support is intimately related to the human life cycle. As people grow and develop, their need for kinds and amounts of social support changes. The availability and accessibility of social support in their culture also might change.
- *Social support is a process.* Social support, its need, options, availability, and accessibility, is directly related to changes in the social and physical environment, as well as to individual life experiences. Social support is a function of time and place. Therefore, it cannot be assessed at one point in time and assumed to be generalizable for an individual over time.
- *Social support is learned and modified by experience.* Social support is learned through modeling by adults and through our own experience. We learn about the availability, accessibility, and restraints of social support through our exposure to sources of support, and based on our individual needs for affiliation, we learn how to give and receive support from these sources. Since learning about social support is usually experiential and individualistic, it is important to consider the cultural context to fully understand why supportive resources are used or not.
- *Social support is part of the adaptive process.* Social support is not only important during times of distress; it affects the quality of connections between people on a daily basis. Some people need more continuous support than others; others seem to avoid supportive ties even in crises.
- *Social support cannot be assumed to be uniform or continuous.* Individuals might exhibit considerable overt support, but this level of support cannot be assumed to exist to the same degree among families or a community as a whole. Some sources of support might not be overt, but available and accessible when called upon. Therefore, to determine how much or to what degree social support exists in families or in a community will require that these entities be observed at different points in time and under different circumstances. Social support exhibits itself along a continuum, which, like a rubber band, stretches and relaxes with the demand exerted upon it.
- *Social support has two sides.* Too little or too much social support creates its own problems. It is generally assumed that social support is protective,

invigorating, and health promoting, and its absence is deleterious. Social support is not a panacea. To be smothered by closeness and its demands can be stressful, and to be alone, free from the demands of others, can be creatively refreshing. Social support and the lack of it each have their limits.

- *Social support and its mechanisms might not always be observable or measurable.* It might be assumed that people like to talk about social support and the amount they need. For some people, demonstrable social support might be restricted to private contexts. Males, in particular, might associate social support with weakness and minimize their need for it. Also, social support has qualitative aspects apart from the numbers of friends one has or the number of organizations one belongs to. To tap the qualitative aspects of social support might involve interviewing other people in addition to selected subjects.
- *Social support might be known by other terms.* Social support is a term that is not in the everyday lexicon of the average person on the street. The ideas of trust and respect for others are concepts that might be more recognizable in the lay world. Social trust comes from norms of reciprocity and networks of engagement. Social trust facilitates cooperation and an attitude of reciprocity between people. Ethnic ties, for example, constitute the social basis of trust in immigrant communities. We tend to engage others with a similar purpose or interest — people who one can depend upon — to accomplish a task or meet a goal. While social trust and social engagement are a part of social support, social support in turn generates and reinforces trust and network ties. The term *social support* might not have the same meaning to a researcher and a subject, and rather than ask questions about its meanings, the subject might answer questions about a phenomenon known to them as something else.

These principles can serve as guidelines for more rigorous study designs that test relationships between social support and the risk, recovery, and survival of persons with a variety of diseases, including CHD. Perhaps the common theme uniting these principles is that social support has a developmental baseline that is moderated by life events and is culturally and situationally defined. Therefore, social support needs to be examined retrospectively, longitudinally, and at periodic intervals to capture its dynamism.

People have always relied on their friends, neighbors, and coworkers as well as family members for social support, but support from outside the family might be increasingly important as high divorce rates persist and high levels of residential mobility take people away from their relatives. Past research suggests that women give and receive more emotional support than do men. Men are unlikely to receive emotional support from male friends and are unlikely to have many female friends, so many rely on female family members for emotional support.[22] Women's relationships depend on emotional closeness, while men's relationships focus on shared activities. This suggests why women might be more likely than men to exchange emotional support. However, it also suggests that men might be more likely than women to exchange instrumental support if the exchange is built around shared activities. Marital status also has strong effects on the exchange of social support. Married couples are able to rely on one another for both emotional and instrumental support. Consequently, they might be less likely to exchange support with friends, neighbors, and coworkers than are the unmarried.[22]

Other factors influence the opportunities to exchange social support with non-kin. Involvement in organizations, the availability of friends, informal socializing with friends, and being employed are all opportunities to give and receive social support outside of the family and expand one's social network. Socioeconomic status affects the form and composition of personal networks; however, the relationship between income and social support has been contradictory. With respect to health, poor health has been shown to constrain the exchange of support with friends, yet research has shown positive effects of social support on health. Poor health limits social contact with friends, but has no effect on contacts with family. Healthier individuals have been found to have larger social networks.[22]

GENDER, EMOTIONS, AND SOCIAL SUPPORT IN THE INCIDENCE AND PROGRESSION OF CHD

Although almost all studies of the relationship between social support and disease have been carried out among adults with high risk factors for a particular disease, or among adults after they were diagnosed with a disease, e.g., a myocardial infarction, there is evidence that there are developmental antecedents of social support in childhood that lay the groundwork for adult experiences. Luecken[23] hypothesized that early parental loss coupled with poor-quality family relationships during childhood would be associated with increased hostility, depression, and low social support in adulthood. She found that subjects who lost a parent and reported poorer-quality family relationships showed higher levels of depressive symptoms and lower social support in adulthood. In families where subjects did not experience parental death but were characterized by low affection, low social support, and high conflict, the subjects showed higher adult hostility scores. These results suggest that children who do not lose a parent, yet are raised with little affection and social support and high levels of conflict, are likely to externalize their feelings through hostility, cynicism, and aggression. Children who experience a parental death in addition to a poor-quality family environment are likely to internalize their feelings through depression and social isolation. These findings, which apply to both genders, indicate that social support has long-standing developmental precursors that are important to consider in understanding the dynamics of adult social support. For example, Allen and his colleagues[24] found that hostility is powerful enough to outweigh the influence of high social support in healthy black and white men and women. But a high degree of outwardly expressed anger and low social support appear to work synergistically and hasten the progression of coronary atherosclerosis among both men and women with coronary heart disease.[25] The lack of social support alone has been found to contribute to the severity of coronary artery disease (CAD) in women.[26] Knox and her associates[27] found that a high ratio of hostility to support more than doubled the odds of myocardial infarction alone. The odds of carotid lesions in high-risk women also increased substantially when hostility was associated with low social support. A similar effect was seen in high-risk men, but to a lesser degree.

The interaction between anger, hostility, and social support appears to be related to the occurrence and severity or progression of CAD. Hostility and anger alone (either expressed or repressed) and low social support alone have been identified as precursors for myocardial infarction. Moderate levels of anger expression seem to be protective against CHD.[28] Hostile and angry people might be successful in generating only support from people like themselves and might therefore lack a positive social support system. Persons with low social support might become hostile and angry at their isolation and project the reasons outside of themselves. All of this can create an unsatisfying cycle, especially if it is a lifelong pattern. Several studies emphasize that negative emotions are not in themselves a problem; rather, it is their chronicity that makes them a significant risk factor.[29,30] Indeed, clinical depression has been shown to be an independent risk factor for CAD for several decades after the onset of depression.[31]

Some prospective evidence suggests that prolonged, unresolved emotional tension can result in physical and mental exhaustion (emotional drain), which in turn can be a contributing factor in provoking a heart attack.[32] Appels,[33] in a large prospective study in the Netherlands, found "vital exhaustion" present in the year prior to a heart attack. Appels found the prevalence of myocardial infarction, defined as unstable angina pectoris plus electrocardiographic signs of ischemia, to be more than four times higher among exhausted and depressed persons than among persons who were not so affected.

GENDER, SOCIAL SUPPORT, AND RECOVERY FROM MYOCARDIAL INFARCTION OR CORONARY ARTERY SURGERY

Before hospital discharge, patients recovering from a myocardial infarction were asked questions about aspects of masculinity, femininity, and social support. They were then followed prospectively by telephone to monitor their recovery. The single greatest predictor of recovery was spouse disclosure. Patients who reported less spouse disclosure during the initial hospitalization were more likely to be rehospitalized, suffer more severe chest pain, and perceive their health as worse. Marriage was found to have greater protective health benefits for men than for women.[34] In a study of males recovering from coronary bypass surgery, it was found that married patients who received higher hospital support took less pain medication and recovered more quickly than their low-support counterparts.[35] Higher support was predictive of better emotional status, perceived quality of life, and compliance, but did not predict cardiac health during follow-up.[36] The cardiac rehabilitation process differs between men and women. Psychosocial well-being and adjustment after a heart attack seem to be worse in women than in men.[37] Women who had coronary artery bypass surgery have been found to be more depressed than men, the depression being significantly related to pain and impairment, while depression among men was related more to the lack of social support than to pain and impairment. Indeed, Barefoot and his associates[39] found that cardiac patients who reported high levels of social support while in the hospital showed more improvement in depressive symptoms, especially among younger patients.

Social support appears to be a salient factor for patients with heart disease in maintaining compliance with their rehabilitation programs. Depression following a heart attack is expected and can negatively affect patients' following of physicians' recommendations to reduce further cardiac risk.[38] Patients who receive support from family and friends are more likely than others to comply with risk factor modification and postcoronary rehabilitation programs. Friis and Taff[41] note that the most promising social support or social network variables isolated from a literature review appear to be the number and intimacy of social ties, satisfaction with social activities, work and financial status, perceived opportunities to discuss problems, and the level of social interaction.

GENDER, SOCIAL SUPPORT, DEPRESSION, AND MORTALITY FROM CHD

Emotions like anger, anxiety, and depression seem to increase CHD incidence and mortality, particularly in women; loneliness, infrequent vacations, and believing oneself prone to CHD have been found to be predictive of fatal and nonfatal CHD.[37] Low social support has been found to increase the incidence of CHD in several prospective studies.[39,40] Lack of social support increases the risk of death once CHD has become manifest.[41,42]

Mortality and morbidity after myocardial infarction are higher in women than in men, and women appear to be more likely to experience a subsequent heart attack or die within a year after their first myocardial infarction. Women undergoing coronary heart bypass surgery or coronary angioplasty have higher hospital mortality rates than men. Women do not possess any survival advantage over men.[37]

The relationship between mortality from CHD and social isolation (or low social support) has been documented in men and women after 10 and 20 years of follow-up. Men and women with scarce social networks had significantly increased mortality rates both from all causes and from CHD. An especially increased mortality was found for men living alone and for men reporting low social participation and inadequate emotional support.[43,44] The relationship between social isolation and increased risk of mortality among CHD patients has also been documented by others; for example, Brummett and his associates[50] found that the only psychological indicator related to social isolation was hostility, with isolated patients having higher hostility ratings. This coincides with findings of the higher mortality experience of socially isolated type A men than of those who are socially integrated.[45] It appears that the personality characteristics of type A in men with CHD and a socially isolated lifestyle are a potentially deadly combination. Similarly, the combination of depression and low social support is associated with a marked increase in mortality among CHD patients.[46] In a study of patients with congestive heart failure, social isolation was found to be a significant predictor of mortality when depressive symptoms, age, and the severity of disease were controlled.[47]

Hopelessness has been identified as a strong, independent predictor of CHD morbidity and mortality in Finnish and American populations. In a population-based study of middle-age Finnish men who underwent carotid ultrasonography and were followed prospectively, it was found that men who reported high levels of hopelessness at baseline and 4 years later had faster progression of carotid atherosclerosis. Progression was greatest among men who reported high levels of hopelessness at both baseline and follow-up.[48] Appels[55] found that unusual or disabling fatigue had stronger predictive power for a first heart attack than depression, irritability, or hopelessness. Similar to Appels' concept of unusual fatigue or vital exhaustion is the concept of emotional drain, which was found to be more evident and pervasive in the lives of patients than in their matched controls. A series of continuing frustrations that are perceived to be unsolvable but keep the body and mind in a state of readiness, along with a lack of supportive relationships, can result in emotional drain and the likelihood of a cardiac event.[32] The ideas of vital exhaustion and emotional drain are not new in the CHD literature. Schmale[56] concluded after an extensive review of the literature that the concept of psychic "giving up" was an antecedent condition to the appearance of symptoms that can lead to a diagnosis of somatic or psychic disease. Giving up was the last straw or final blow of those who could no longer cope after a period of episodes with illness and conflict and the persistence of helplessness or hopelessness. Wolf[57] suggested that autonomic responses, including potentially fatal cardiac disturbances, could be initiated from the higher centers of the brain in individuals who are in some way alienated from their environmental support or otherwise at the "end of their rope."

SUMMARY

House[58] pointed out that our knowledge regarding how and why the lack of social ties are risky for health is still limited. The deleterious effects of the lack of social ties on health have been recognized and documented qualitatively and quantitatively, using many different research techniques and study designs, in many different cultures. The opposite side of the coin has been examined, that is, how and why social ties are protective of health and longevity.[49] We know *why* social ties are important. They shape the quality of our lives. Social cooperation is an essential part of man's survival as a species, just as it has been in the survival of subhuman primates. Group living is an adaptation that provides protection, cooperation, competition, and communication to improve the chances for survival. Yet, *how* community and group ties promote health is not fully understood, and *how* the lack of social ties is harmful to health remains a neurophysiological black hole. Collecting more evidence is not sufficient to answer the how questions. The evidence must be the right kind. Future evidence should be targeted to discovering mechanisms. One approach toward discovering mechanisms is through intervention studies.

Cwikel and Israel[60] reviewed 17 intervention studies that involved some type of social support or social network approach in the area of physical health problems. They concluded that:

- Social support and social network interventions exhibit greater effects for those people who have recently experienced life crises.
- Studies that used a combination of different types of social support in the intervention were more effective.
- The provision of social support by peers, significant others, and professionals can affect the level of adherence to medical regimens.
- Studies that incorporated both affective and appraisal support had positive results.
- Stronger effects were noted when interventions provided more emotional than informational support.
- Some of the more successful interventions used lay counselors or peers to deliver the intervention.
- The presence of a spouse can inhibit successful interaction about emotionally laden issues.

A second approach toward uncovering mechanisms is studying people's reactions to real-life events over time. We can learn much about what the brain sees through event mapping, that is, by focusing on environmental stimuli and people's responses to them. These natural experiments will enable us to better understand how an individual appraises an event and to investigate the antecedent of appraisal in the person and situation.

The pathophysiological links between behavioral factors and cardiovascular diseases appear to involve sympathoadrenomedullary activity. Many pathophysiological processes are known to cause hypertension, myocardial infarction, and sudden death. The basic disease processes do not cause signs or symptoms by themselves. Clinical manifestations occur only when complications are added to the basic disease processes. Behavioral factors can influence both the basic disease processes and the clinical manifestations.

REFERENCES

1. Angell, M., Disease as a reflection of the psyche. *N. Engl. J. Med.*, 12, 1570, 1985.
2. Scheidt, S., The current status of heart-mind relationships. *J. Psychosom. Res.*, 48, 317, 2000.
3. Krantz, D.S. and McCeney, M.K., Effects of psychological and social factors on organic disease: a critical assessment of research on coronary heart disease. *Am. Rev. Psychol.*, 53, 341, 2002.
4. Wolf, S., Social environment and health: the struggle to document a truism. *Integ. Phys. Behav. Sci.*, 28, 115, 1993.
5. Lynch, J.J., *A Cry Unheard: The Medical Consequences of Loneliness*. Baltimore, MD: Bancroft Press, 2000.
6. Bruhn, J.G., Thurman, A.E., Chandler, B.C. and Bruce, T.A., Patients' reactions to death in a coronary care unit. *J. Psychosom. Res.*, 14, 65, 1970.
7. Wolf, S., Psychosocial forces and neural mechanisms in disease: defining the question and collecting the evidence. *Integ. Phys. Behav. Sci.*, 30, 85, 1995.
8. Mendes de Leon, C.F., Depression and social support in recovery from myocardial infarction: confounding and confusion. *Psychosom. Med.*, 61, 738, 1999.

9. Heitzmann, C.A. and Kaplan, R.M., Assessment of methods for measuring social support. *Health Psychol.*, 7, 75, 1988.
10. Winemiller, D.R., Mitchell, M.E., Sutliff, J. and Cline, D.J., Measurement strategies in social support: a descriptive review of the literature. *J. Clin. Psychol.*, 49, 638, 1993.
11. Barrera, M., Destructions between social support concepts, measures, and models. *Am. J. Commun. Psychol.*, 14, 413, 1986.
12. Bruhn, J.G. and Philips, B.U., Measuring social support: a synthesis of current approaches. *J. Behav. Med.*, 7, 151, 1984.
13. Coyne, J.C. and De Longis, A., Going beyond social support: the role of social relationships in adaptation. *J. Consult. Clin. Psychol.*, 54, 454, 1986.
14. Bruhn, J.G., People need people: perspectives on the meaning and measurement of social support. *Integ. Phys. Behav. Sci.*, 26, 325, 1991.
15. Bruhn, J.G., Beyond discipline: creating a culture for interdisciplinary research. *Integ. Phys. Behav. Sci.*, 30, 331, 1995.
16. Tennant, C., Life stress, social support and coronary heart disease. *Aust. N.Z. J. Psychiatr.*, 33, 636, 1999.
17. Greenwood, D.C., Muir, K.R., Packham, C.J. and Madeley, R.J., Coronary heart disease: a review of the role of psychosocial stress and social support. *J. Public Health Med.*, 18, 221, 1996.
18. Berkman, L.F., The relationship of social networks and social support to morbidity and mortality, in *Social Support and Health*, Cohen, S. and Syme, S.L. (Eds.). New York: Academic Press, 1985, Chapter 12.
19. Bruhn, J.G. and Wolf, S., The mind as a process. *Integ. Phys. Behav. Sci.*, 38, 75, 2003.
20. Damasio, A., *Looking for Spinoza: Joy, Sorrow, and the Feeling Brain*. New York: Harcourt, 2003.
21. Wegner, D.M., *The Illusion of Conscious Will*. Cambridge, MA: MIT Press, 2002.
22. Liebler, C.A. and Sandefur, G.D., Gender differences in the exchange of social support with friends, neighbors, and co-workers at midlife. *Soc. Sci. Res.*, 31, 364, 2002.
23. Luecken, L., Attachment and loss experiences during childhood are associated with adult hostility, depression, and social support. *J. Psychosom. Res.*, 49, 85, 2000.
24. Allen, J., Markovitz, J., Jacobs, D.R. and Knox, S.S., Social support and health behavior in hostile black and white men and women in CARDIA. *Psychosom. Med.*, 63, 609, 2001.
25. Angerer, P., Siebert, V., Kothay, W., Mühlbauer, D., Mudra, H. and von Schacky, C., Impact of social support, cynical hostility and anger expression on progression of coronary atherosclerosis. *J. Am. Coll. Cardiol.*, 36, 1781, 2000.
26. Orth-Gomer, K., Horsten, M., Wamala, S.P., Mittleman, M.A., Kirkeeide, R., Svane, B., Ryden, L. and Schenck-Gustafsson, K., Social relations and extent and severity of coronary artery disease. *Eur. Heart J.*, 19, 1648, 1998.
27. Knox, S.S., Adelman, A., Ellison, R.C., Arnett, D.K., Siegmund, K., Weidner, G. and Privince, M.A., Hostility, social support, and carotid artery atherosclerosis in the National Heart, Lung, and Blood Institute Family Heart Study. *Am. J. Cardiol.*, 86, 1086, 2000.
28. Eng, P.M., Fitzmaurice, G., Kubansky, L.D., Rimm, E.B. and Kawachi, I., Anger expression and risk of stroke and coronary heart disease among male health professionals. *Psychosom. Med.*, 65, 100, 2003.
29. Barefoot, J.C., Dahlstrom, G. and Williams, R.B., Hostility, CHD incidence, and total mortality: a 25-year follow-up study of 255 physicians. *Psychosom. Med.*, 45, 59, 1983.
30. Siegman, A.W., Cardiovascular consequences of expressing, experiencing, and repressing anger. *J. Behav. Med.*, 16, 539, 1993.

31. Ford, D.E., Mead, L.A., Cheng, P.P., Cooper-Patrick, L., Wang, N. and Klag, M.J., Depression is a risk factor for coronary artery disease in men. *Arch. Intern. Med.*, 158, 1422, 1998.
32. Bruhn, J.G., McCrady, K.E. and du Plessis, A., Evidence of "emotional drain" preceding death from myocardial infarction, *Psychiatr. Dig.*, 29, 34, 1968.
33. Appels, A., The year before myocardial infarction, in *Biobehavioral Bases of Coronary Heart Disease*, Dembroski, T.M., Schmidt, T.H. and Blumchen, G. (Eds.). Basel: Karger, 1983, Chapter 2.
34. Helgeson, V.S., The effects of masculinity and social support on recovery from myocardial infarction. *Psychosom. Med.*, 53, 621, 1991.
35. Kulik, J.A. and Mahler, H.I., Social support and recovery from surgery. *Health Psychol.*, 8, 221, 1989.
36. Kulik, J.A. and Mahler, H.I., Emotional support as a moderator of adjustment and compliance after coronary artery bypass surgery: a longitudinal study. *J. Behav. Med.*, 16, 45, 1993.
37. Brezinka, V. and Kittel, F., Psychosocial factors of coronary heart disease in women: a review. *Soc. Sci. Med.*, 42, 1351, 1995.
38. Con, A.H., Linden, W., Thompson, J.M. and Ignaszewski, A., The psychology of men and women recovering from coronary artery bypass surgery. *J. Cardiopulm. Rehabil.*, 19, 152, 1999.
39. Barefoot, J.C., Brummett, B.H., Clapp-Channing, N.E., Siegler, I.C., Vitaliano, P.P., Williams, R.B. and Mark, D.B., Moderators of the effect of social support on depressive symptoms in cardiac patients. *Am. J. Cardiol.*, 86, 438, 2000.
40. Ziegelstein, R.C., Depression in patients' recovery from a myocardial infarction. *JAMA*, 286, 1621, 2001.
41. Friis, R. and Taff, G.A., Social support and social networks, and coronary heart disease rehabilitation, *J. Cardiopulm. Rehabil.*, 6, 132, 1986.
42. Orth-Gomer, K. and Johnson, J.V., Social network interaction and mortality: a six-year follow-up study of a random sample of the Swedish population. *J. Chron. Dis.*, 40, 949, 1987.
43. Berkman, L.F., Summers, L. and Horwitz, R.I., Emotional support and survival after myocardial infarction. A prospective, population-based study of the elderly. *Am. Intern. Med.*, 117, 1003, 1992.
44. Eaker, E.D., Prinsky, J. and Castelli, W.P., Myocardial infarction and coronary death among women: psychosocial predictors from a 20-year follow-up of women in the Framingham Study. *Am. J. Epidemiol.*, 135, 854, 1992.
45. Wingard, D.L. and Cohn, B.A., Coronary heart disease mortality among women in Alameda County, 1965 to 1973, in *Coronary Heart Disease in Women*, Eaker, E.D., Packard, B., Wenger, N.K., Clarkson, T.B. and Tyroler, H.A. (Eds.). New York: Haymarket Doyma, 1987.
46. Chandra, V., Szklo, M., Goldberg, R. and Tonascia, J., The impact of mental status on survival after an acute myocardial infarction: a population-based study. *Am. J. Epidemiol.*, 117, 320, 1983.
47. Williams, R.B., Barefoot, J.C., Califf, R.M., Haney, T.L., Saunders, W.B., Pryor, D.B., Hlatky, M.A., Siegler, J.C. and Mark, D.B., Prognostic importance of social and economic resources among medically treated patients with angiographically documented coronary artery disease. *JAMA*, 267, 520, 1992.
48. Orth-Gomer, K., Rosengren, A. and Wilhelmson, L., Lack of social support and incidence of coronary heart disease in middle-aged Swedish men. *Psychosom. Med.*, 55, 37, 1993.

49. Orth-Gomer, K., Unden, A. and Edwards, M., Social isolation and mortality in ischemic heart disease: a 10-year follow-up study of 150 middle-aged men. *Acta Med. Scand.*, 224, 205, 1988.
50. Brummett, B.D., Barefoot, J.C., Siegler, I.C., Clapp-Channing, N.E., Lytle, B.L., Bosworth, H.B., Williams, R.B. and Mark, D.B., Characteristics of socially isolated patients with coronary artery disease who are at elevated risk for mortality. *Psychosom. Med.*, 63, 267, 2001.
51. Orth-Gomer, K. and Unden, A., Type A behavior, social support, and coronary risk: interaction and significance for mortality in cardiac patients. *Psychosom. Med.*, 52, 59, 1990.
52. Frasure-Smith, N., Lespérance, F., Gravel, G., Masson, A., Juneau, M., Talajic, M. and Bourassa, M.G., Social support, depression, and mortality during the first year after myocardial infarction. *Circulation*, 101, 1919, 2000.
53. Murberg, T.A. and Bru, E., Social relationships and mortality in patients with congestive heart failure. *J. Psychosom. Res.*, 51, 521, 2001.
54. Everson, S.A., Kaplan, G.A., Goldberg, D.E., Salonen, R. and Salonen, J.T., Hopelessness and 4-year progression of carotid atherosclerosis. *Arterioscler. Thromb. Vasc. Biol.*, 17, 1490, 1997.
55. Appels, A., Kop, W.J. and Schouten, E., The nature of the depressive symptomatology preceding myocardial infarction. *Behav. Med.*, 26, 86, 2000.
56. Schmale, A.H., Giving up as a final common pathway to changes in health. *Adv. Psychosom. Med.*, 8, 20, 1972.
57. Wolf, S., The end of the rope: the role of the brain in cardiac death. *Can. Med. Assoc. J.*, 97, 1022, 1967.
58. House, J.S., Social isolation kills, but how and why? *Psychosom. Med.*, 63, 273, 2001.
59. Patrick, D.L. and Wickizer, T.M., Community and health, in *Society and Health*, Amick, B.C., Levine, S., Tarlov, A.R. and Walsh, D.C. (Eds.). New York: Oxford University Press, 1995, Chapter 3.
60. Cwikel, J.M. and Israel, B.A., Examining mechanisms of social support and social networks: a review of health-related intervention studies, *Public Health Rev.*, 15, 159, 1987.

13 Social Support, Life Events, and Depression in HIV Disease

John Green and Ashley Frize

CONTENTS

The last decade has seen a revolution in the treatment of HIV disease. The coming of combination therapy (highly active antiretroviral therapy (HAART)) has led to a major increase in life expectancy and a reduction in morbidity for those with the disease. People who could once have expected to become disabled and die rapidly after diagnosis are now able to continue to live more or less normal lives, albeit somewhat interrupted by frequent hospital visits and often tiresome medication regimes. At the same time, the disease has spread widely across the world and continues to do so. Treatment is expensive and there is as yet no effective vaccine.

The seriousness and high incidence of the disease has led to an unprecedented research effort that has far outstripped expenditure on any other infectious disease in history. Part of that research effort has been into the links between stress, psychological distress, and HIV, reflecting the modern awareness that physical diseases usually have psychological consequences. However, other issues have also driven research in this area: the possibility that psychological factors might affect physical health and mortality in some way and the recognition that since HIV, like just about every other infectious disease, is spread by people's behavior, it is important to identify and quantify such links. Finally, there has been an interest in whether HIV disease can provide information at a theoretical level about the impact of stress on immune functioning generally.

Before looking at the extensive literature, it is important to consider some of the constraints and difficulties that researchers have had in looking at these topics.

0-8493-1820-3/05/$0.00+$1.50

BACKGROUND ISSUES

In looking at the effects of stress on HIV disease, it is important to have clearly defined outcomes. It is not always obvious what they should be. HIV is a disease that primarily attacks the immune system; therefore, it might seem logical to choose immune system functioning as one of the outcomes. However, the immune system is immensely complicated, a collection of many different systems. There is no single good measure of immune system functioning, nor could such a measure exist. Most research has been on T lymphocytes, particularly CD4+ and CD8+ cells. There has also been interest in natural killer cell activity. All three types of cells play a part in the body's response to viral infection. However, there are many other aspects of immune system functioning that have not been studied, including other important parts of the cellular immunity systems and the efficiency of the innate immune system.

The favorite target for studies on the immune system in HIV has been CD4+ levels. The virus directly infects CD4+ cells, and the level of these cells in the blood reflects the extent of the damage that HIV has caused to the patient's immune system, at least in a rather gross way. Thus, CD4+ count is a marker of disease progression and gross falls in CD4+ count are associated with increased risk of opportunistic infections and tumors and with ill health generally. CD4+ levels were, in the past, the main measure of the effectiveness of treatment and of disease stage. More recently, viral load, the amount of virus present, has taken over as the main clinical index of success of treatment because it is a better predictor of clinical endpoints and more rapidly responsive to antiviral treatment. Nonetheless, CD4+ counts are still routinely collected and used and, because they are routinely collected, are a convenient index for use in studies of everything from the effects of diet to the impact of psychological variables on HIV disease. However, CD4+ levels are a fairly gross measure of immune functioning and probably a better measure of the extent of viral activity than of immunity per se.

Unfortunately, CD4+ levels are also responsive to a host of environmental factors, including exercise, smoking, and transient infections. Not only do these environmental influences create a background of statistical noise that makes it difficult to detect the effects of stress, but they also make it difficult to interpret the meaning of any linkages that can be established between CD4+ levels and stress. It seems likely that some degree of change in CD4+ levels can occur without any impact on overall health. It has, for instance, proved difficult to associate immune changes in athletes, including changes in CD4+ levels associated with high levels of exercise, with any change in the ability of the body to fight off disease. A modest association between stress and CD4+ levels might in theory be of no practical importance at all to the integrity of an individual's immune system.

In theory, if stress affected the immune functioning of people with HIV disease, one might expect to see higher viral loads in people under stress than in people not under stress. Little psychosocial research has used viral load as an index. Moreover, the single largest factor in determining viral load in patients in the West today is the treatment that they are receiving. If stress is substantially correlated with failure of adherence to medication regime, then it is likely that this effect would swamp out any effects of psychosocial factors on viral load (and indeed with CD4+ levels).

Simply establishing a correlation between immune measures such as CD4+ levels or viral load and stress is not in itself enough to establish that stress influences these measures. CD4+ counts and viral loads, which patients are made aware of and whose significance they understand, are themselves sources of stress. The patient who sees their CD4+ count rapidly declining or their viral load rapidly increasing is likely to make the not unreasonable assumption that their treatment is failing and that they might become ill.

Perhaps the gold standard in terms of outcome is mortality. A number of studies have used mortality as their endpoint. However, mortality has a number of problems as a measure of the impact of continuous variables such as stress. The coming of combination therapy has reduced the death rate from HIV disease considerably. Studies that use mortality as their endpoint require large numbers of patients or a long follow-up. Particularly today, death rates from AIDS are likely to be linked primarily to success or failure of treatment, and therefore treatment adherence is likely to be a critical factor. Individuals struggling with treatment adherence might both be more distressed and have worse outcomes.

Finally, it is worth remarking that in our opinion, efforts to use diseases that attack the immune system, such as HIV, as models on which to test theoretical hypotheses about the direct effects of stress on immune system functioning are misguided. HIV itself directly attacks the immune system, and this attack is so powerful as to likely drown out the relatively small amount of variance that might be expected to be attributable to stress, except in large or lengthy studies. Treatment adds additional "noise" into the system since patients have differential responses to treatment, further adding to the difficulties of identifying the effects of psychosocial variables. Once one adds the need to partial out those effects of stress mediated indirectly by lifestyle factors, then the possibility of generating false negatives or false positives becomes substantial. Whether health and disease are influenced by stress is a question of importance in its own right, but there are better models for looking at theoretical issues about the linkages between stress and immune functioning than HIV; indeed, it is hard to think of a worse one.

Linked to the issue of stress is the issue of social support. While it might be thought fairly straightforward to elucidate the impact of social support on HIV disease, it has its own problems. One difficulty is in deciding which aspects of social support ought to be measured. It can be, for instance, difficult to decide whether the size of a social network or its intensity is likely to be the most important factor to be measured. If intensity is chosen as the measure, then there is a question of whether actual intensity, for instance, the amount of episodes of social contact over some period, or the degree to which the individual feels supported should be the measure used. Social support has both practical and emotional elements and can include, for instance, things like other people doing shopping or acting as carers for the person with HIV. It is not always easy to see which of these is likely to be the most important when planning a study. Where size of the social network is selected as a variable to be measured, it can be difficult to know where to draw the boundaries of the social network; in practical terms, how much support does one have to have from an individual in order for them to be included in your social network? There is also the issue of actual vs. potential social network; for instance, the patient can have many friends but be unwilling to draw on them as a source of support either because to do so would necessitate disclosure of one's HIV status or because one is unwilling to call on friends for psychological reasons. The latter is perhaps particularly likely to occur when an individual is depressed. Finally, it is worth considering that different measures of social support tend to be intercorrelated, to some extent at least. Simply because emotional social support or specific HIV-related support turn out to be related to stress does not mean that it is not practical help with nutrition or getting to the hospital for appointments that is the crucial factor.

Of course, the effects of stress on the individual with HIV disease are unlikely to be limited to purely physical ones. The psychological well-being of the patient is also a matter worthy of consideration. If those individuals with HIV disease who are under stress experience a sharply reduced quality of life relative to those who are not under stress because, for instance, they are more likely to become depressed, then that in itself would suggest that we ought to make efforts to intervene to reduce the impact of stress. Even if stress had no impact on immune functioning and made no difference to survival or physical morbidity in people with HIV, it might still be an important consideration in their care.

Three issues have dominated work on stress and HIV disease: depression, life events, and social support. Although other issues such as coping style, optimism, and mood more generally have also attracted attention, we have concentrated on these three issues because they have by far the best evidence base.

DEPRESSION AND HIV

The relationship between stress and depression is a complex one. Depression might be both a result of stress and a cause of stress. Similarly, it might result from low levels of social support and also be a cause of low levels of social support, since social withdrawal is a common symptom of depression. More subtly, it might render what emotional social support an individual has less rewarding because of anhedonia. For these reasons, and presumably because it is with anxiety the most measured psychological factor in medicine, the impact of depression has attracted particular attention.

It is clear that depression is more common in individuals with HIV infection than in the population at large and in most studies than in controls (Cruess et al., 2003; Turrina et al., 2001). Levels seem to be elevated across the board with socially disadvantaged women (Catz et al., 2002), those attending primary care (Komiti et al., 2003), drug users (Perdue et al., 2003), gay men (Perdue et al., 2003), mothers living with HIV (Murphy et al., 2002b), older people (Heckman et al., 2002), and women (Richardson et al., 2001; Morrison et al., 2002), all showing the effect, and the finding is worldwide (Martin Suarez et al., 2002; Sebit et al., 2002; Chandra et al., 2003). As might be expected, usage of psychotropic medication, particularly antidepressants but also anxiolytics and hypnotics, is extremely common among those with HIV infection (Vitiello et al., 2003).

The question then arises as to why people with HIV are more prone to depression. At first glance, the answer is simple: they are often ill, are faced with a potentially life-threatening illness, and have a stigmatized disease that places severe limitations on their sex lives. However, the issue looks less straightforward when examined in detail. The introduction of combination therapy has meant that in the Western world, at least, life expectancy has rocketed and the incidence of ill health has plummeted. However, somewhat surprisingly, rates of depression in individuals with HIV reported today do not differ a great deal from those reported prior to the introduction of effective antiviral regimes, although treatment does seem to produce some degree of improvement in some studies (Brechtl et al., 2001). If it were solely ill health or the apprehension of imminent death that is producing such high rates of depression, then one would expect to have seen a very marked drop in depression rates over the past few years and much more marked differences than the modest ones between those taking combination therapy and those not taking it (Starace et al., 2002b).

One possibility is that some depression can be a side effect of anti-HIV medication (Blanch et al., 2001). While depression is a possible side effect of some antiviral regimes, there is no evidence that this is a major factor. It is also possible that the virus itself in some way directly causes depression. It is neuropathic and leads to the release of, for instance, interferon, which when administered exogenously can produce anxiety and mood disturbance (Rockstroh et al., 2002). There is some evidence that depression and neuropsychological impairment might be linked in some individuals, although it is difficult to interpret this finding (Vazquez-Justo et al., 2003).

Another possible connection between HIV and depression is fatigue. Fatigue is a common feature of viral illnesses generally and is very common in HIV (Milikin et al., 2003). If fatigue predisposes individuals to become depressed, or if its symptoms lead to misdiagnosis of individuals as being depressed when they are not, then that might elevate rates of actual or apparent depression. Sullivan and Dworkin (2003) reported that a third of individuals with HIV had significant fatigue, and this was positively related to depression, disease staging, and anemia, but not to CD4+ count or viral load. Barroso et al. (2002) reported that depression was predicted by psychosocial factors while fatigue was predicted by both psychosocial and physical factors. More generally, there is a problem with many commonly used depression scales in that the symptoms of depression that make up the scales frequently overlap to some extent with symptoms common in physical ill health. There is thus a danger that as HIV disease progresses and individuals have more physical symptoms, their scores on depression scales will rise without any change in mood.

Another possibility is that those with HIV are drawn from populations where depression is prevalent anyway. Almost all of the studies that have reported on demographic factors in HIV populations have reported that among those with HIV, the poor and disadvantaged have higher levels of depression. If these risk factors are more common in individuals with HIV disease than in the population at large, then they might as a group have a higher incidence of depression. Drug users are particularly at risk of HIV infection through sharing injection equipment and probably because they tend to have sex with other drug users, and rates of depression and other mental health problems are high in uninfected drug users relative to the general population. In one large study of women with HIV and behaviorally similar women who were uninfected, both groups showed quite high rates of depression and adverse life events, but there was no difference between groups (Moore et al.,

1999). Richardson et al. (2001) reported that while depression was more common in HIV+ individuals, it was also very common in controls who were otherwise similar. It is often much more difficult to draw samples of controls for studies than samples of patients, since the latter have to keep coming in for treatment and precise matching can be a major problem.

Another possibility is that even within particular risk populations those individuals who are depressed are more prone to contracting HIV. Again, this would elevate depression rates in those with HIV not only in comparison to the general population, but also relative to controls. The evidence for this proposition is somewhat mixed (Crepaz and Marks, 2002), but there is probably sufficient positive evidence to suggest that it is plausible. Perdue et al. (2003) reported that drug users who were depressed were more likely to share syringes and depressed gay men reported more partners. Blumberg and Dickey (2003) found that individuals in the population who suffered from depression or anxiety disorders were more likely to have engaged in risky sexual behavior than those who did not have these problems. Depression was significantly associated with a greater probability of unsafe sex in adolescents (Murphy et al., 2002a), while greater anxiety was associated with sexual activity per se. Beck et al. (2003) reported that depression was associated with increased risky behavior in gay men and that the connection was mediated by perceptions that sexual risk was not controllable. Similar findings were reported by Semple et al. (2000).

It seems likely that one reason why risky behaviors might be related to depression is the issue of control. Depressed individuals frequently feel that they have little control over events and are pessimistic about the possibility of their behavior influencing the outcome of negative events.

The association between depression and risk behaviors carries through into those who are already infected. Kalichman et al. (2002a) reported that depression, anxiety. and personality problems were associated with recent unsafe sexual activity in individuals with HIV. Other studies have also found associations between depression and unsafe sexual activity in seropositives (Desquilbet et al., 2002).

There can be other factors in the high rates of depression seen in those with HIV disease. For instance, HIV+ individuals report high rates of past sexual assault, and past sexual assault is associated with an increased risk of depression (Kalichman et al., 2002b). It can also be the case that individuals who are acutely depressed are more likely to seek medical assistance or HIV testing. This would cause elevated rates of depression (and subsequent decline over time) in individuals recruited soon after diagnosis (Savetsky et al., 2001).

Depression is a particularly nasty condition that is of great importance in its own right and that merits treatment to relieve suffering regardless of any other effects that it might have. If there is indeed a connection between depression and unsafe sexual activity in those with HIV disease, then that is also of considerable practical importance. There are additionally two other issues of interest: depression has been linked to poor adherence to antiretroviral medication, and it has been suggested that depression might lead to a more rapid deterioration in physical health in those with HIV and to earlier death.

Adherence, taking the right medication at the right time and in the right quantities, is particularly important in HIV disease (Bartlett, 2002). Poor adherence is related to poorer prognosis, not only because if you do not take the medication, then it cannot help you, but also because intermittent suboptimal antiviral treatment is thought to encourage the development of drug-resistant virus and so make later treatment more problematic. There is also the problem that resistant virus is potentially transmissible to other, drug-naïve individuals.

A review by Starace et al. (2002a) concluded that there was strong evidence that depression was linked to poor adherence even though there was no definitive study. Adherence has been reported to be poor in those with severe mental illness, including severe depression, with poor adherence associated with higher viral load (Wagner et al., 2003). In a large U.S. survey of people with HIV, both depression and anxiety were associated with decreased medication adherence. Alcohol and illicit drug usage also predicted nonadherence (Tucker et al., 2003). These differences were independent of other demographic variables. In a study of French drug users, injection drug use, depression, and social isolation were related to nonadherence (Carrieri et al., 2003). There is some evidence that appropriate psychiatric treatment might improve adherence (Turner et al., 2003). Women who are depressed are less likely to use antiviral therapy, but treatment for their mental health problems increases usage (Cook et al., 2002).

The possible connection between depression and disease progression and survival is one of both practical and theoretical importance. While earlier studies tended not to identify a convincing linkage (Zorilla et al., 1996), two more recent large studies have suggested that a linkage might exist.

In the large U.S. multicenter AIDS (MACS) study, somatic symptoms of depression were a significant predictor of disease progression and survival (Farinpour et al., 2003), although as noted earlier, there are problems in interpreting the physical symptoms of depression. They interacted with age and IQ in predicting outcomes. In a large study of female HIV-positive individuals, depression was related to both a steeper decline in CD4++ count and a greater mortality rate (Ickovics et al., 2001). The death rate of those with chronic depression was double that of women without depression, and the effect was greater in women who had lower CD4++ counts.

Some caution needs to be exercised in interpreting these studies (Leserman, 2003). Perhaps the main difficulty is in being sure which way the arrow of causation points. It is possible that the connection is simply that those who see their health improve on treatment are less likely to become or stay depressed. This is a highly plausible mechanism. In one study, individuals who experienced a reduction in viral load in response to treatment showed reduced depression and distress, while those whose viral load rose showed signs of increasing distress (Kalichman et al., 2002a). There is even some evidence to suggest that simply being treated can impact mood (Sebit et al., 2002), an effect familiar to any clinician. Depression has been reported to be more strongly related to subjective assessment of disease status rather than to objective measures and is also associated with reporting more health problems (Jones et al., 2001).

Ultimately, the only way to be absolutely sure whether depression affects prognosis is likely to be to carry out a randomized control trial (RCT) to assess the effects of treatment of depression on physical health outcomes. Such a study would face formidable practical and ethical problems.

SOCIAL SUPPORT

Social support is another variable that has attracted considerable interest from a theoretical point of view and also because many agencies seek to provide social support to individuals with HIV. There are some difficulties in that several studies have found linkages between social support and depression, making it difficult to decide which is primary. There is the possibility that social support, depression, and life events are all mutually linked, although few studies have looked at all three, making it difficult to be sure what linkages exist and how they operate.

There is some evidence that social support and coping influence depression and quality of life independently of life events (Safren et al., 2002). There is also evidence that there are links between depression and social support, particularly with the existence of and quality of the primary relationship. Not being in a relationship, or being in an unhappy or dysfunctional one, has been linked to depression (Komiti et al., 2003). In another study, Richardson et al. (2001) found, perhaps not surprisingly, that women were more likely to be depressed if they were in an unhappy relationship. Women who were depressed were reported to have higher stress and lower social support and to use less active coping strategies (Catz et al., 2002). Among mothers living with HIV, depression was associated with poorer family cohesion and functioning and with problems in getting everyday tasks done, although cause and effect are difficult to separate (Murphy et al., 2002b).

Adherence seems also to be linked to social support. Adherence among prisoners has been reported to be related to trust in the treatment and in the doctor, and nonadherence to social isolation and fear of side effects (Altice et al., 2001). Among French drug users, social instability was associated with poorer compliance with antiretroviral therapy (Bouhnik et al., 2002). Demas et al. (2002) found that HIV-positive mothers with less social support were less likely to maintain the correct antiviral regime to prevent neonatal infection. Older people who showed psychiatric symptomatology had lower social support and less access to social services (Heckman et al., 2002). In a study of French injection drug users, depression and social isolation were all related to nonadherence (Carrieri et al., 2003). On the other hand, a possible linkage to risky behavior seems less clear. Bachanas et al. (2002) found no evidence that social support was linked to unsafe sexual behavior in African-American adolescent girls.

It would be helpful to know whether social support generally is an important factor, or whether social support specifically related to HIV is the critical factor and whether some types of social support, for instance, a primary relationship, are more important than others, or whether they are interchangeable and it is simply the overall level of support that is important. In one study that addressed sources of support (Schrimshaw, 2003), it appeared that both friends and family can provide support, and to some extent these appear to be interchangeable (Wagner et al., 2003).

Clearly, HIV-specific social support cannot be provided if the individual does not tell anyone about his or her status, and this has led to an interest in disclosure. Many individuals are unable or unwilling to disclose their status, thus limiting access to HIV-specific support (Kalichman et al., 2003). Where disclosure does occur, it is likely to be selective; few individuals disclose their status across the board. Disclosure is a very complex area; for instance, Green et al. (2003) reported that in the case of genital herpes, individuals disclosed to sexual partners largely on the basis of their predictions of the partners' likely reaction. Nondisclosure might be as much about the person to whom disclosure might be made (or at least perceptions about them) as about the person making the disclosure.

While nondisclosure can be associated with increased risk of HIV and STI infection, it is not always so. In a study of young men across six U.S. cities (Anonymous, 2001), infection rates were lower for those who did not disclose their sexuality. Ullrich et al. (2003) found that gay men who were less willing to disclose their sexual identities had more social constraints, more depressive symptoms, and lower CD4+ counts. On the other hand, a small study from India failed to establish an association between disclosure of HIV and psychological functioning or morbidity, although there was some impact on quality of life (Chandra et al., 2003).

One potential way of trying to sort out the impact of social support is to experimentally vary this and to measure the outcomes. Unfortunately, the evidence from intervention studies has been mixed, and most have been small and their impact on the target variable has often been less than optimal. For instance, Weiss et al. (2003) compared educational groups against support groups, but the interventions failed to differentially affect perceived social support. Distress and coping did not differ between conditions. The labor-intensive nature of this sort of study tends to limit their size and therefore their power to detect changes in both social support and more distant variables such as distress, morbidity, and behavior.

LIFE EVENTS

The impact of life stresses, as measured by incidence and severity of life events, on the progression of HIV has attracted some interest. Clearly, adverse life events related to the infection are likely to be common. Getting HIV can mean being exposed to prejudice, frequently becoming ill and having to go to the hospital, losing significant relationships, losing employment, restriction on sexual behavior, and a whole range of other changes. However, there is also evidence that adverse life events can be more common not just in those with HIV, but in those at higher risk for HIV who are not infected (Moore et al., 1999). In one study of individuals testing for HIV, negative life events were uncommon after testing, although there was a raised incidence of relationship breakdown in those who tested positive (Grinstead et al., 2001).

Leserman et al. (1999, 2000) reported on a small series of gay men with HIV disease followed for up to 7 years. They found that stressful life events elicited at interview, depression, and lower social support predicted faster progression to AIDS in seropositives. Interestingly, cortisol levels were also a predictor, while the lifestyle factors they studied did not seem to be predictors. Naturally, over the length of the study, a small sample was reduced further by loss to follow-up, but the study was notably well conducted. In a study of children, those with more negative life events had a greater probability of immune suppression (Howland et al., 2000), with life events predicting the development of suppression. On the other hand, immunological parameters were not predicted by negative life events in women in another study, although pessimism was a predictor (Byrnes et al., 1998).

OVERVIEW

Up until recently, the evidence that progression of HIV disease was linked to life events or to stress was not particularly convincing, and what positive evidence there was rested, in large part, on relatively small studies (Zorilla et al., 1996). More recent studies do suggest that depression, social support, and perhaps life events can influence immune system functioning and, more informatively, morbidity and mortality. However, the available evidence is still rather sketchy and incomplete and cannot be described as remotely conclusive. The nature of the area means that large studies or long follow-ups or both are required to answer questions about the linkages between psychosocial variables and HIV disease, and these are expensive and time-consuming to conduct. Long studies also mean that progress is inevitably slow. If it takes 7 years to get an interesting finding, then it takes another 7 to confirm or disconfirm it.

It is very difficult to be sure from published studies that, say, depression is actually causing increased morbidity and mortality. Patients are aware of the progress they are making in terms of their treatment, and it might be that their mood reflects their health rather than the other way round. Perhaps the process works both ways and mood and health are interlinked in a circular fashion. Physical health might influence ability to get or utilize social support — for instance, if you are suffering from fatigue you might be less likely to want to go out to see friends — and it would not be a surprise if those who are in worse health have more life events, for instance, if they were less likely to be able to keep a job. In the case of depression, there is the problem of the extent to which physical symptoms get wrongly labeled as symptoms of depression, potentially increasing the size of any apparent linkages.

Assuming for a moment that either depression, social support, life events, or any combination of these factors really does influence morbidity and mortality or immune functioning, then it would be foolhardy in the state of current knowledge to assume that this was some sort of direct psychoneuroimmunological effect (although it *might* be in part). There is good evidence to suggest that mood and social support at least influence adherence to antiviral therapy and that adherence to antiviral therapy has a very large influence on general health, survival, and immunological and viral markers. These factors might also influence other lifestyle factors of importance — everything from smoking to nutrition to exercise to how soon people seek help if they develop an opportunistic infection. Any of these or none of these might influence physical health and prognosis; we simply have too little data to be sure.

On the other hand, there is good evidence to suggest that depression is very common in individuals with HIV disease, that they are subject to an unusually high incidence of adverse life events that they find distressing, and that they tend to have suboptimal social support. These things are important issues in their own rights; they make a major impact on the quality of individuals' lives and, as such, are good grounds for intervention. There is a danger in overly concentrating on potential physical health outcomes of these issues and missing the fact that they are major issues in their own rights. Linked to that is the increasing evidence that distress generally can be linked to an increase in behaviors that put people at risk of acquiring HIV infection and possibly of behaviors that put others at risk by those who already have the infection. Overall, there are very pressing reasons for believing that it is important to treat depression in those with HIV infection, to try to help them to minimize or cope with adverse life events, and to help them develop, maintain, and optimize their usage of social support.

REFERENCES

Altice FL, Mostashari F, Friedland GH. (2001). Trust and the acceptance of and adherence to antiretroviral therapy. *Journal of Acquired Immune Deficiency Syndromes: JAIDS*, 28:47–58.

Anonymous. (2003). HIV/STD risks in young men who have sex with men who do not disclose their sexual orientation: six U.S. cities, 1994–2000. *MMWR: Morbidity and Mortality Weekly Report*, 52:81–86.

Bachanas PJ, Morris MK, Lewis-Gess JK, Sarett-Cuasay EJ, Sirl K, Ries JK, Sawyer MK. (2002). Predictors of risky sexual behavior in African American adolescent girls: implications for prevention interventions. *Journal of Pediatric Psychology*, 27:519–530.

Barroso J, Preisser JS, Leserman J, Gaynes BN, Golden RN, Evans DN. (2002). Predicting fatigue and depression in HIV-positive gay men. *Psychosomatics*, 43:317–325.

Bartlett JA. (2002). Addressing the challenges of adherence. *Journal of Acquired Immune Deficiency Syndromes: JAIDS*, 29(Suppl 1):S2–S10.

Beck A, McNally I, Petrak J. (2003). Psychosocial predictors of HIV/STI risk behaviours in a sample of homosexual men. *Sexually Transmitted Infections*, 79:142–146.

Bing EG, Burnam MA, Longshore D, Fleishman JA, Sherbourne CD, London AS, Turner BJ, Eggan F, Beckman R, Vitiello B, Morton SC, Orlando M, Bozzette SA, Ortiz-Barron L, Shapiro M. (2001). Psychiatric disorders and drug use among human immunodeficiency virus-infected adults in the United States. *Archives of General Psychiatry*, 58:721–728.

Blanch J, Martinez E, Rousaud A, Blanco JL, Garcia-Viejo MA, Peri JM, Mallolas J, De Lazzari E, De Pablo J, Gatell JM. (2001). Preliminary data of a prospective study on neuropsychiatric side effects after initiation of efavirenz. *Journal of Acquired Immune Deficiency Syndromes: JAIDS*, 27:336–343.

Blanch J, Rousaud A, Hautzinger M, Martinez E, Peri JM, Andres S, Cirera E, Gatell JM, Gasto C. (2002). Assessment of the efficacy of a cognitive-behavioural group psychotherapy programme for HIV-infected patients referred to a consultation-liaison psychiatry department. *Psychotherapy and Psychosomatics*, 71:77–84.

Blumberg SJ, Dickey WC. (2003). Prevalence of HIV risk behaviors, risk perceptions, and testing among U.S. adults with mental disorders. *Journal of Acquired Immune Deficiency Syndromes: JAIDS*, 32:77–79.

Bouhnik AD, Chesney M, Carrieri P, Gallais H, Moreau J, Moatti JP, Obadia Y, Spire B. (2002). Nonadherence among the HIV-infected, *Journal of Acquired Immune Deficiency Syndromes: JAIDS*, 31(Suppl 3):S149–S153.

Brechtl JR, Breitbart W, Galietta M, Krivo S, Rosenfeld B. (2001). The use of highly active antiretroviral therapy (HAART) in patients with advanced HIV infection: impact on medical, palliative care, and quality of life outcomes. *Journal of Pain and Symptom Management*, 21:41–51.

Byrnes DM, Antoni MH, Goodkin K, Efantis-Potter J, Asthana D, Simon T, Munajj J, Ironson G, Fletcher MA. (1998). Stressful events, pessimism, natural killer cell cytotoxicity, and cytotoxic/suppressor T cells in HIV+ black women at risk for cervical cancer. *Psychosomatic Medicine*, 60:714–722.

Carrieri MP, Chesney MA, Spire B, Loundou A, Sobel A, Lepeu G, Moatti JP. (2003). Failure to maintain adherence to HAART in a cohort of French HIV-positive injecting drug users. *International Journal of Behavioral Medicine*, 10:1–14.

Catz SL, Gore-Felton C, McClure JB. (2002). Psychological distress among minority and low-income women living with HIV. *Behavioral Medicine*, 28:53–60.

Chandra PS, Deepthivarma S, Jairam KR, Thomas T. (2003). Relationship of psychological morbidity and quality of life to illness-related disclosure among HIV-infected persons. *Journal of Psychosomatic Research*, 54:199–203.

Ciesla JA, Roberts JE. (2001). Meta-analysis of the relationship between HIV infection and risk for depressive disorders. *American Journal of Psychiatry*, 158:725–730.

Cohen M, Hoffman RG, Cromwell C, Schmeidler J, Ebrahim F, Carrera G, Endorf F, Alfonso CA, Jacobson JM. (2002). The prevalence of distress in persons with human immunodeficiency virus infection. *Psychosomatics*, 43:10–15.

Cook JA, Cohen MH, Burke J, Grey D, Anastos K, Kirstein L, Palacio H, Richardson J, Wilson T, Young M. (2002). Effects of depressive symptoms and mental health quality of life on use of highly active antiretroviral therapy among HIV-seropositive women. *Journal of Acquired Immune Deficiency Syndromes: JAIDS*, 30:401–409.

Crepaz N, Marks G. (2002). Are negative affective states associated with HIV sexual risk behaviors? A meta-analytic review. *Health Psychology*, 20:291–299.

Cruess DG, Evans DL, Repetto MJ, Gettes D, Douglas SD, Petitto JM. (2003). Prevalence, diagnosis, and pharmacological treatment of mood disorders in HIV disease. *Biological Psychiatry*, 54:307–316.

Demas PA, Webber MP, Schoenbaum EE, Weedon J, McWayne J, Enriquez E, Bamji M, Lambert G, Thea DM. (2002). Maternal adherence to the zidovudine regimen for HIV-exposed infants to prevent HIV infection: a preliminary study. *Pediatrics*, 110:35–40.

Desquilbet L, Deveau C, Goujard C, Hubert JB, Derouineau J, Meyer L, PRIMO Cohort Study Group. (2002). Increase in at-risk sexual behaviour among HIV-1-infected patients followed in the French PRIMO cohort. *AIDS*, 16:2329–2333.

Farinpour R, Miller EN, Satz P, Selnes OA, Cohen BA, Becker JT, Skolasky RL Jr, Visscher BR. (2003). Psychosocial risk factors of HIV morbidity and mortality: findings from the Multicenter AIDS Cohort Study (MACS). *Journal of Clinical and Experimental Neuropsychology*, 25:654–670.

Green J, Ferrier S, Kocsis A, Shadrick J, Ukuomunne O, Murphy S. (2003). Determinants of disclosure of genital herpes to partners. *Sexually Transmitted Infections*, 79:42–44.

Grinstead OA, Gregorich SE, Choi KH, Coates T. (2001). Positive and negative life events after counselling and testing: the Voluntary HIV-1 Counselling and Testing Efficacy Study. *AIDS*, 15:1045–1052.

Heckman TG, Heckman BD, Kochman A, Sikkema KJ, Suhr J, Goodkin K. (2002). Psychological symptoms among persons 50 years of age and older living with HIV disease. *Aging and Mental Health*, 6:121–128.

Howland LC, Gortmaker SL, Mofenson LM, Spino C, Gardner JD, Gorski H, Fowler MG, Oleske J. (2000). Effects of negative life events on immune suppression in children and youth infected with human immunodeficiency virus type 1. *Pediatrics*, 106:540–546.

Ickovics JR, Hamburger ME, Vlahov D, Schoenbaum EE, Schuman P, Boland RJ, Moore J. (2001). Mortality, CD4 cell count decline, and depressive symptoms among HIV-seropositive women: longitudinal analysis from the HIV Epidemiology Research Study. *Journal of the American Medical Association: JAMA*, 285:1466–1474.

Jones DJ, Beach SR, Forehand R. (2001). Disease status in African American single mothers with HIV: the role of depressive symptoms. *Health Psychology*, 20:417–423.

Kalichman SC, Difonzo K, Austin J, Luke W, Rompa D. (2002a). Prospective study of emotional reactions to changes in HIV viral load. *AIDS Patient Care and Standards*, 16:113–120.

Kalichman SC, DiMarco M, Austin J, Luke W, DiFonzo K. (2003). Stress, social support, and HIV-status disclosure to family and friends among HIV-positive men and women. *Journal of Behavioral Medicine*, 26:315–332.

Kalichman SC, Sikkema KJ, DiFonzo K, Luke W, Austin J. (2002b). Adjustment in survivors of sexual assault living with HIV-AIDS. Journal of Traumatic Stress, 15:289–296.

Komiti A, Judd F, Grech P, Mijch A, Hoy J, Williams B, Street A, Lloyd JH. (2003). Depression in people living with HIV/AIDS attending primary care and outpatient clinics. *Australian and New Zealand Journal of Psychiatry*, 37:70–77.

Leserman J. (2003). HIV disease progression: depression, stress, and possible mechanisms. *Biological Psychiatry*, 54:295–306.

Leserman J, Jackson ED, Petitto JM, Golden RN, Silva SG, Perkins DO, Cai J, Folds JD, Evans DL. (1999). Progression to AIDS: the effects of stress, depressive symptoms and social support. *Psychosomatic Medicine*, 6, 397–406.

Leserman J, Petitto JM, Golden RN, Gaynes BN, Gu H, Perkins DO, Silva SG, Folds JD, Evans DL. (2000). Impact of stressful life events, depression, social support, coping, and cortisol on progression to AIDS. *American Journal of Psychiatry*, 157:1221–1228.

Martin Suarez I, Cano Monchul R, Perez de Ayala P, Aguayo Canela M, Cuesta F, Rodriguez P, Pujol de la Llave E. (2002). Quality of life, psychological and social aspects in patients with advanced HIV disease. *Anales de Medicina Interna*, 19:396–404.

Millikin CP, Rourke SB, Halman MH, Power C. (2003). Fatigue in HIV/AIDS is associated with depression and subjective neurocognitive complaints but not neuropsychological functioning. *Journal of Clinical and Experimental Neuropsychology*, 25:201–215.

Moore J, Schuman P, Schoenbaum E, Boland B, Solomon L, Smith D. (1999). Severe adverse life events and depressive symptoms among women with, or at risk for, HIV infection in four cities in the United States of America. *AIDS*, 13:2459–2468.

Morrison MF, Petitto JM, Ten Have T, Gettes DR, Chiappini MS, Weber AL, Brinker-Spence P, Bauer RM, Douglas SD, Evans DL. (2002). Depressive and anxiety disorders in women with HIV infection. *American Journal of Psychiatry*, 159:789–796.

Murphy DA, Durako SJ, Moscicki AB, Vermund SH, Ma Y, Schwarz DF, Muenz LR. (2002a). No change in health risk behaviors over time among HIV infected adolescents in care: role of psychological distress. *Journal of Adolescent Health*, 29(Suppl):57–63.

Murphy DA, Marelich WD, Dello Stritto ME, Swendeman D, Witkin A. (2002b). Mothers living with HIV/AIDS: mental, physical, and family functioning. *AIDS Care*, 14:633–644.

Perdue T, Hagan H, Thiede H, Valleroy L. (2003). Depression and HIV risk behavior among Seattle-area injection drug users and young men who have sex with men. *AIDS Education and Prevention*, 15:81–92.

Richardson J, Barkan S, Cohen M, Back S, Fitzgerald G, Feldman J, Young M, Palacio H. (2001). Experience and covariates of depressive symptoms among a cohort of HIV infected women. *Social Work in Health Care*, 32:93–111.

Rockstroh JK, Mudar M, Lichterfeld M, Nischalke HD, Klausen G, Golz J, Dupke S, Notheis G, Stein L, Mauss S. (2002). Pilot study of interferon alpha high-dose induction therapy in combination with ribavirin for chronic hepatitis C in HIV-co-infected patients. *AIDS*, 16:2083–2085.

Safren SA, Radomsky AS, Otto MW, Salomon E. (2002). Predictors of psychological well-being in a diverse sample of HIV-positive patients receiving highly active antiretroviral therapy. *Psychosomatics*, 43:478–485.

Savetsky JB, Sullivan LM, Clarke JM, Stein MD, Samet JH. (2001). Evolution of depressive symptoms in human immunodeficiency virus-infected patients entering primary care. *Journal of Nervous and Mental Disease*, 189:76–83.

Schrimshaw EW. (2003). Relationship-specific unsupportive social interactions and depressive symptoms among women living with HIV/AIDS: direct and moderating effects. *Journal of Behavioral Medicine*, 26:297–313.

Sebit MB, Chandiwana SK, Latif AS, Gomo E, Acuda SW, Makoni F, Vushe J. (2002). Neuropsychiatric aspects of HIV disease progression: impact of traditional herbs on adult patients in Zimbabwe. *Progress in Neuro-Psychopharmacology and Biological Psychiatry*, 23:451–456.

Semple SJ, Patterson TL, Grant I. (2000). Psychosocial predictors of unprotected anal intercourse in a sample of HIV positive gay men who volunteer for a sexual risk reduction intervention. *AIDS Education and Prevention*, 12:416–430.

Simoni JM, Ng MT. (2001). Trauma, coping, and depression. *AIDS Care*, 12:567–580.

Starace F, Ammassari A, Trotta MP, Murri R, De Longis P, Izzo C, Scalzini A, d'Arminio Monforte A, Wu AW, Antinori A. (2002a). Depression is a risk factor for suboptimal adherence to highly active antiretroviral therapy. *Journal of Acquired Immune Deficiency Syndromes: JAIDS*, 31(Suppl 3):S136–S139.

Starace F, Bartoli L, Aloisi MS, et al. (2002b). Cognitive and affective disorders associated to HIV infection in the HAART era: findings from the NeuroCONA study: cognitive impairment and depression in HIV/AIDS. The NeurolCONA Study. *Acta Psychiatrica Scandinavica*, 106:20–26.

Sullivan PS, Dworkin MS. (2003). Prevalence and correlates of fatigue among persons with HIV infection. *Journal of Pain and Symptom Management*, 25:329–333.

Tucker JS, Burnam MA, Sherbourne CD, Kung FY, Gifford AL. (2003). Substance use and mental health correlates of nonadherence to antiretroviral medications in a sample of patients with human immunodeficiency virus infection. *American Journal of Medicine*, 114:573–580.

Turner BJ, Laine C, Cosler L, Hauck WW. (2003). Relationship of gender, depression, and health care delivery with antiretroviral adherence in HIV-infected drug users. *Journal of General Internal Medicine*, 18:248–257.

Turrina C, Fiorazzo A, Turano A, Cacciani P, Regini C, Castelli F, Sacchetti E. (2001). Depressive disorders and personality variables in HIV positive and negative intravenous drug-users. *Journal of Affective Disorders*, 65:45–53.

Ullrich PM, Lutgendorf SK, Stapleton JT. (2003). Concealment of homosexual identity, social support and CD4 cell count among HIV-seropositive gay men. *Journal of Psychosomatic Research*, 54:205–212.

Vazquez-Justo E, Rodriguez Alvarez M, Ferraces Otero MJ. (2003). Influence of depressed mood on neuropsychologic performance in HIV-seropositive drug users. *Psychiatry and Clinical Neurosciences*, 57:251–258.

Vitiello B, Burnam MA, Bing EG, Beckman R, Shapiro MF. (2003). Use of psychotropic medications among HIV-infected patients in the United States. *American Journal of Psychiatry*, 160:547–554.

Wagner GJ, Kanouse DE, Koegel P, Sullivan G. (2003). Adherence to HIV antiretrovirals among persons with serious mental illness. *AIDS Patient Care and Standards*, 17:179–186.

Weiss JL, Mulder CL, Antoni MH, de Vroome EM, Garssen B, Goodkin K. (2003). Effects of a supportive-expressive group intervention on long-term psychosocial adjustment in HIV-infected gay men. *Psychotherapy and Psychosomatics*, 72:132–140.

Zorilla EP, McKay JR, Luborsky LP, Schmidt K. (1996). Relation of stressors and depressive symptoms to clinical progression of viral illness. *American Journal of Psychiatry*, 153:626–635.

14 Interpersonal Communication: The Key to Unlocking Social Support for Preventive Stress Management

Marilyn Macik-Frey, James Campbell Quick, and Jonathan D. Quick

CONTENTS

0-8493-1820-3/05/$0.00+$1.50

INTRODUCTION

Interpersonal communication is a key element in human interactions and a fundamental process for socialization and the development of relationships. In fact, it is that which makes us uniquely human and has been a fascination of scholars for centuries. In the context of preventive stress management, interpersonal communication is strongly linked to social support, but until recently, it has taken a secondary role in theoretical frameworks. This chapter shifts the focus from the effects of social support in preventive stress management to those processes that result in the effects, that is, communication processes. This shift is in the same vein as that proposed by Albrecht et al.[1] in the communications literature, but in this chapter we build upon their ideas to suggest incorporating aspects of communication and interpersonal communication skills acquisition into the area of prevention in stress management.

In the first edition of this handbook, Quick et al.[2] focused on social support in the context of attachment theory, the formation and maintenance of secure interpersonal attachments, and then proposed a framework for transcendent attachment. By using natural scientific research and scripture from the Holy Bible, the first chapter explored a secure attachment relationship with God, or whatever language the reader might use for a higher spiritual power. The core thesis was that self-reliance is a paradoxical form of interdependent, rather than independent, behavior. Subsequent research by Joplin et al.[3] explored the relationships between interpersonal attachment orientations, health, and social support. The adverse health and social support effects of insecure attachments, in contrast to the secure attachments of a self-reliant orientation, were manifest in that research.

This chapter refocuses attention to the horizontal set of human relationships we have in this world, yet brings central attention to another aspect of interpersonal behavior, i.e., interpersonal communication rather than interdependent attachments. Specifically, we acknowledge that social support has positive implications for mental and physical health, yet understand less about the mechanisms by which relationships achieve their effects. It is well documented that social support is a complex process with variability in outcomes, behaviors, relationships, and contexts. It is less understood why this variability occurs. Why are some attempts at support perceived negatively while others are perceived positively? What are the mechanisms that underlie the type of social support that affects health positively? Can the process be identified and taught so that a larger population experiences social support benefits? This chapter proposes that interpersonal communication is the key to finding valid and practical answers to these questions.

Figure 14.1 presents our conceptual model of interpersonal communication and social support in a stressful context. The stressful context, strain, and social support elements in the model reflect the well-established framework for examining the direct and buffering effects of social support on stressors, strain, and the stressor–strain relationship. What we have added to this core, and the central concern of this chapter, are the constructs of interpersonal communication and the moderating variables that help explain how interpersonal communication is the key to unlocking social support for preventive stress management. The model includes four moderators: cognitive complexity, emotional intelligence, gender, and personality. We show

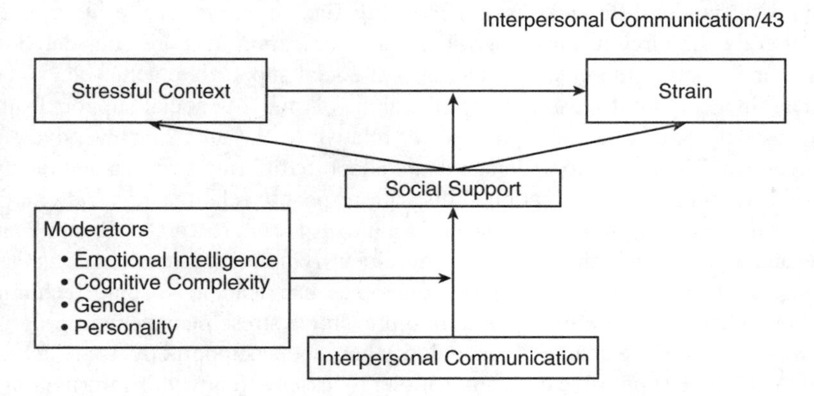

FIGURE 14.1 Interpersonal communication and social support in a stressful context.

that these four moderators are related to the three dimensions of communication competence: cognitive, affective, and behavioral dimensions.

Communication competence and those variables that impact this competence might be the critical factors that explain social support variability. Understanding the dynamic nature of communication provides key insights into when and how supportive communication can be the pathway to the benefits social support offers. Finally, if communication is indeed the key to social support, then those strategies that effectively improve communication competence can also improve successful social support, decrease the negative outcomes of stress, and improve the health and well-being of the interactants.

This chapter has four major sections. The first section reviews social support in the context of stress management, health, and well-being, a principle focus of the study of social support for years and a strong component of preventive stress management (see Quick and Quick[4] for an original formulation of the concepts of prevention in addressing organizational stress and Quick et al.[5] for a complete presentation of the theory of preventive stress management in organizations). The second section introduces a recent shift in focus from the effects of social support to the underlying process that results in the relationships that produce those effects, specifically interpersonal communication. Building on the ideas of Albrecht et al.,[1] this section suggests that rather than conceptualize interpersonal communication as a part of social support, it might be more reasonable to think of social support as a component of interpersonal communication, that is, defining social support as the result of effective supportive communication. Thus, the communication competences of the provider and recipient of social support are critical aspects of the success. This section forms the intellectual heart of the chapter.

The next section analyzes individual differences that moderate the relationship between interpersonal communication and the resultant outcome, which is positive when the communication is perceived as supportive or negative when the communication is perceived as increasing stress, obligation, or conflict. These moderators might explain individual differences in communication competence in the support role. The four moderating variables addressed are emotional intelligence, cognitive complexity, gender differences, and personality. Each might influence either directly or indirectly the circumstances in which communication acts are considered supportive and whether the positive outcomes of social support are achieved.

The final section discusses the implications of studying social support from an interpersonal communications perspective relative to the area of preventive stress management. The ability to understand and adapt to differing communication styles and to learn better communication skills with respect to relationships and emotions and social support can potentially serve as a means to link research with application in the area of stress, health, and well-being.[6] Identifying communication competence dimensions that affect social support outcomes can lead to specific techniques, training, and strategies to incorporate into preventive stress management programs. The conclusions of the chapter further clarify how social support effects are achieved through effective supportive communication processes and how this information can be used to improve the means by which individuals give and receive support in times of stress through targeted communication competence strategies.

In overview, we accept that social support is a real phenomenon that has positive effects on health and is one means for preventive stress management. One's sense of social support is a direct result of effective interpersonal communication. Interpersonal communication competence can be affected by emotional intelligence, cognitive complexity, gender, and personality. The effects are variable and not fully understood, but research evidence supports their importance. Some evidence suggests, and we assert, that interpersonal communication skills can be learned. Therefore, developing communication competence as a key to unlocking social support is a worthy goal because of the positive effects of social support on people and organizations.

SOCIAL SUPPORT IN PREVENTIVE STRESS MANAGEMENT

Social support is considered an important component of preventive stress management and has significant positive effects on health and well-being. House et al.[7] point out that socially isolated and less socially integrated individuals suffer greater psychological and physiological health consequences and are more likely to die than those who have social support. Multiple research studies support this conclusion and suggest a growing need to understand the mechanisms by which social support affects health and well-being. Figure 14.2 depicts the skeletal framework for these constructs, with social isolation having direct negative effects on morbidity and mortality, while social support is hypothesized to have a direct inverse effect on social isolation. That is, increases in social support reduce the experience of social isolation.

Definitions and Measurement of Social Support

Definitions

Social support is a concept that is generally understood in an intuitive sense. Yet as House[8] notes, early work on social support sometimes lacked any explicit definition of the concept. Over the last two decades of work in the field, however, theorists

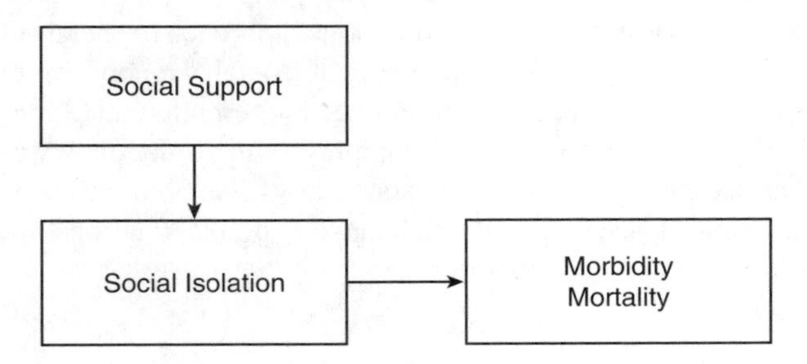

FIGURE 14.2 Social isolation and social support.

and researchers have put forward a wide variety of complementary definitions and concepts of social support. These concepts can be described as perceptual, developmental, dynamic, structural, and functional.

In one of the earliest major reviews on social support, Cobb[9] takes a perceptual approach, defining social support as the individual belief that one "is cared for and loved, esteemed and valued, and belongs to a network of communication and mutual obligation." By contrast to the perceptual approach, a developmental approach to social support is reflected in Bowlby's[10,11] work on attachment theory. Attachment theory suggests that secure attachments in childhood are rooted in instinctive human behavior. These attachments become a basis for an adult's ability to form effective social support relationships.

Social support has also been described in dynamic terms. House[8] summarizes earlier work in the field that defined social support in terms of interpersonal transactions. Later, Shumaker and Hill[12] defined social support as "an exchange of resources between at least two individuals perceived by the provider or recipient to be intended to enhance the well-being of the recipient."

Several authors describe social support in structural terms. That is, what are the types and sources of social support? In an oft-cited construct of social support, House[8] described four main categories of social support:

1. Emotional support, which generally comes from family and close friends, is the most commonly recognized form of social support. It includes empathy, concern, caring, love, and trust.
2. Appraisal support involves transmission of information (as opposed to affect) in the form of affirmation, feedback, or social comparison. This information is often evaluative and can come from family, friends, coworkers, or community sources.
3. Informational support includes advice, suggestions, or directives that assist the person in responding to personal or situational demands.
4. Instrumental support is the most concrete direct form of social support, encompassing help in the form of money, time, in-kind assistance, and other explicit interventions on a person's behalf.

These four classes or types of social support actually combine elements of perceptual, dynamic, and functional definitions of social support.

Finally, several authors have taken a functional approach to social support. Quick and colleagues[13] describe the five functions of social support for executives as protective, informational, evaluative, modeling, and emotional. Using role theory, Zey[14] describes 12 supporting-cast roles representing functional ways in which individuals might support a person: advisor, catalyst, celebrator, cheerleader, constructive critic, contact, esteem builder, financier, public relations specialist, role model, sponsor, and technical supporter.

Measures

As there are many definitions, descriptions, and functions ascribed to the concept of social support, there are also a variety of ways in which social support is operationalized and measured. This leads to problems, as noted by writers who find a lack of any consistent method for measuring social support.[15,16] One of the earliest measures of social support in the workplace was a brief questionnaire developed by House and Wells,[17] whose three central questions were:

1. How much can each of the following people be relied on when things get tough at work? Immediate supervisor or boss, other people at work, spouse, friends, relatives.
2. How much is each of these same people willing to listen to your work-related problems?
3. How much is each of these same people helpful to you in getting your job done?

The majority of subsequent research on social support has used this genre of self-report questionnaire aimed at identifying supportive relationships and assessing the degree of support from, type of support in, and quality of each relationship. There are three exceptions to this general measurement approach. First, Fleury[18] used interviews to explore the role of social networks in motivating health behavior change. Second, Kulik and Mahler[19] used the number of hospital visitations as an archival measure of marital support for hospitalized patients. Third, Gerin et al.[20] used an experimental manipulation in a laboratory study in which one confederate attacked the subject as a negative social relationship and one confederate was support neutral.

Health Consequences of Social Support: Explanation of the Effect

The general relationship between social support and health is supported in a broad array of research suggesting that a wide range of diseases and causes of death are associated with lack of social support.[21] House et al.[7] reviewed the evidence on social support and health, with particular attention to the health risk of social isolation. They found that the socially isolated individual is less psychologically and less physically healthy than his or her counterpart in supportive social relationships. In addition, the socially isolated individual is at greater risk of death from all causes.

Their extensive meta-analysis indicated that positive health outcomes, particularly longer life span, are associated with social support. House and his associates concluded that social isolation is a risk factor for both mortality and morbidity. This was first identified by Lynch[22] in his examination of the medical consequences of loneliness, with particular attention to the effects on the cardiovascular system and heart disease, then confirmed in the House et al.[7] research and Lynch's[23] own subsequent research.

Five prospective studies examined the age-adjusted mortality rate for men and women linked with their levels of social integration (for details, see Quick et al.[2]). In each study, the increased risk of mortality, for both sexes, was associated with lower levels of social integration. To illustrate the nature of these studies, consider the monumental research study conducted by Berkman and Syme[24] in Alameda County, California. The researchers tracked the health histories of 7,000 non-Japanese residents for 9 years. Information was gathered on marital status, organization memberships, and religious service attendance. Berkman and Syme found that individuals with fewer social relationships had higher mortality rates from all causes — three times higher than those who had more social relationships. These results held even when controlling for factors such as age, race, and smoking behavior.

While there is a strong connection between social relationships and health, it is not altogether clear what the mechanisms are for the health consequences of social support. Three possible mechanisms have been considered, two direct effects and one indirect effect. First, social support might have a direct effect upon stressors and demands by either altering the stressor or modifying one's response to it. [8] Second, social support might have a direct effect upon health outcomes by improving one's physical or psychological well-being. Third, social support might buffer the adverse effects of stressors and demands upon the individual's health outcomes. In the stress-buffering model, support might influence the stressor–strain connection by altering cognitive appraisal of the stressor, or by dampening health-damaging psychological processes.[25,26]

There is not strong, consistent empirical evidence to support any one of these three possible mechanisms over the other; at best, the research has yielded mixed results. Whereas some studies have found evidence for a buffering effect (c.f. Astrand et al.[27] and Johnson et al.[28]), still other studies have found only significant main effects or no buffering effects[29]. Carlson and Perrewé[30] looked at four models for explaining the mechanism behind the effects of social support in the context of work–family conflict. Each of the four models looks at social support from different perspectives, as a moderating, intervening (mediating), antecedent, or independent variable. All four models are well documented in the research, but this was the first attempt to study them in combination as part of a single analysis. Their analysis found that the antecedent model (social support being an antecedent to perceived role stressors and time demands) showed the best fit with their data over all other models and combinations of models. However, the statistical tools used have limitations in terms of making conclusive best-fit determinations and their results, although compelling and comprehensive, still leave questions as to what might be missing.

However, although the precise mechanism might not be well understood or specified, there is an impressive amount of evidence from epidemiological studies that shows social support playing a very positive role in enhancing individual health. Thus, research shows that social support is important, and given the absence of a clear understanding of the mechanism, we turn to the consideration of social support as a fundamental form of interpersonal communication.[1]

Social Support and Interpersonal Communication

Sarason et al.[31] suggest that social support is most easily understood as a heterogeneous construct made up of homogenous parts, and the meaning is evolving over time. Albrecht et al.[1] described this evolution of the definition of social support from emphasis on individual's responses, to the study of processes of exchange, and then into interpersonal terms. The most recent transition is to that of studying interactional processes, which by their definition are components of interpersonal communication.[1,32,33] According to Albrecht et al.,[1] social support is a fundamental form of human communication that is a result of ordinary and extraordinary relationships, or life events, and leads to multiple emotional and physical well-being outcomes. Supportive communication is the key to creating and sustaining interpersonal relationships[33,34] and the basis for creating social support in times of stress. Albrecht and Adelman[32,35] suggested a shift in the focus of the study of supportive behaviors from the effects on health and well-being to the mechanisms by which these effects are produced. The focus of these researchers and this chapter is on communication processes, communication competence, the variables that impact them, and how they affect the perception and benefits of social support.

INTERPERSONAL COMMUNICATION

According to Burgoon and Ruffner,[36] interpersonal communication is a transactional, symbolic process of mutual influence embedded within relationships and social networks. Communication is also defined as a transfer and exchange of information and understanding from one person to another through meaningful symbols, that is, a process of sharing ideas, attitudes, values, opinions, and facts.[37] Social support as a communication phenomenon is then defined by Albrecht and Adelman[32] as "verbal and nonverbal communication between recipients and providers that reduces uncertainty about the situation, the self, the other, or the relationship, and functions to enhance a perception of personal control in one's life experience" (p. 19).

We take this communications perspective on social support a step farther to suggest that the desired outcome of uncertainty reduction and personal control through verbal and nonverbal communication is a function of the level of communication competence of both the provider and the recipient and the resultant interaction. Communication competence has been defined as the perceived ability to communicate ideas, values, and intent as well as understand another's perspective across a variety of communication interactions.[38] It has three dimensions: cognitive, affective, and behavioral. The cognitive dimension involves the knowledge and flexibility to perceive and express a wide range of information in a variety of contexts. The affective dimension involves the ability to empathize, understand and control emotion, and adapt to the emotional tone of the context. The behavior

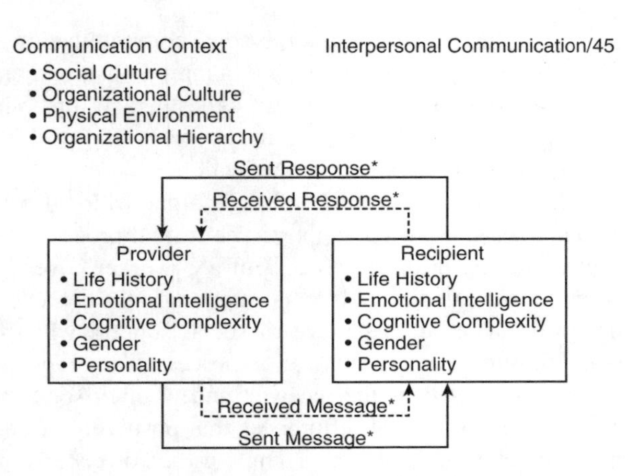

FIGURE 14.3 Process model of interpersonal communication.

dimension is the task performance and involves the form, content, and method of performing the communication.

Communication competence is impacted by multiple variables, in particular, personality differences, emotional intelligence, cognitive complexity, and gender differences. Thus, the level of positive social support experienced is proposed to be directly and positively related to the level of communication competence of the interactants. The important and key distinction of this focus over others for social support is in the dynamic interaction between the intent and skill of the provider to support and the skill to elicit and perceive support by the receiver. To truly understand social support, the entire communication exchange must be addressed.

The process model of interpersonal communication presented in Figure 14.3 uses the communication models of Adler[39] and Nelson and Quick[40] as its point of departure and builds on these by incorporating key variables related to communication competence. The resulting process model suggests that communication is a mutual, reciprocal process of a provider sending a message and a recipient responding. The model explicitly recognizes that the sent and received messages, as well as the sent and received responses, might not be coincident. Any sent–received discrepancy might be of consequence in the process of unlocking social support. In addition, the provider's and recipient's life history, cognitive complexity, emotional intelligence, gender, and personality are moderating variables in the interpersonal communication process that can also play a role in any sent–received discrepancy. Finally, contextual variables for the interpersonal communication process include the social culture, organizational culture, physical environment, and hierarchical relationship of the provider and recipient, that is, the power differential between them.

While theory and research in interpersonal communication overlap some with theory and research in social support, the constructs are distinct, as we suggest in Figure 14.1. However, we also assert that they are linked and that interpersonal communication unlocks social support because it is the pathway or delivery system through which one receives and experiences social support. Thus, in Figure 14.3, the provider uses the words, actions, and deeds of interpersonal communication to convey social support to the recipient. If interpersonal communication is the pathway, the process, and the bridge between two people in a relationship, then it serves also as the key to the social support that one or the other person, or both people, need at any given point in time. Therefore, social support is the positive outcome of effective and competent interpersonal communication.

In Payne,[41] for example, formal and informal organizational processes within the work environment serve as social support. The formal process of implementing work behavior rules and the informal process of a coworker covering a shift for a few hours are examples provided of such social support. In the context of this chapter, these formal and informal processes serve as social support when they convey a supportive message through the communication process. They represent a symbolic message that is then interpreted by the receiver, and whether social support results is a function of numerous individual differences that positively or negatively affect communication competence and exchange. Thus, if the coworker's offer to cover a shift is perceived as a signal of lack of confidence on the part of the coworker rather than as a supportive gesture, then the offer could result in increased stress rather than the intended support.

This breakdown in supportive communication could be a result of personality difference between the provider and receiver, gender differences, or other factors that negatively affect the competence of the two to complete the intended communication. Likewise, if the overall climate of the organization is punitive, the implementation of rules could be perceived as communicating lack of trust and respect, furthering feelings of loss of control and increasing distress. Again, the effectiveness of this supportive communication is a direct function of the competence of the leaders of the organization to communicate a positive intent in a manner that facilitates the perception of the symbol or action as supportive by the workers. It is also a function of the workers' ability and willingness to understand and appreciate the intention of the provider.

The operational forms of social support described by House[8] of emotional, appraisal, informational, and instrumental support can all be adequately delivered through interpersonal communication processes. In order for each to be considered support, the specific intent must be adequately communicated by the provider and perceived as supportive by the receiver. As in the previous example, poorly communicated messages can result in more rather than less distress despite good intention, a finding well documented in the research.[2,32] We speculate that the study of communication processes and competence could also serve to explain and possibly reduce this negative outcome.

We are suggesting that positive intent is at the heart of social support, and therefore, positive communication is a natural pathway to social support. However, one of the dilemmas in this notion centers on House's concept of appraisal support, which is evaluative and critical by nature. If appraisal support aims to provide corrective feedback by the provider to the recipient, then the former's intent is positive and the latter's experience might be negative. This is the classic dilemma in performance appraisals, in which Meyer et al.[42] found a high percentage of defensive responses by recipients to providers' critical evaluations. Within our framework, the challenge for the provider and the recipient both, because communication is a mutual, reciprocal interpersonal process, is to stay focused on positive intent and supportive responses for the other.

Even cases of instrumental support when tangible physical resources are exchanged, such as providing housing, can be viewed as examples of communicative exchanges for social support. The symbolic meaning attached to the giving of the object communicates support to the recipient if the action is perceived as genuine and intended to help the receiver regain some control or reduce uncertainty about the future. The moderators discussed later in this chapter influence whether this physical resource results in a message of support being communicated. Thus, if the provider of this resource is an anonymous donor that requests nothing in return and expresses that the housing is intended to help the recipient "get back on his or her feet," the recipient might interpret this symbolic gesture as supportive, as it reduces uncertainty and provides increased control while preserving the dignity and self-respect of the recipient. Suppose, in contrast, the provider of the housing is a social agency that requires the recipient to stand in long lines, fill out complicated forms, and endure repeated personally intrusive interviews, and indicates the housing is only temporary and can be withdrawn at any time. Then the symbolic meaning or communication to the recipient is one of less control and uncertainty. In such a case, the agency's communication processes or competencies lack the understanding, empathy, and implementation to provide support despite the intended goal of assistance.

Supportive communication, based on the more comprehensive nature of interpersonal communication, extends the idea of social support from perceived caring and value by the recipient to a broader definition encompassing the total communication processes. These processes include not only expressions of care and concern but also active listening, empathizing, legitimizing, exploring emotions, encouraging, appreciating, reassuring, respecting, showing confidence, and providing information or advice, as well as many other verbal and nonverbal behaviors.[33,43] By studying social support through the interpersonal communication process, we are able to tap into the vast research in communication to better understand how social support effects occur. Individual differences in communication skills are well substantiated[44] and can be a key determinant of when an interaction or relationship is considered supportive. Analyzing moderating factors that affect communication skills can help determine ways to improve supportive communication attempts and maximize the benefits to health and well-being that result from successful social support.

Since research shows that similar behaviors and interactions vary considerably in their ability to provide support in any given situation, and at times might even increase distress,[2,33,35,45] there is an ongoing need to develop a model or framework to determine why these variations occur. The Optimal Matching Model (OMM) developed by Cutrona and Russell[46] is one such attempt. The OMM matches supportive behaviors and specific types of stress with the premise that if optimal matching can be determined, the positive outcomes of social support can be maximized. For example, this matching model would lead to specifying certain supportive behaviors for stressors such as death of a coworker, illness of coworkers, or major downsizing events at work. The Optimal Matching Model suggests that the support offered must be relevant or meaningful to the recipient in relation to the specific stress experienced. Cutrona and her colleagues reviewed an extensive list of studies to determine the type of support that works best in which situations and found patterns from which to develop the model. Burleson[33] suggests that the OMM has not held up well to empirical testing and the variability in findings is still not clearly explained. This variability might be attributable to the model's attempt at generalization vs. an attempt to account for individual differences or idiosyncratic variances across individuals. The significant variances in human behavior, especially in organizations, are often overlooked or not accounted for by management.[47]

Our model presented in Figure 14.1 suggests two additions to further expand this theory. First, we incorporate interpersonal communication as the mechanism for social support achieving its positive direct and buffering effects in stressful contexts. Second, we introduce individual differences as moderators. These moderators affect communication competence and therefore the pathway from interpersonal communication to social support. Thus, our model incorporates individual variance and individual differences. The interaction of the context, which we capture in Figure 14.3, with the type of stressor, individual communication competence, and type of support might help us better understand the variability in social support effects that research continues to struggle to understand. The following section explores the moderators of emotional intelligence, cognitive complexity, gender, and personality differences with respect to communication skills. How do these moderators influence social support and preventive stress management?

MODERATING VARIABLES OF COMMUNICATION COMPETENCE AND SOCIAL SUPPORT

Both communication competence and social support vary considerably depending upon the context, skills, and motives of the interactants. We suggest that this variability is at least partially explained by four moderators that can impact the communication competence of the individuals. These four moderators — emotional intelligence, cognitive complexity, gender, and personality — are presented in Figure 1. Specifically, these moderators influence the cognitive knowledge of multiple communication options, the ability to determine the most appropriate response, the behavioral skill and flexibility to perform the chosen option,[38] and the motivation to do so. We begin the discussion with emotional intelligence and cognitive complexity, which are related to the affective and cognitive dimensions of communication competence, respectively. We follow with a discussion of gender differences in communication and how these differences might also explain social support inconsistencies. Finally, we discuss the effect of individual personality differences on communication competence and how this relates to social support.

EMOTIONAL INTELLIGENCE

Salovey and Mayer,[48] credited with originating the term, define emotional intelligence (EI) as a set of competencies that refer directly to the way an individual deals with emotions, a key determinant of how they also deal with stress. The components of EI include the ability to be self-aware of emotions, to express them appropriately, to judge sincere vs. insincere expressions of emotions, to distinguish and prioritize different emotions, and to assess problems from multiple emotional perspectives. EI components also include the ability to understand complex dual emotions and natural transitions from one emotion such as fear to another such as anger or hostility and to connect or disconnect from an emotion depending upon its usefulness to the situation. More emotionally intelligent individuals are reported to cope better with stressful situations because they "accurately perceive and appraise their emotional states, know how and when to express their feelings, and can effectively regulate their mood states."[49]

The EI ability most relevant to communication of support is the ability to know *how and when* to express feelings. However, it is unclear from the research whether most scholars of EI would consider strong interpersonal communication a logical consequence of this emotional skill or if it is possible to know how and when to express emotion, but not possess the communication abilities to do so effectively. Studies using measurement of actual behaviors compared to self-report might shed some light on this distinction.

Despite the unanswered questions surrounding EI, in the context of providing supportive communication (social support) in times of stress, EI might play a key part. We propose that EI represents the affective dimension of communication competence — the ability to experience empathy and emotion and manage them effectively in communicative exchanges. Therefore, it is proposed that the level of EI of an individual will be positively correlated with communication competence and increased social support.

The idea that a person possesses the ability to understand his or her own emotions and manage them successfully suggests that in the role of *recipient* of social support, he or she would be more likely to seek social support and to know how to request the type of support that would be most effective for his or her emotional situation. He or she would also be a better judge of the supportive message and appreciate the intent of the provider even when the communication skill or message is not optimal. Thus, it is proposed that the person high in emotional intelligence would be less likely to suffer adverse reactions to poorly provided supportive communication when it was indeed given with good intent because of his or her superior ability to appreciate the emotion of the provider. In contrast, the low emotional intelligent person would be expected to have a higher incidence of misreading the provider's intent or the message and have resultant higher adverse stress effects of poor social support. This low EI person can also have difficulty understanding when and how to seek social support because of poor ability to understand the emotions surrounding his or her stress and poor ability to verbalize what he or she feels.

From a *provider* of social support perspective, the high EI individual would potentially be a strong source of supportive communication. He or she would have an increased ability, over low EI individuals, to identify the needs of distressed others and have the skill to determine the best strategies to use in a show of support. These individuals would also be more likely to understand the negative reactions to support attempts and adjust their behavior to remedy the problem. On the negative side, the provider of support with high EI might be more prone to suffering adverse effects of the interactions due to dependency of the distressed person, depletion of resources, and personal distress based on high empathy and internalization of the stress situation. For example, a high EI person providing support to a bereaved individual might become the key confidant to that person and the relationship might demand an unrealistic amount of time. Also, the experience of supporting the person in his or her time of grief can result in increased stress, sadness, and depression for the provider who understands and empathizes with the emotions.

Currently, the research in EI tends to center around developing reliable and valid measurement devices, clearly defining the construct, determining if it can be taught and how it fits within specific social contexts such as the work setting, education, and, most important for this discussion, stress management. However, little reference is made to the relationship of EI to communication in general or to supportive communication in particular. The proposed interaction relationships between EI and communicative support for providers and recipients of social support need to be studied to differentiate speculation from reality. Matthews and Zeidner[50] indicate that no clear EI construct has been identified in the stress domain, but that the adaptive cognitions might be associated with some personality trait or traits that support the EI construct in a lesser sense. This chapter proposes that EI's correlation with stress, that is, high EI is related to better coping with stress,[49] might be explained, at least in part, by increased interpersonal communication competence related to supportive messages.

In summary, we suggest that high EI contributes to greater communication competence on the affective dimension, both for the provider and the recipient (see Figure 14.3). Conversely, we suggest that low EI reduces communication competence on the affective dimension and thus interferes with communication being an effective pathway to the provision of social support. Therefore, the level of EI of the provider and recipient of social support moderates the communication competence of both individuals in the relationship and impacts the delivery and experience of social support in a stressful context.

Cognitive Complexity

Cognitive complexity is a construct for describing how individuals process social information. Some do so in a simplistic manner while others do so in a multidimensional processs, i.e., cognitively complex.[51] Cognitive complexity is defined in degree and relates to "the ability to perceive behavior in a multidimensional manner."[52] Cognitively complex individuals have increased listening comprehension,[53] better listener-adapted communication[54] and higher communication effectiveness,[54] and are better at comforting communication.[43] The concept of the ability to specifically analyze and process multiple communication, relational, and behavioral aspects of an interaction is suggestive of the communication competence dimension referred to previously as the cognitive dimension.

Burleson,[33] in his discussion of emotional support skill, incorporates the idea of cognitive complexity. He suggests that for comforting messages to be of high quality, they require complex behaviors that result from sophisticated cognitive processes. Generation of a successful supportive message begins with goal generation. Successful providers of support develop detailed cognitive representations of the stress stituation. That is, they "attend to and process information about the target [distressed other] (e.g., aspects of the other's cognitive and emotional state), the social context (e.g., situationally relevant roles and rules), and the interactional setting (e.g., potential for privacy)."[55] Burleson[33] equates these skills with interpersonal cognitive complexity and social perceptive ability and cites research findings showing that these constructs are correlated with the use of sophisticated emotion-focused forms of support. Although the term *EI* is not specifically mentioned, the skills and behaviors described seem to allude to aspects of the EI construct as well.

The relationship between cognitive complexity, social perceptive ability, and EI needs further clarification, but for our discussion purposes, cognitive complexity is proposed to represent the skills necessary for the cognitive dimension of communication competence, while EI represents the skills necessary for the affective dimension. Thus, cognitive complexity moderates the relationship between communication and the positive outcome of social support through the cognitive dimension of communication competence. That is, the higher the cognitive complexity of the interactants to a communication exchange, the more likely the perception and ultimate benefits of social support will be felt. Conversely, lower levels of cognitive complexity of one or both interactants in a supportive exchange are proposed to have a negative effect on the outcome of social support. Therefore, we propose that cognitive complexity has a rather direct influence on an individual's communication competence through the cognitive dimension.

Gender

Gender differences in communication skills, emotion, and stress response have been extensively studied with a complex and somewhat confusing pattern of findings. In general, differences are found in specific aspects of communication behavior, in particular in relation to expression of emotion, but there also appears to be more similarity than difference, and this confounding finding makes interpretation of the literature difficult.[56–58] Also, the explanation of why differences exist between genders in communication skills is debatable, and the debate sometimes becomes outright confrontational. Some would suggest that there are inherent differences between the genders that explain the findings, while others would support a theory of socialization differences resulting in gender-specific behaviors. Part of the controversy centers on placing judgmental value and importance on the differences that are found. Most do agree that communication differences exist between genders; the debate begins with the magnitude or importance of the differences and the explanations of why they occur.[59]

To begin the discussion of gender differences in communication in relation to social support, we must first address the current use of the term *gender* vs. *sex*. In contemporary literature, sex and gender are sometimes used interchangeably or one term is used over another at the preference of the researcher. However, it is becoming increasingly common to see a distinction made between the terms. Sex is typically defined as the biological determination of being male or female, while gender is defined as the social and cultural meaning associated with biological sex.[60,61] We have chosen to use the term *gender* in our discussion of social support and communication because these concepts are so tightly intertwined with socialization and culture, although its use does not preclude the possibility that some of the differences discussed might have a biological component.

Gender Differences in Communication of Support

General differences between genders in communication skills related to social support are well documented. Men and women use different interaction goals to prioritize and pursue support[62] and vary in the behaviors employed to achieve these goals. However, it is important to view these differences in light of the equally compelling research regarding similarities. That is, values of both genders appear to be quite similar in what they consider as a supportive message, how important support is within a relationship, and to which gender they prefer to supply support.[62,63]

Burleson and Gilstrap[61] point out that those interaction goals used to prioritize and pursue support situations differ between genders. Interaction goals are the highly proximal generative mechanisms employed in message production.[64] Barbee and Cunningham[65] categorize interaction goals into a four-part typology that includes a distinction between problem-focused and emotion-focused goals, and a distinction between approach and avoidance of the support situation. Combinations of these factors result in the following communicative behavior options available to the provider of support:[61]

Emotion-Focused
1. Escape — avoiding a distressed other's emotions
2. Solace — approaching or addressing a distressed other's emotions

Problem-Focused
3. Dismiss — avoiding the issue of the distressed person's problem
4. Solve — approaching or focusing on the distressed person's problem

Research shows that men and women give highest priority to approach-oriented, emotion-focused (solace) strategies. Both genders also agree on the level of importance to be given to the solve strategy. However, the relative degree of importance differs. Women reported that the solace strategy is significantly more important to them than it is to men, and men felt solve was more important than women.[62] Therefore, although solace is considered the best support strategy focus by both genders, women see it as even more important in their communication paradigm. Further, women are more likely to pursue solace and are less likely to choose escape than men, men are more likely to choose solve than women, and both genders are equally likely to use dismiss per self-report.[61]

Instrumentality and expressivity are personality traits that have been shown to differ significantly by gender. In general, women are higher in expressivity (which coincides with the emotion focus) and men are higher in instrumentality (which coincides with problem focus).[66] Women are more likely to choose emotion-focused forms of communication such as comforting and ego support. Men are more likely to opt for instrumental forms of communication such as informing and persuading.

Taylor et al.[67] identified a fundamental difference between genders in primary responses to stress or threat. Their research indicates that in addition to fight and flight, the traditionally accepted principal reactions to stress, women also show a high inclination to "tend and befriend" during times of extreme stress. This behavior pattern suggests that women turn to emotional support more readily when in stress (recipient) and are more likely to direct their energy to nurturing and friendship (provider), which indicates a reciprocal social support pattern. These findings suggest a potential for women to have strong reciprocal tendencies in social supportive communication during stress. That is, the tend-and-befriend pattern suggests women possess a greater tendency to be both recipient and, more importantly, provider of social support than men. It is unclear whether the difference in response to stress provides women a greater opportunity to develop the communication competencies necessary for effective social support or whether their higher skill in communication competence leads naturally to this tend-and-befriend response, but the general consensus is that women are stronger in receipt and provision of social support.

Explanations of Why Gender Differences Exist

The research clearly shows some differences in the emotional support behaviors of males and females, but the explanation for why these differences occur is quite varied. Two competing perspectives of relevance to this chapter are the different cultures perspective and the skill specialization perspective. Kunkel and Burleson[62] provide an analysis and comparison of both perspectives with an admitted bias toward the latter while emphasizing that the different cultures view is more prevalently held in both lay and academic literature. First, the different cultural perspective suggests that males and females vary in language, socialization, emotional experiences, and communication styles to such a degree that they represent two distinct cultures.[68–70] Inherent in this explanation is that men and women live in different emotional worlds, and as such, different values and standards exist for males and females regarding the importance and communication of social support. Alternatively, the specialization perspective focuses on the idea that men and women are more similar than they are different and that they do value and hold the same standards in terms of social support and supportive communication, but differ in terms of skills.[61,62] Kunkel and Burleson[62] suggest that this skill differential most likely results from socialization differences whereby females are encouraged to express and manage emotions more so than males and, through practice and increased exposure, develop greater skill in the area of nurturing, providing support, and comforting. Likewise, males develop greater proficiency in persuasive, informative, and narrative skills in general.

The fundamental difference between the two perspectives is that for the specialization perspective, the specific skills themselves are equally valued by both genders, but abilities differ. The different cultures perspective suggests that the specific communication skills that are valued and used vary with gender.[68,69] The perspective one adopts has implications for the intervention premise later in the chapter. If one assumes that the genders operate as different cultures, then communication competence for one might not equate to communication competence for the other. However, the finding that both men and women value similar interaction patterns for social support (i.e., solace) and that both prefer to receive social support from women[62,63] does not support the cultural differentiation. Further, if we were to accept two communication paradigms for social support, one for men and one for women, then it would also require that in therapeutic and preventive strategies for stress management, skills to be emphasized would differ greatly and would be gender specific. Our bias, therefore, is to accept the idea that men and women operate within the same cultural value system in relation to social support and communication, but exhibit varying degrees of competence in specific communication behaviors.

In conclusion, gender differences in communication of social support exist, but just as with the other moderators of supportive communication, they can play a part in the more complex interaction of factors, but are unlikely to be a primary explanation of the differences that are seen. In very general terms, women are higher in supportive communication competencies. However, the within-gender differences far exceed the between-gender differences and suggest that the gender factor is but one element among a much more complex interaction of factors that determine when communicative behavior is supportive and when it is not.

Personality

The relationship of different personality dimensions or traits and the broad construct of stress and coping has been the emphasis of much research in the stress domain. Personality variables have been found to affect both stress appraisal and stress response.[71,72] Some of the most often cited personality variables related to stress are perceived control, hardiness, type A behavior pattern (TABP), anger and hostility, sense of coherence, self-esteem, power motivation, and positive and negative affectivity, including extraversion, neuroticism, and trait anxiety. An important personality dimension in the study of the stress process and one that is related to the more narrowly defined topic of social support and stress is that of perceived control[72] or locus of control. For a general review of the relevant personality research, see Schaubroeck and Ganster,[73] and for more detailed information on specific personality traits and stress, reference the collection of articles contained in Cooper and Payne.[74] Although the focus of the research stream is on the stress response in general, many of the findings can be analyzed with respect to the more specific areas of interpersonal communication, personality differences, and social support.

From an interpersonal communications perspective, individual personality differences of the *provider* and the *recipient* of social support are important,[75] as well as factors of the reciprocity and overall nature of the relationship.[76] This complex mix might be a key to successful and healthy support vs. that which results in negative effects such as overdependence, learned helplessness, anxiety, impression management problems, and feelings of obligation. See Albrecht et al.[1] for a review of the literature on negative effects of social support. For the purposes of this chapter, it is important to realize that the process of social support is more than the effect on the recipient, but includes a complex interaction of the perceptions and behaviors of the *provider*, the perceptions and behaviors of the *recipient*, and the characteristics of the *relationship* within which the communication takes place.

The primary differences related to providers' communication of social support are suggested to be interpersonal sensitivity or perceptiveness and interpersonal behavior skills such as effective listening.[77] This perceptiveness might be tied to the trait of high self-monitoring and allow an individual to better assess appropriate behaviors.[78] Personality might affect both the provider's assessment of a particular situation and his or her response to it. For example, locus of control might shape the provider's perception of whether assistance will be of any help to the distressed individual. An internal orientation (belief that events are controlled by one's own actions) vs. an external orientation (belief that events in life are controlled by outside forces) could make a potential provider of social support more or less likely to provide supportive communication. Further, the locus-of-control orientation might influence the choice of communication behaviors that would determine the effectiveness or ineffectiveness of the support. An externally oriented individual might assess the situation of a distressed other as being beyond the control of either party and choose to withhold any supportive communication based on the perception that it will do no good. Or the externally oriented person might choose to attempt supportive communication, but the message might only reinforce that the situation is out of the support recipient's control, furthering the distress.

Another illustration involves the type A personality, which is defined by Blaney and Ganellen[79] as "an individual who constantly tries to take control, seeks out challenges, and is highly committed to his or her work." This trait, although incorporating the same constructs as hardiness, control, commitment, and challenge, does so in apparently markedly different ways. It is proposed that type A individuals will assess a distressed person's situation and if they perceive the need to help, might apply overly aggressive and controlling components to the messages they convey. This same type A person might choose often to avoid offering social support because of its interference with his or her drive to accomplish personal goals and limited focus on others who are not directly related to those goals. Other traits of type A include excessive speed, impatience, time urgency, and competitiveness,[80] all of which are predicted would deter a provider from offering social supportive communication in most situations and significantly affect its effectiveness if offered. Studies that assess the impact of personality on communication skills and social support are limited and, from the aspect of the provider of supportive information, almost nonexistent. A need for more analysis of this dimension is necessary to complete the communication process and fully understand social support.

The personality of the recipient of social support might also affect the success or failure of the communication interaction. The type A behavior pattern, as defined by Friedman and Rosenman,[80] might not only be less likely to seek support, but also act as a barrier to development of supportive relationships. Spielberger[81] found that high levels of experienced and expressed anger interfere with interpersonal relationships for this group. As with the provider of social support, the recipient might also be impacted by locus of control. Studies have shown that of all personality variables found to affect stress, control perception is most often cited[72] and appears to have the strongest effect.[82] Internally oriented individuals, believing that their actions and decisions influence what happens to them, might be more likely to seek out support and use supportive relationships. Sandler and Lakey[83] found that a buffering effect against stress resulted from supportive relationships, but only for individuals with an internal locus of control.

Quick et al.[84] would characterize healthy executives with internal loci of control as self-reliant, a paradoxical term characterizing their capacity for interdependence in contrast to independence. Subsequent research with executives, basic military trainees, and military officer candidates found that the self-reliant personalities were ones able to form and maintain secure interpersonal attachments, while those with overdependent or codependent personalities experienced various difficulties in interpersonal communication.[13,85] More recently, Peterson et al.[85] intensively studied 17 CEOs and their top management teams (TMTs) using independent, qualitative observational data that were then subjected to the group dynamics q-sort method designed to permit rigorous, quantitative comparisons of data derived from qualitative sources. Peterson and his research team found CEO personality to affect the interpersonal dynamics in TMTs, which in turn had an impact on organizational performance. The five dimensions of CEO personality considered were conscientiousness, emotional instability, agreeableness, extraversion, and openness. We are suggesting that these personality attributes might have moderating effects in the interpersonal communication–social support link.

In summary, we propose that personality differences moderate communication competence and thus ultimately the successful delivery of social support. We suggest that the behavioral dimension of communication competence is linked to personality differences and that these differences help explain variations in socially supportive exchanges. In essence, the personalities of the provider and recipient of a supportive exchange and their interaction impact the behavioral choices of each and partially explain why some communication exchanges are supportive and others are not, regardless of intent. We cannot draw a general conclusion that similar personalities are more likely to have better communication and therefore social support as a result of these similarities. Nor can we draw a general conclusion that complementary personalities are more likely to have better communication and social support as a result of their differences. Hence, personality is an important moderator of communication and social support.

The preceding section on moderator variables outlines ways in which emotional intelligence, cognitive complexity, gender, and personality differences affect the interpersonal communication of social support. We propose that for communication exchanges to be supportive, the interactants must exhibit a critical level of communication competence. Each of the three dimensions of communication competence can be linked to one of more of these moderators. That is, emotional intelligence is expected to positively impact the affective dimension of communication competence. Cognitive complexity is most closely related to the cognitive dimension, while gender and personality are most closely linked to the behavioral dimension. Thus, our model incorporates the interaction of these variables with communication exchanges to explain how variations in the perception and experience of social support occur.

COMPREHENSIVE MODEL OF THE RELATIONSHIP OF COMMUNICATION AND SOCIAL SUPPORT

Supportive communication is important in the realm of preventive stress management and personal health because understanding the processes by which it occurs can improve people's lives. Thus far in the chapter we have provided information on various important parameters in the relationship between communication competence and, ultimately, successful social support by isolating specific moderators. However, the processes at work when support is provided are highly complex, multifactorial, and interactive.[8,87] Therefore, there appears to be value in breaking the complex process into components for study to uncover new knowledge in a more manageable way, but the ultimate end must be to integrate this information into a comprehensive model that offers a broader understanding of this social phenomenon. It is not likely that cognitive complexity, emotional intelligence, gender, or personality will provide a complete understanding of the pathway between communication competence and social support. However, these moderators in combination with other factors such as context, type of stressor, cultural differences, contextual relevance, opportunity, motivation, and expectations can lead to this more comprehensive model.

Several researchers have developed a comprehensive theory or model to explain social support,[8,9] but these models focus on the outcomes, types, or effects of social support. There is relatively little theoretical framework for the communicative processes and factors affecting those outcomes. A better understanding of how successful communication results in positive social support effects and what constitutes competence in supportive communication could lead to skills training and other interventions to improve social support.

Burleson and Gilstrap[61] suggest a model that combines biological sex, gender-based personality traits, and interaction goals in support situations. Their model is a mediational model in which personality traits mediate the effects of biological sex on the interaction goals of the support situation. Cutrona and Russell's[46] Optimal Matching Model, discussed earlier in this chapter, is also a comprehensive attempt to match situational variables with specific types of behaviors of support. Expansion of this model to include communication competence can further account for the variation seen. We propose that the provider must have the intent to communicate a positive supportive message to a recipient and that the message must be delivered and interpreted with clear intent and congruence of meaning to result in the positive effects of social support (i.e., decreased stress, improved health and well-being). The key to this interaction is the communication competence of the interactants, which is influenced by the cognitive complexity, emotional intelligence, personality, and gender of the participants. Figures 14.1 and 14.3 capture our provisional concept for a comprehensive model that shows the complex, multidimensional, and interactive processes that must occur to achieve social support.

BUILDING COMMUNICATION COMPETENCE TO INCREASE SOCIAL SUPPORT FOR PREVENTIVE STRESS MANAGEMENT

Research on the relationship of communication competence and social support, especially in stressful contexts, is important because we need to understand how communication competence can contribute to preventive stress management through enhanced social support while averting distress and strain. Successful training in understanding of communication differences and in communication competence skill acquisition has important implications for improving the amount of social support available as well as the effectiveness. If specific communication competence skills and behaviors that increase the success of supportive communication can be identified, these same skills can be targeted in training programs. Empirical research to determine the specific components and efficacy of resulting training agendas is needed.

Burleson[33] suggests that social perception processes, emotional sensitivity, prosocial values, support self-efficacy, willingness to communicate, and aspects of procedural memory might be targets for training to improve emotional support. He further suggests that the quantity and quality of emotional support offered to others is often quite poor. At a minimum, he suggests that training programs focus on development of rhetorical skills for conveying supportive intentions (e.g., clearly and effectively conveying positive intent), dealing with the target's public "face" or status (e.g., providing support without causing the target to suffer decreased self-esteem or sense of self-efficacy), and learning to use person-centered messages (e.g., reflecting an awareness of and adaptation to the subjective, affective, and relational aspects of communicative contexts). Burleson[33] alludes to the success of training in communication skills for public presentations, conflict management, interviewing, decision making, and other communication targets as support for the idea that similar results should be possible with training in communicative support skills.

We further suggest that training in communicative competence skills for social support needs to address the difference in ability that might be related to cognitive complexity skills, emotional intelligence, personality, and gender differences, as well as awareness of these abilities in others. Although some individuals might be inherently strong in supportive communication skills due to these moderating characteristics, those who are not might benefit from training targeting their weaknesses. Also, any preventative or therapeutic intervention strategy to improve social support needs to address these factors in relationship to the entire communication event. The uniqueness of the provider, the recipient, and the context must be understood to create the highest potential to positively affect social support outcome. Cognitive complexity, like EI, can also be an inherent trait with dimensions that might be developed in individuals through targeted training.

Salovey and Mayer[48] suggest that emotional intelligence is not a fixed trait, but can change through maturation, developmental growth, and suitable training. Many training programs are currently being used to increase the skills generally considered to compose EI, but little empirical support for their efficacy exists.[50] Most of these training programs identify specific components felt to be a part of the general concept of EI and train those specific skills. As this chapter would suggest, a more effective method targeting communicative competence related to social support might require more comprehensive and integrated training of individual differences awareness, communication, and EI skills. Focusing the training toward a more specific outcome such as perceived social support might provide a means to determine effective methods of improving the EI skill.

From the personality perspective, training in supportive communication might focus on specific skills such as learned optimism, or it might also be helpful for perception such as learning about and understanding how to interact with differing personality types. Both skills and perception training should focus on both the receiver and the provider of supportive communication for the best result. The increased knowledge of individual differences related to communication can increase overall communicative attempts and success of social support. Thus, components of personality traits that influence supportive communication's success and failure could be a key focus of stress prevention management programs.

Gender differences and training issues are complicated by the controversies surrounding this area of study. If the different cultures perspective is followed, the training might involve learning gender-specific strategies for understanding the other's culture and how best to communicate within that context. However, if the skills specialization perspective were accepted, then the same skills would be targeted regardless of gender. The inclusion of differences related to gender is ultimately needed, but the identification of what these differences are and how to teach this information is still being debated. The relatively new information related to tend-and-befriend female tendencies in response to stress is an intriguing shift in long-held beliefs and might prove to spur additional thinking in the area of gender differences and stress.

CONCLUSION

Social support is an important factor in preventive stress management, and it has been shown to positively affect health and well-being. The mechanism through which the benefits of social relationships and social support are achieved is not clearly understood. In fact, there appears to be a great deal of variability related to social support attempts with both negative and positive outcomes. In our quest to unlock the secret of how to better harness the benefits of social support, we must first find the key to explain what it is and how it works. Understanding the nature of social support and the factors that explain the variability in outcomes is required to develop a comprehensive model of the phenomenon. A clear model of the mechanism of social support can then lead to improvements in the prevention and management of stress.

This chapter proposes that the key to unlocking the mystery of social support is interpersonal communication. Specifically, we propose that social support results from the successful communication of a supportive message or symbol. Both social support and interpersonal communication competence are impacted by many of the same factors. Our thesis is that interpersonal communication is the pathway or bridge to social support and that communication competence can be the enabling force to enhance the effectiveness and efficiency of this pathway. Our review of the literature found that communication competence differs in individuals based on the moderating variables of emotional intelligence, cognitive complexity, gender, and personality. So, too, we found that the outcomes of social support attempts are impacted by these moderating variables. In our model presented in Figure 14.1, the affective dimension of communication competence corresponds to emotional intelligence, the cognitive dimension to cognitive complexity, and the behavioral dimension to personality and gender differences. Our model, as extended in Figure 14.3, encompasses the entire communication event beginning with the context within which the communication interaction occurs, followed by the interacting effects of the moderating variables on both the provider and the recipient of the communication. This model is proposed to help explain why variability in social support outcomes occurs, but it can also serve as a basis for identifying aspects of communication competence to target in attempts to improve social support.

Previous empirical research and professional practice in the communication field related to training and improving interpersonal communication competence can serve as a foundation for development of supportive communication training in a variety of organizational contexts, especially high-stress work environments such as emergency rooms, the trading floor of stock exchanges, or military combat zones. The health and well-being benefits of social support are well documented and suggest the need to further understand and incorporate this phenomenon into preventive stress management. Facilitating supportive communication competence might well be the key to making this happen.

ACKNOWLEDGMENTS

The authors express their appreciation for support from the Center for Research on Organizational and Managerial Excellence (CROME) in the completion of this work. They thank Debra L. Nelson, Pamula L. Perrewé, and Sheri Schember Quick for helpful comments in earlier drafts of the chapter. They also thank Marilyn Saba for her help in the preparation of the text and references, and Deepa S. Iyer and Sheelam Maurya for the preparation of the figures in the chapter.

REFERENCES

1. Albrecht, T.L., Burleson, B.R., and Goldsmith, D., Supportive communication, in *Handbook of Interpersonal Communication*, 2nd ed., Knapp, M.L., and Miller, G.R., Eds., Sage Publications, Thousand Oaks, CA, 1994.
2. Quick, J.D., et al. Social support, secure attachments, and health, in *Handbook of Stress, Medicine, and Health*, Cooper, C.L., Ed., CPR Press, Boca Raton, FL, 1996, Chapter 14.
3. Joplin, J.R.W., Nelson, D.L., and Quick, J.C., Attachment behavior and health: relationships at work and home, *J. Org. Behav.*, 20, 783–796, 1999.
4. Quick, J.C., and Quick, J.D., Reducing stress through preventive management, *Human Resour. Manage.*, 18, 15–22, 1979.
5. Quick, J.D., Quick, J.C., and Nelson, D.L., The theory of preventive stress management in organization, in *Theories of Organizational Stress*, Cooper, C.L. Ed., Oxford University Press, New York, 1998, Chapter 12.
6. Adelman, M.B., and Albrecht, T.L., Intervention strategies for building support, in *Communicating Social Support*, Albrecht, T.L., and Adelman, M.B., Eds., Sage Publications, Newbury Park, CA, 1987, Chapter 12.
7. House, J.S., Landis, K.R., and Umberson, D., Social relationships and health, *Science*, 241, 540–545, 1988.
8. House, J.S., *Work Stress and Social Support*, Addison-Wesley, Reading, MA, 1981.
9. Cobb, S., Social support as a moderator of life stress, *Psychosom. Med.*, 38, 300–314, 1976.
10. Bowlby, J., *Attachment and Loss*, Vol. I, *Attachment*, rev. ed., Basic Books, New York, 1982.

11. Bowlby, J., *A Secure Base*, Basic Books, New York, 1988.
12. Shumaker, S.A., and Hill, D.R., Gender differences in social support, and physical health, *Health Psychol.*, 10, 102–111, 1991.
13. Quick, J.C., Nelson, D.L., and Quick, J.D., *Stress and Challenge at the Top: The Paradox of the Successful Executive*, John Wiley & Sons, Chichester, England, 1990.
14. Zey, M.G., *Winning with People*, Jeremy P. Tarcher, Los Angeles, 1990.
15. Bloom, J.R., The relationship of social support and health, *Soc. Sci. Med.*, 30, 635–637,1990.
16. Callaghan, P., and Morrissey, J., Social support and health: a review, *J. Adv. Nurs.*, 18, 203–210, 1993.
17. House, J.S., and Wells, J.A., Occupational stress, social support, and health, in *Reducing Occupational Stress: Proceedings of a Conference,* McLean, A., Black, G., and Colligan, M., Eds., DHEW (NIOSH) Publication 78-140, 1978, pp. 8–29.
18. Fleury, J., An exploration of the role of social networks in cardiovascular risk reduction, *Heart Lung*, 22, 134–144, 1993.
19. Kulik, J.A., and Mahler, H.I.M., Social support and recovery from surgery, *Health Psychol.*, 8, 221–238, 1989.
20. Gerin, W., Pieper, C., Levy, R., and Pickering, T.G., Social support in social interaction: a moderator of cardiovascular reactivity, *Psychosom. Med.*, 54, 324–336, 1992.
21. Bruhn, J.G., Social support and heart disease, in *Handbook of Stress, Medicine, and Health*, Cooper, C.L., 2nd ed., CRC Press, Boca Raton, FL, 1996, pp. 253–268.
22. Lynch, J.J., *The Broken Heart: The Medical Consequences of Loneliness*, Basic Books, New York, 1977, Chapter 1.
23. Lynch, J.J., *A Cry Unheard: New Insights into the Medical Consequences of Loneliness*, Bancroft, Baltimore, 2000.
24. Berkman, L.F., and Syme, S.L., Social networks, host resistance, and mortality: a nine-year follow-up study of Alameda County residents, *Am. J. Epidemiol.*, 109, 186–204, 1979.
25. Cohen, S., Stress, social support, and the buffering hypothesis, *Psych. Bull.*, 98, 310–357, 1992.
26. Schwarzer, R., Hahn, A., and Fuchs, R., Unemployment, social resources, and mental and physical health: a three-wave study of men and women in stressful life transition, in *Job Stress in a Changing Workforce*, Keita, G.P., and Hurrell, J.J., Eds., American Psychological Association, Washington, DC, 1994, pp. 75–88.
27. Astrand, N.E., Hanson, B.S., and Isacson, S.O., Job demands, job decision latitude, job support, and social network factors as predictors of mortality in a Swedish pulp and paper company, *Brit. J. Ind. Med.*, 46, 334–340, 1989.
28. Johnson, J.R., Hall, E.M., and Theorrell, T., Combined effects of job strain and social isolation on cardiovascular disease morbidity and mortality in a random sample of the Swedish male working population, *Scand J. Work Environ. Health*, 19, 21–28, 1989.
29. Ganster, D., Interventions for building healthy organizations: suggestions from the stress research literature, in *Job Stress Interventions*, Murphy, L.R., Hurrell, Jr., J.J., Sauter, S.L., and Keita, G.P., Eds., American Psychological Association, Washington, DC, 1995, pp. 323–336.
30. Carlson, D.S., and Perrewé, P.L., The role of social support in the stressor-strain relationship: an examination of work-family conflict, *J. Manage.*, 25, 513–540, 1999.
31. Sarason, B.R., Sarason, I.G., and Pierce, G.R., Traditional views of social support and their impact on assessment, in *Social Support: An Interactional View*, Sarason, B.R., Sarason, I.G., and Pierce, G.R., Eds., John Wiley & Sons, New York, 1990, Ch. 14.

32. Albrecht, T.L., and Adelman, M.B., Rethinking the relationship between communication and social support: an introduction, in *Communicating Social Support*, Albrecht, T.L., and Adelman, M.B., Eds., Sage Publications, Newbury Park, CA, 1987, pp. 13–16.
33. Burleson, B.R., Emotional support skill, in *Handbook of Communication and Social Interaction Skills*, Green, J.O., and Burleson, B.R., Eds., Lawrence Erlbaum Associates, Mahway, NJ, 2003, Chapter 14.
34. Burleson, B.R., Comforting as social support: relational consequences of supportive messages, in *Personal Relationships and Social Support*, Duck, S., and Silver, R., Eds., Sage, London, 1990, pp. 66–82.
35. Albrecht, T.L., and Adelman, M.B., Dilemmas of supportive communication, in *Communicating Social Support*, Albrecht, T.L., and Adelman, M.B., Eds., Sage Publications, Newbury Park, CA, 1987, Chapter 11.
36. Burgoon, J., and Ruffner, M., *Human Communication*, Holt, Rinehart & Winston, New York, 1978.
37. Wood, J.T., Clarifying the issues, *Pers. Relation.*, 4, 221–228, 1997.
38. Query, J.L., and James, A.C., The relationship between interpersonal communication competence and social support groups in retirement communities, *Health Commun.*, 1, 165–184, 1989.
39. Adler, N.J., *International Dimensions of Organizational Behavior*, 4th ed., South-Western/Thompson Learning, Mason, OH, 2000, pp. 74–77.
40. Nelson, D.L., and Quick, J.C., *Organizational Behavior: Foundations, Realities, and Challenges*, 4th ed., Thompson Learning/South-Western, Mason, OH, 2003, pp. 256–257.
41. Payne, R., Organizational stress and social support, in *Current Concerns in Occupational Stress*, Cooper, C.L., and Payne, R., Eds., Wiley, New York, 1980, pp. 269–298.
42. Meyer, H.H., Kay, E., and French, J.R.P., Split roles in performance appraisal, *Harvard Bus. Rev.*, 43, 123–129, 1965.
43. Burleson, B.R., Age, social-cognitive development, and the use of comforting strategies, *Commun. Monogr.*, 51, 140–153, 1984.
44. Knapp, M.L., Miller, G.R., and Fudge, K., Background and current trends in the study of interpersonal communication, in *Handbook of Interpersonal Communication*, 2nd ed., Knapp, M.L., and Miller, G.R., Eds., Sage Publications, Thousand Oaks, CA, 1994, Chapter 1.
45. Coyne, J.C., Ellard, J.H., and Smith, D.A., Social support, interdependence, and the dilemmas of helping, in *Social Support: An Interactional View*, Sarason, B.R., Sarason, I.G., and Pierce, G.R., Eds., John Wiley & Sons, New York, 1990.
46. Cutrona, C.E., and Russell, D.W., Type of social support and specific stress: toward a theory of optimal matching, in *Social Support: An Interactional View*, Sarason, B.R., Sarason, I.G., and Pierce, G.R., Eds., John Wiley & Sons, New York, 1990.
47. Buckingham, M., *First, Break All the Rules*, Simon & Schuster, New York, 1999.
48. Salovey, P., and Mayer, J.D., Emotional intelligence, *Imagination Cognit. Personality*, 9, 185–211,1990.
49. Salovey, P., Bedell, B.T., Detweiler, J.B., and Mayer, J.D., Coping intelligently: emotional intelligence and the coping process, in *Coping: The Psychology of What Works*, Snyder, C.R., Ed., Oxford University Press, New York, 1999, p. 161.
50. Matthews, G., and Zeidner, M., Emotional intelligence, adaptation to stressful encounters, and health outcomes, in *The Handbook of Emotional Intelligence*, Bar-On, R., and Parker, J.D.A., Eds., Jossey-Bass, New York, 2000, pp. 459–489.

51. Schroder, H.M, Driver, M.J., and Streufert, S., *Human Information Processing*, Holt, Rinehart & Winston, New York, 1967, pp. 109–125.
52. Schneier, C.E., Operational utility and psychometric characteristics of behavioral expectations scales: a cognitive reinterpretation, *J. Appl. Psychol.*, 62, 541, 1977.
53. Beatty, M.J., and Payne, S.K., Listening comprehension as a function of cognitive complexity: a research note, *Commun. Monogr.*, 51, 85–89, 1984.
54. Hale, C.L., Cognitive complexity-simplicity as a determinant of communication effectiveness, *Commun. Monogr.*, 47, 304–311, 1980.
55. Burleson, B.R., Emotional support skill, in *Handbook of Communication and Social Interaction Skills*, Green, J.O., and Burleson, B.R., Eds., Lawrence Erlbaum Associates, Mahway, NJ, 2003, Chapter 14.
56. Aries, E., *Men and Women in Interaction: Reconsidering the Differences*, Oxford University Press, New York, 1996.
57. Canary, D.J., and Hause, K.S., Is there any reason to research sex differences in communication? *Commun. Q.*, 41, 129–144, 1993.
58. Wright, P.W., Toward an expanded orientation to the study of sex differences in friendship, in *Sex Differences and Similarities in Communication: Critical Essays and Empirical Investigations of Sex and Gender Interaction*, Canary, D.J., and Dindia, K., Eds., Lawrence Erlbaum Associates, Mahwah, NJ, 1998, Chapter 2.
59. Canary, D.J., and Dindia, K., Eds., *Sex Differences and Similarities in Communication: Critical Essays and Empirical Investigations of Sex and Gender Interaction*, Lawrence Erlbaum Associates, Mahwah, NJ, 1998a, pp. ix–xi.
60. Canary, D.J., and Dindia, K., Prologue: recurring issues in sex differences and similarities in communication, in *Sex Differences and Similarities in Communication: Critical Essays and Empirical Investigations of Sex and Gender Interaction*, Canary, D.J., and Dindia, K., Eds., Lawrence Erlbaum Associates, Mahwah, NJ, 1998, pp. 1–17.
61. Burleson, B.R., and Gilstrap, C.M., Explaining sex differences in interaction goals in support situations: some mediating effects of expressivity and instrumentality, *Commun. Rep.*, 15, 43–55, 2002.
62. Kunkel, A.W., and Burleson, B.R., Social support and the emotional lives of men and women: an assessment of the different cultures perspective, in *Sex Differences and Similarities in Communication*, Canary, D.J., and Dindia, K., Eds., Lawrence Erlbaum Associates, Mahwah, NJ, 1998, pp. 101–125.
63. Burleson, B.R., Kunkel, A.W., Samter, W., and Werking, K.J., Men's and women's evaluations of communication skills in personal relationships: when sex differences make a difference — and when they don't, *J. Soc. Pers. Relations*, 13, 201–224, 1996.
64. Miller, L.C., Cody, M.J., and McLaughlin, M.L., Situations and goals as fundamental constructs in interpersonal communication research, Knapp, M.L., and Miller, G.R., Eds., in *Handbook of Interpersonal Communication*, 2nd ed., Sage Publications, Thousand Oaks, CA, 1994, Chapter 5.
65. Barbee, A.P., and Cunningham, M.R., An experimental approach to social support communications: interactive coping in close relationships, Burleson, B.R., Ed., in *Communication Yearbook*, Vol. 18, Sage, Thousand Oaks, CA, 1995, pp. 381–413.
66. Feingold, A., Gender differences in personality: a meta-analysis, *Psychol. Bull.*, 116, 429–457, 1994.
67. Taylor, S.E., Klein, L.C., Lewis, B.P., Grunewald, R.A., and Updegraff, J.A., Biobehavioral responses to stress in females: tend-and-befriend, not fight-or-flight. *Psychol. Rev.*, 107, 411–429, 2000.

68. Wood, J.T., and Dindia, K., What's the difference? A dialogue about differences and similarities between women and men, in *Sex Differences and Similarities in Communication: Critical Essays and Empirical Investigations of Sex and Gender Interaction*, Canary, D.J., and Dindia, K., Eds., Lawrence Erlbaum Associates, Manwah, NJ, 1998, Chapter 1.
69. Tannen, D., *You Just Don't Understand: Women and Men in Conversation*, William Morrow, New York, 1990.
70. Noller, P., Gender and emotional communication in marriage: different cultures or differential social power? *J. Lang. Soc. Psychol.*, 12, 132–152, 1993.
71. Payne, R., Individual differences in the study of occupational stress, in *Causes, Coping and Consequences of Stress at Work*, Cooper, C.L., and Payne, R., Eds., Wiley & Sons, Chichester, England, 1988, Chapter 7.
72. Cox, T., and Ferguson, E., Individual differences, stress and coping, in *Personality and Stress: Individual Differences in the Stress Process*, Cooper, C.L., and Payne, R., Eds., John Wiley & Sons, Chichester, England, 1991, Chapter 2.
73. Schaubroeck, J., and Ganster, D.C., Associations among stress-related individual differences, in *Personality and Stress: Individual Differences in the Stress Process*, Cooper, C.L., and Payne, R., Eds., John Wiley & Sons, Chichester, England, 1991, Chapter 3.
74. Cooper, C.L., and Payne, R., *Personality and Stress: Individual Differences in the Stress Process*, Wiley & Sons, Chichester, England, 1991.
75. Vinokur, A., Schul, Y., and Caplan, R., Determinants of perceived social support: interpersonal transactions, personal outlook, and transient affective states, in *J. Pers. Soc. Psychol.*, 53, 1137–1145, 1987.
76. Antonucci, T.C., and Jackson, J.S., The role of reciprocity in social support, in *Social Support: An Interactional View*, Sarason, B.R., Sarason, I.G., and Pierce, G.R., Eds., John Wiley & Sons, New York, 1991, Chapter 7.
77. Dunkel-Schetter, C., and Bennett, T.L., Differentiating the cognitive and behavioral aspects of social support, in *Social Support: An Interactional View*, Sarason, B.R., Sarason, I.G., and Pierce, G.R., Eds., John Wiley & Sons, New York, 1990, Chapter 11.
78. Snyder, M., and Cantor, N., Thinking about ourselves and others: self-monitoring and social knowledge, *J. Pers. Soc. Psychol.*, 51, 125–139, 1980.
79. Blaney, P.H., and Ganellen, R. J., Hardiness and social support, in *Social Support: An Interactional View*, Sarason, B.R., Sarason, I.G., and. Pierce, G.R., Eds., John Wiley & Sons, New York, 1991, p. 300.
80. Friedman, M.D., and Rosenman, R.H., *Type A Behavior and Your Heart*, Knopf, New York, 1974.
81. Spielberger, C.D., State-trait anger expression inventory: revised research edition, in *Psychological Assessment Resources*, Odessa, FL, 1991.
82. Cohen, S., and Edwards, J.R., Personality characteristics as moderators of the relationship between stress and disorder, in *Advances in the Investigation of Psychological Stress*, Neufeld, W.J., Ed., Wiley, New York, 1989, Chapter 7.
83. Sandler, I.N., and Lakey, B., Locus of control as a stress moderator: the role of control perceptions and social support, *Am. J. Commun. Psychol.*, 10, 65–78, 1982.
84. Quick, J.C., Joplin, J.R.S., Nelson, D.L., Mangelsdorff, A.D., and Fiedler, E., Self-reliance and military service training outcomes, *Mil. Psychol.*, 8, 279–293, 1996.
85. Peterson, R.S., Smith, B., Martorana, P.V., and Owens, P.D., The impact of CEO personality on TMT dynamics: one mechanism by which leadership affects organizational performance, *J. Appl. Psychol.*, in press.

15 Emotional Processing of Traumatic Events*

Richard B. Slatcher and James W. Pennebaker

CONTENTS

Traumatic experiences and other emotional upheavals, by definition, are profoundly stressful. Divorce, death of a loved one, loss of a job, chronic disease — these are but a few of the many emotional upheavals that can shake one's world in the course of a lifetime. Uncovering the psychological and social factors that underlie the processing of traumatic events has been a central goal in much of our research for almost two decades.

Individuals cope with traumatic experiences in varying ways. While some are able to quickly process their traumatic experiences and move on with relative ease, others might sink into periods of depression and anxiety that can last months or even years. Traumatic events negatively affect health and psychological well-being, but they also have the ability to transform one's social world.

A critical dimension of coping with trauma is the degree to which individuals discuss or psychologically confront emotional upheavals after their occurrence. People have an inherent need to disclose the details of their upsetting experiences

* Preparation of this manuscript was aided by a grant from the National Institutes of Mental Health (MH52391).

0-8493-1820-3/05/$0.00+$1.50

with others (Derlega, 1984; Jourard, 1971). In fact, one study has found that people share over 95% of all emotional experiences on the day that those experiences occur, usually within just a few hours of the experience (Rimé, 1995). Although a great majority of emotional experiences are shared, there are certain emotional experiences that individuals find difficult to share with others — sexual abuse, including rape, being fired from one's job, having a stigmatizing disease such as prostate or breast cancer, marital infidelity, and so on. Under such circumstances, individuals often try to inhibit thoughts and feelings about their experience to put them out of their mind. Ironically, such concerted attempts at thought suppression can lead to greater rumination and increased thoughts about the very experience that they are trying to erase from memory (Wegner, 1994). Such rumination, especially if it continues for extended periods, can consume large stores of cognitive and emotional resources, increase stress, and reduce immune system functioning.

Multiple laboratories, including our own, have found that writing or talking about emotional experiences is associated with improvements in mental and physical health and a host of other positive outcomes. Dating back to the work of Franz Alexander (1950), psychologists and other psychosomatic researchers have been intrigued by the salutatory benefits of self-disclosure. Since the original writing study (Pennebaker & Beall, 1986), research surrounding the effects of writing about emotional experiences has progressed at a remarkable rate. Of particular importance are a number of studies that have begun to shed light on the cognitive, linguistic, and social bases of the benefits of writing (Lepore & Smyth, 2002; Smyth, 1998).

Despite the rapid growth of writing studies, a large number of questions remain unanswered. To what extent does writing about an emotional event bring about changes in people's psychological and social worlds? Are some people more likely than others to benefit from emotional writing? What are the cognitive, linguistic, and social mechanisms that contribute to the positive outcomes derived from writing about emotional topics? In this chapter, we will briefly discuss our writing paradigm and give an overview of some of the relevant findings of other researchers. The chapter will conclude with a discussion of some of the underlying processes that might help to explain some of the powerful effects of self-disclosure.

THE WRITING PARADIGM

BACKGROUND

Our first writing studies were based on the premise that giving people the opportunity to write about previously undisclosed traumatic experiences might improve physical health. The procedure was relatively simple and straightforward (Pennebaker, 1997). Participants were brought into the lab and told that they would be taking part in an experiment wherein they would write about an assigned topic for three or four consecutive days, for 15 to 20 minutes each day. Those in the experiment were assured that their writing would be anonymous and that they would not receive any feedback from the researchers of the study. Those in the experimental condition were asked to write about their deepest thoughts and feelings about the most traumatic event of their lives. Participants assigned to the control condition were asked to write about superficial topics, such as how they use their time (Pennebaker, 1989).

The writing studies have yielded astonishing results. Most surprising is the content of the writing itself. Participants — from children to the elderly, from honor students to maximum security prisoners — disclose a remarkable range and depth of traumatic experiences. Rape, family violence, lost loves, deaths, and tragic failures have been common themes in all of the studies, with approximately half of all participants writing about experiences that most people would agree are truly traumatic. If nothing else, the writing paradigm illustrates people's readiness to disclose deeply personal aspects of their lives when given the opportunity. Even though a large number of participants report crying or being deeply upset by the experience, the overwhelming majority report that the process of writing is both valuable and meaningful. In fact, 98% of experimental participants have said that, given the choice, they would participate in a writing study again (Pennebaker, 1989).

While the nature of the writing itself is interesting, the real value of expressive writing is its influence on physical health. In our first writing study (Pennebaker & Beall, 1986), we followed the students' illness visits to the university health center in the months before and after the experiment. Compared to controls, those who wrote about emotional upheavals reduced their number of health center visits by half in the 2 months after writing.

Later writing studies from multiple labs supported the initial findings. Not only did those who wrote about traumatic experiences visit their doctor less often, but they also reported fewer physical symptoms and exhibited enhanced immune system functioning (as measured by various objective physiological measures). Joshua Smyth (1998), in a meta-analysis of 13 experimental writing studies from five labs, reported that disclosive writing was associated with improved physical and mental health, including drops in doctor visits (d =.42), changes in physiological functioning, including improved immune and hormonal function (d =.68), and reports of better psychological well-being (d =.66).

More recently, dozens of additional studies have been published, accepted for publication, or submitted that further demonstrate the effects of writing. Although the majority of replications and extensions have been conducted with college students, an increasing number are finding that writing about emotional topics is associated with reductions in pain behavior and medication use among chronic pain sufferers (Kelley et al., 1997; Smyth et al., 1999), fewer health visits to the infirmary of maximum security psychiatric prisoners (Richards et al., 2000), reduction of the number of days cystic fibrosis patients spend in the hospital (Taylor et al., 2003), fewer doctor appointments and self-reported symptoms among women with breast cancer (Stanton et al., 2002), fewer doctor visits and lower levels of depression among persons with type 1 diabetes (Bodor, 2003), fewer doctor visits, improved cardiac status, and greater adherence to rehabilitation activities for those recovering from a myocardial infarction (Wilmott et al., 2003), and reduced rates of depression among victims of crime (Schoutrop et al., 1997).

Research also indicates that the health benefits of emotional writing might not be confined to writing about traumatic experiences. Studies by Laura King and colleagues have examined how writing about positive experiences can improve physical health. In one study (King, 2001), participants were randomly assigned to write about their most traumatic life event, their best possible future self, both of these topics, or a nonemotional control topic. Those who wrote about their best possible selves had an increase in subjective well-being. At the 5-month follow-up, those who wrote about their best possible selves as well as those who wrote only about their traumas were both significantly lower in illness than participants in the control groups. In another study (Burton & King, 2004), people who wrote about intensely positive experiences had enhanced positive mood and fewer health center visits than controls. While more confirming evidence in this area is still needed, these studies demonstrate that perhaps one can enjoy the health benefits of writing without the emotional costs associated with writing about trauma.

Additional Outcomes of Writing

In the late 1980s and 1990s, most writing studies focused on objective health measures, such as health center visits, medication use, medical costs, and various biological markers. An increasing number of experiments soon began to demonstrate that writing about emotional topics could potentially affect nonhealth outcomes. For example, studies found that students who write about coming to college subsequently evidenced improved grades (Cameron & Nicholls, 1998; Pennebaker & Francis, 1996). Men laid off from their jobs who wrote about their experiences found jobs more quickly than those who did not write or who wrote about time management (Spera et al., 1994).

Emotional writing can bring about positive changes in close relationships as well. In one recent study from our lab (Slatcher & Pennebaker, 2003), individuals in committed romantic relationships were asked to write about their deepest thoughts and feelings about their relationship. Those in the control condition were asked to write about time management. Two months later, those who wrote about their relationship were much more likely to still be with their romantic partner. Similarly, Lepore and Greenberg (2002) found that students assigned to expressively write about a recent relationship breakup were more likely to reunite with their ex-partner than were control participants who wrote about nonemotional topics.

Having demonstrated that simply expressing one's thoughts and emotions in writing is a powerful therapeutic tool, many researchers are now investigating the mediators, moderators, and overall parameters of this relationship. The explanations for the experimental success of the writing paradigm are still in dispute (e.g., Sloan & Marx, 2004). Furthermore, the writing–health link appears to influence individuals along multiple levels. The following section of this chapter will discuss some of the intriguing and oftentimes unexpected findings emerging from various labs that have begun to address the underlying mechanisms of emotional writing.

Underlying Mechanisms

While there is now solid evidence that translating emotional experiences into language can be healthy, one of the more intriguing aspects of this phenomenon has been trying to develop theories that best explain it. Over the years, theoretical views in this area have evolved tremendously. Originally, our theories were based primarily on a model of inhibition. While the inhibition model continues to provide a number of valuable insights, many labs, including our own, are investigating the importance of cognitive and linguistic processes. Most recently, we have begun to explore the active role that writing plays on the social dynamics of people who write. Each of these theoretical positions is briefly outlined below.

Inhibitory Processes

One of the first theories to explain the effectiveness of disclosure dealt with inhibition. Specifically, it was proposed that not talking about emotional upheavals was a form of inhibition. That is, actively holding back thoughts, emotions, or behaviors was a form of stress that exacerbated a number of adverse biological processes, such as increased cortisol production and immune suppression (Traue & Deighton, 1999). According to the inhibition model, writing about an emotional topic should allow individuals to organize and assimilate previously inhibited thoughts and feelings, thus bypassing the need for further inhibition (Pennebaker, 1989). Indeed, several correlational studies have hinted that such processes can be at work (Cole et al., 1996; Gross & Levenson, 1997; Major & Gramzow, 1999). These ideas also are consistent with Wegner's (1994) work on thought suppression and ironic processing. By actively attempting to control ongoing thoughts, individuals actually end up monitoring more information at higher rates.

Despite the promise of inhibition models, direct tests of changes in inhibition among people who write about emotional topics have yielded disappointing results. For example, participants who claim that they have not previously disclosed their traumas have not differed in health outcomes vs. those who have disclosed their traumas (Greenberg & Stone, 1992). In addition, individuals have great difficulty answering (or even understanding) questions that ask them the degree to which they are actively inhibiting their thoughts, emotions, or behaviors (Pennebaker et al., 1988). Thus, at this point, the inhibition model should be considered unproven and still not adequately tested.

Cognitive Processes

Another explanation for the effects of writing is that the act of converting emotions and images into words changes the way a person organizes and thinks about an emotional experience. During an emotional upheaval, part of the distress caused by the trauma results not just from the events themselves but also from the person's reaction to them. By integrating thoughts and feelings, one can then construct more easily a coherent narrative of an experience. Once this integration takes place, the event can be summarized, stored, and forgotten more efficiently.

The various explicit and implicit cognitive models have focused on different facets of cognitive and narrative construction. Smyth and his colleagues (1999), for example, have assumed that writing fundamentally organizes an upsetting experience. As an indirect test of this, the authors had people write about a trauma in either an organized or unstructured way. Only the organized writing resulted in health and mood improvements.

Using a different analysis strategy of looking directly at the ways individuals write about emotional topics, several researchers are now finding support for the idea that constructing a narrative over the course of writing helps individuals to better integrate the experience. Specifically, by looking at word usage (e.g., an increasing use of cognitive words over the days of writing), health improvements are efficiently predicted. These word patterns have now been reported in multiple studies (Campbell & Pennebaker, 2003; Keough et al., 1998; Klein & Boals, 2001; Pennebaker & Francis, 1996; Pennebaker et al., 1997; Petrie et al., 1998).

Social Integration

Self-disclosure, by nature, is an inherently social activity. The ultimate purpose of language is to communicate ideas and thoughts with other people. The fact that writing about emotional topics can improve health suggests that talking about emotional topics with other people serves the same purpose (Pennebaker & Graybeal, 2001; Mehl & Pennebaker, 2003). When someone talks to other people about his or her experiences, it alerts them to the person's psychological state and ultimately allows him or her to remain socially tied to them. Conversely, people who have traumatic experiences and do not tell their friends are more likely to live in a detached, isolated state. Consistent with this approach, Rimé (1995) argues that disclosure in the first days or weeks after a trauma has the power to change the quality of a person's social network by bringing people closer together. Disclosure, then, serves as a force of social integration. Rimé suggests that even private disclosure (as with writing) helps free a person from the stress of a nondisclosed event, which ultimately allows for greater social integration.

Rimé's work, as well as some of our own, is consistent with many of the social integration ideas first suggested by Durkheim (1951) wherein mental health was viewed as the result of the relationship between individuals and their social worlds. Durkheim and, more recently, a growing number of social support researchers (e.g., Cohen et al., 2000; Cutrona, 1989; Pierce et al., 1992) have argued that individuals' relations with others must be viewed from both the individuals' needs and those of their potential social network. But with a few notable exceptions (e.g., Bradbury & Fincham, 1992; Dunkel-Schetter et al., 1992), most work that attempts to look at social support and integration has relied exclusively on self-reports rather than on objective changes in peoples' social interactions or relationships.

Social integration remains a somewhat ambiguous concept in psychology — we are yet unable to precisely label or measure its causes and constituents. Commonly, social integration is conceptualized as a sense of belonging, cohesion, confidence, and security with others (e.g., Antonovsky, 1993). The problem is that most attempts to tap this construct have relied on people's self-reports. There is good reason to believe that more objective indicators of social integration are needed — measures that tap the degree to which people are fluidly talking with one another. This could include measures of linguistic synchrony between people (e.g., Niederhoffer & Pennebaker, 2002), general interaction patterns, and the ways people naturally approach their social worlds (Mehl & Pennebaker, 2003a). Future research on social integration and writing must thus explore the obvious and subtle ways that social behaviors shift in the days and weeks after expressive writing.

Other Explanatory Models

While the inhibitory, cognitive, and social integration models have been the dominant theories of the last few years, other explanations for the effectiveness of emotional writing have been examined. One problem is that many of these approaches are examining the disclosure–health relationship from different levels of analysis. Thus, several models could all be true. In addition to the inhibitory and cognitive approaches, some additional explanations for the writing paradigm have been suggested (see also a recent review by Sloan & Marx, 2004).

Habituation

Greenberg et al. (1996) reported the results of a fascinating project wherein previously traumatized students wrote about either their own personal trauma or someone else's trauma as though it were their own or, in a third group, superficial topics. The authors found that writing about an imaginary trauma was as effective as writing about one's own trauma. They argue that the mere writing of an emotional topic helps to habituate the person to the emotions aroused by the topic (cf. Mendolia & Kleck, 1993).

Individual Differences

An ongoing debate in the writing–health research area concerns the degree to which individual differences might moderate the benefits of translating experiences into words. Most studies drawing on normal populations have failed to find consistent personality markers. However, studies drawing extreme samples of high and low hostility (Christensen & Smith, 1993) and alexithymia (Paez et al., 1999; Solano et al., 2003) suggest that those naturally more hostile and unable to verbalize their feelings might benefit more than low hostile or alexithymic individuals (for a review, see Lumley et al., 2002). Similarly, Smyth's (1998) meta-analysis indicates that males might benefit more from writing than females.

Explorations into Language

Language, by its very nature, is a social tool. Many of the behavioral effects associated with writing — better grades, fewer illnesses, ability to get better jobs, etc. — are indirectly and directly social. What several studies are now indicating is that the cognitive changes that can result from writing change the writers' relationships with others in their social worlds. Whereas the immediate effect of writing is to change how an individual thinks about trauma, the salutary effects are likely to be linked to the social changes that result from these cognitive changes.

In postexperiment interviews with participants from our first writing studies, it was clear that they were gaining more through the writing than simply disclosing would suggest. In listening to the language that participants used to recount their experiences — such as "realize," "understand," "come to terms," "getting past," and so forth — writing was fostering a better understanding of both themselves and the situations about which they wrote. On an intuitive level, an individual's cognitive reorganization was crucial for the positive outcomes that were emerging. To further investigate this idea, we wanted to find an empirical way to examine the writers' essays more closely to see if language use could predict improvements in health among those who had written about emotional topics.

Development of Tools to Analyze Language

To develop a standardized way of measuring the ways people use words that express emotions and thoughts, we developed a computer program called the Linguistic Inquiry and Word Count (LIWC) that could analyze essays in text format. LIWC was developed by having groups of judges evaluate the degree to which over 2,000 words or word stems were related to each of several dozen categories. Although there are now over 70 word categories in the most recent version of the LIWC program (LIWC2001, Pennebaker et al., 2001), only four were of primary interest to us. Two of the categories were emotion dimensions and the other two were cognitive. The emotion categories included negative emotion words (e.g., sad, angry) and positive emotion words (e.g., happy, laugh). The two cognitive categories, causal words (e.g., because, reason) and insight words (e.g., understand, realize), were intended to capture the degree to which participants were actively thinking in their writing. For each essay that a person wrote, we were able to quickly compute the percentage of total words that these and other linguistic categories represented.

LIWC allowed us to go back to previous writing studies and link word usage among individuals in the experimental conditions with various health and behavioral outcomes. Analyzing the use of negative and positive emotion words, two important findings were revealed (Pennebaker et al., 1997). First, the more that people used positive emotion words, the more their health improved. Negative emotion word use also predicted health changes but in an unexpected way. Individuals who used a moderate number of negative emotions in their writing about upsetting topics evidenced the greatest drops in physician visits in the months after writing. That is, those people who used a very high rate of negative emotion words and those who used very few were the most likely to have continuing health problems after participating in the study. In many ways, these findings are consistent with others in the literature. Individuals who tend to use very few negative emotion words are undoubtedly most likely to be characterized as repressive copers — people who Weinberger et al. (1979) have defined as having poor ability at being able to identify and label their emotional states. Those who overuse negative emotion words might well be the classic high neurotic or high negative affect (Watson & Clark, 1984) individuals. These individuals are people who ponder their negative emotions in exhaustive detail and who might simply be in a recursive loop of complaining without attaining closure. Indeed, this can be exacerbated by the inability of these individuals to develop a story or narrative.

Although the findings concerning emotion words use were intriguing, the results surrounding the cognitive word categories were even more robust. Recall that in our studies, people wrote for 3 to 5 days, 15 to 30 minutes per day. As they wrote, they gradually changed what they said and how they said it. The LIWC analyses showed strong and consistent effects for changes in insight and causal words over the course of writing. Specifically, people whose health improved, who got higher grades, and who found jobs after writing went from using relatively few causal and insight words to using a high rate of them by the last day of writing. In reading the essays of people who showed this pattern of language use, it became apparent that they were constructing a story over time. Building a narrative, then, seemed to be critical in reaching understanding. Interestingly, those people who started the study with a coherent story that explained some past experience did not benefit from writing (see Gergen & Gergen, 1988; Mahoney, 1995; Meichenbaum & Fong, 1993).

An alternative computer-based approach to linguistic analysis relies on more inductive ways of establishing the pattern of word use. One particularly promising strategy is latent semantic analysis (LSA) (e.g., Landauer & Dumais, 1997). A technique such as LSA is akin to a factor analysis of individual words. By establishing the factor structure of a large number of writing samples, it is possible to learn how any new writing samples are similar to one another.

Across a series of style-based LSA analyses, we have discovered that particles or function words are related to a variety of social and psychological processes (Pennebaker et al., 2003). Particles include pronouns, prepositions, articles, conjunctions, and auxiliary verbs. These words are markers of people's linguistic styles and tell us how people talk rather than the content of what they are saying. Overall, the use of particles in general and pronouns in particular has been found to correlate highly with health improvements. In essence, the more that individuals shift in their use of pronouns from day to day in writing, the more their health improves. Indeed, across three separate studies, pronoun shifts among trauma writers correlated between .3 and .5 with changes in physician visits (Campbell & Pennebaker, 2003).

Closer inspection of these data suggest that healthy writing is associated with a relatively high number of self-references on some days but not on others. Alternatively, people who always write in a particular voice — such as first-person singular — simply do not improve. Although our LSA studies are still in the early stages, they are suggesting that the ability to change perspective in dealing with an emotional upheaval might be critically important. The data also indicate that pronouns can be an overlooked linguistic dimension that could have an important meaning for researchers in health and social psychology.

Exploring Language and Emotional Expression in the Real World

In our most recent studies, we are investigating whether writing could facilitate social integration, whether one of the health benefits of writing enables individuals to better connect with their social group. Do people begin to interact differently with others, or perhaps see themselves in a new light, after writing about an emotional topic? To explore these ideas, we have attempted to capture how people naturally talk and interact with others by developing the electronically activated recorder (EAR) — a simple tape recorder with an attached computer chip that records for 30 seconds every 12 minutes. The EAR is a lightweight and nonintrusive device worn by participants for two consecutive days. A small external microphone allows researchers to hear pieces of conversations, as well as determine where participants are and what they are doing (Mehl et al., 2000).

In the first study (Mehl & Pennebaker, 2003a), participants wore the EAR for two consecutive days, 2 weeks prior to as well as 2 weeks after having participated in a routine writing study. Transcriptions of the conversations yielded promising results in terms of participants' physical behaviors, as well as their language as analyzed by LIWC. Compared to participants in the control condition, where they were asked to write about time management, trauma writers began talking to their friends more, laughing more, and using significantly more positive emotions in their daily language. Trauma writers also demonstrated significant drops in their resting levels of both diastolic and systolic blood pressure. Similarly, writing about emotion appears to have encouraged participants to use more present-tense words and less past tense. Interestingly, these effects were far stronger for men, who are naturally less socially integrated than women.

More recently, EAR was used to analyze social interactions during the days surrounding the terrorist attacks of September 11, 2001 (Mehl & Pennebaker, 2003b). In this study, participants wore the EAR for 10 days, from September 11 to 21. Prebaseline data were available for all participants. In examining participants' interactions, an intriguing trend emerged. While participants did not change in their overall amount of interactions after 9/11, they gradually shifted from group conversations to dyadic interactions. In a set of exploratory analyses, this natural shift toward dyadic encounters tended to predict better subsequent psychological adjustment in the form of fewer 9/11 intrusions and avoidance behaviors. Consistent with our previous discussion of social integration, this suggests that dyadic interactions can facilitate psychological coping during traumatic events. Following an emotional upheaval, one-on-one encounters can provide the intimacy needed to reaffirm one's shaken worldviews, reevaluate and calibrate one's beliefs and opinions, and help come to terms with what happened by gradually developing a personal narrative.

In addition to the EAR system, we have found instant messaging (IM) to be an effective tool in examining social interactions outside of the lab. For many, IM is quickly replacing e-mail as their preferred mode of online dyadic communication (Pew Internet and American Life Project, 2003). Unlike e-mail, IM allows its users to chat with each other in real time so that a conversation can unfold much in the same way that spoken conversation does. In a recent study (Slatcher & Pennebaker, 2003), we collected 10 days of instant messages from undergraduate couples. On days 4 to 6 of the study, one person from each couple either wrote about their deepest thoughts and feelings about their relationship or completed a time management exercise. In the instant messages that followed the writing assignments, those who wrote about their relationships used significantly more emotion words than those who wrote about time management. Further, the partners of those in the relationship writing condition used significantly more emotion words as well. Three months later, those couples who wrote about their relationship were more likely to still be dating each other. These findings lend strong support to the idea that the effects of emotional expression extend to people's interpersonal relationships, thus helping them to become more integrated into their social networks.

CONCLUSIONS

Traumatic events have the ability to negatively affect nearly every aspect of one's life. In addition to making us depressed, anxious, and sick, they change the ways in which we interact with friends, loved ones, and others with whom we come into contact on a daily basis. As we have discovered through our own research, the social impact of emotional upheavals is profound. By choosing to share or inhibit our thoughts and feelings about a traumatic event, we have the power not only to determine how we cognitively and emotionally process the event, but also to shape the ways in which we interact with others and how others perceive us. If, for example, one chooses to retreat into himself after the death of a loved one, various social consequences might follow. Not only is this person giving up an opportunity for social support, but by not talking with people about the event, he might cause others to misconstrue the reasons for his retreat.

On the other hand, if people choose to disclose a traumatic event to others, they might strengthen personal relationships with others and help themselves to better cognitively process the event. It is becoming clear that this process of social integration is key to moving past trauma and developing a more coherent social world. Further, it suggests that we should be focusing on models of integration and coherence in far greater detail. By social integration, we propose that people are able to talk more openly about their thoughts and feelings, spend more time with others, use more emotion words, and laugh more with one another on a daily basis.

The benefits of social integration extend beyond interpersonal relationships. The more socially integrated people are, the more they should be able to remain focused on various daily tasks and goals and spend less time ruminating about emotional events. This process seems to occur not only in the case of personal trauma, but during shared trauma as well — such as the terrorist attacks of September 11 — during which social sharing can help to maintain our shared beliefs and perceptions of the world. This approach to social integration is much more active and dynamic than traditional views of social support. In line with Durkheim (1951) and others, we assume that traumatized individuals are active in selecting and taking part in their social worlds.

Recent research suggests that looking at language in a real-world context will help us to clarify the role that social integration plays in helping people to process and move past traumatic events. Using computer-aided technology such as the EAR system, instant messaging, and LIWC, it is now possible to measure social and linguistic behaviors among individuals for several weeks or even months. In doing so, we hope to gain more insight into how emotional upheavals alter our social worlds. Tracking how people naturally talk and interact should help us to refine and better understand the underlying processes that account for the now well-established psychological and health benefits of self-disclosure.

REFERENCES

Alexander, F. (1950). *Psychosomatic Medicine*. New York: Norton.

Antonovsky, A. (1993). Complexity, conflict, chaos, coherence, coercion and civility. *Social Science and Medicine*, 37, 969–974.

Bodor, N. Z. (2003). The Health Effects of Emotional Disclosure for Individuals with Type 1 Diabetes. Unpublished doctoral dissertation, University of Texas, Austin.

Bradbury, T. N., & Fincham, E. D. (1992). Attributions and behavior in marital interaction. *Journal of Personality and Social Psychology*, 63, 613–628.

Burton, C. M., & King, L. A. (2004). The health benefits of writing about intensely positive experiences. *Journal of Research in Personality*, 38, 150–163.

Cameron, L. D., & Nicholls, G. (1998). Expression of stressful experiences through writing: Effects of a self-regulation manipulation for pessimists and optimists. *Health Psychology*, 17, 84–92.

Campbell, R. S., & Pennebaker, J. W. (2003). The secret life of pronouns: Flexibility in writing style and physical health. *Psychological Science*, 14, 60–65.

Christensen, A. J., & Smith, T. W. (1993). Cynical hostility and cardiovascular reactivity during self-disclosure. *Psychosomatic Medicine*, 55, 193–202.

Cohen, S., Underwood, L. G., & Gottlieb, B. H. (2000). *Social Support Measurement and Intervention: A Guide for Health and Social Scientists*. New York: Oxford University Press.

Cole, S. W., Kemeny, M. E., Taylor, S. E., & Visscher, B. R. (1996). Elevated physical health risk among gay men who conceal their homosexual identity. *Health Psychology*, 15, 243–251.

Cutrona, C. E. (1989). Ratings of social support by adolescents and adult informants: Degree of correspondence and prediction of depressive symptoms. *Journal of Personality and Social Psychology*, 57, 723–730.

Derlega, V. (1984). Self-disclosure and intimate relationships. In V. Derlega (Ed.), *Communication, Intimacy and Close Relationships* (pp. 1–9). Orlando, FL: Academic Press.

Dunkel-Schetter, C., Blasband, D. E., Feinstein, L. G., & Herbert, T. B. (1992). Elements of supportive interactions: When are attempts to help effective? In S. Spacapan & S. Oskamp (Eds.), *Helping and Being Helped in the Real World* (pp. 83–114). Newbury Park, CA: Sage.

Durkheim, E. (1951). *Suicide*. New York: Free Press.

Gergen, K. J., & Gergen, M. M. (1988). Narrative and the self as relationship. In L. Berkowitz (Ed.), *Advances in Experimental Social Psychology*, Vol. 21 (pp. 17–56). New York: Academic Press.

Greenberg, M. A., & Stone, A. A. (1992). Emotional disclosure about traumas and its relation to health: Effects of previous disclosure and trauma severity. *Journal of Personality and Social Psychology*, 63, 75–84.

Greenberg, M. A., Stone, A. A., & Wortman, C. B. (1996). Health and psychological effects of emotional disclosure: A test of the inhibition-confrontation approach. *Journal of Personality and Social Psychology*, 71, 588–602.

Gross, J. J., & Levenson, R. W. (1997). Hiding feelings: The acute effects of inhibiting negative and positive emotion. *Journal of Abnormal Psychology*, 106, 95–103.

Jourard, S. M. (1971). *Self Disclosure: An Experimental Analysis of the Transparent Self*. New York: Wiley Interscience.

Keough, K. A., Garcia, J., & Steele, C. M. (1998). Reducing Stress and Illness by Affirming the Self. Unpublished manuscript.

Kelley, J. E., Lumley, M. A., & Leisen, J. C. (1997). Health effects of emotional disclosure in rheumatoid arthritis patients. *Health Psychology*, 16, 331–340.

King, L. A. (2001). The health benefits of writing about life goals. *Personality and Social Psychology Bulletin*, 27, 798–807.

Klein, K., & Boals, A. (2001). Expressive writing can increase working memory capacity. *Journal of Experimental Psychology: General*, 130, 520–533.

Landauer, T. K., & Dumais, S. T. (1997). A solution to Plato's problem: The latent semantic analysis theory of acquisition, induction, and representation of knowledge. *Psychological Review*, 104, 211–240.

Lepore, S. J., & Greenberg, M. A. (2002). Mending broken hearts: Effects of expressive writing on mood, cognitive processing, social adjustment and health following a relationship breakup. *Psychology and Health*, 17, 547–560.

Lepore, S. J., & Smyth, J. (2002). *The Writing Cure*. Washington, DC: American Psychological Association.

Lumley, M. A., Tojek, T. M., & Macklem, D. J. (2002). Effects of written emotional disclosure among repressive and alexithymic people. In S. Lepore & J. Smyth (Eds.), *The Writing Cure* (pp. 75–95). Washington, DC: American Psychological Association.

Mahoney, M. J. (Ed.). (1995). *Cognitive and Constructive Psychotherapies: Theory, Research, and Practice*. New York: Springer Publishing.

Major, B., & Gramzow, R. (1999). Abortion as stigma: Cognitive and emotional implications of concealment. *Journal of Personality and Social Psychology*, 77, 735–745.

Mehl, M. R., & Pennebaker, J. W. (2003a). The sounds of social life: A psychometric analysis of students' daily social environments and natural conversations. *Journal of Personality and Social Psychology*, 84, 857–870.

Mehl, M. R., & Pennebaker, J. W. (2003b). The social dynamics of a cultural upheaval: Social interactions surrounding September 11, 2001. *Psychological Science*, 14, 579–585.

Mehl, M. R., Pennebaker, J. W., Crow, D. M., Dabbs, J., & Price, J. (2001). The electronically activated recorder (EAR): A device for sampling naturalistic daily activities and conversations. *Behavior Research Methods, Instruments, and Computers*, 33, 517–523.

Meichenbaum, D., & Fong, G. T. (1993). How individuals control their own minds: A constructive narrative perspective. In D. M. Wegner & J. W. Pennebaker (Eds.), *Handbook of Mental Control* (pp. 473–490). Englewood Cliffs, NJ: Prentice Hall.

Mendolia, M., & Kleck, R. E. (1993). Effects of talking about a stressful event on arousal: Does what we talk about make a difference? *Journal of Personality and Social Psychology*, 64, 283–292.

Niederhoffer, K. G., & Pennebaker, J. W. (2002). Linguistic style matching in social interaction. *Journal of Language and Social Psychology*, 21, 337–360.

Paez, D., Velasco, C., & Gonzales, J. L. (1999). Alexithymia as dispositional deficit in self-disclosure and cognitive assimilation of emotional events. *Journal of Personality and Social Psychology*, 77, 630–641.

Pennebaker, J. W. (1989). Confession, inhibition, and disease. In L. Berkowitz (Ed.), *Advances in Experimental Social Psychology*, Vol. 22 (pp. 211–244). New York: Academic Press.

Pennebaker, J. W. (1997). Writing about emotional experiences as a therapeutic process. *Psychological Science*, 8, 162–166.

Pennebaker, J. W., & Beall, S. K. (1986). Confronting a traumatic event: Toward an understanding of inhibition and disease. *Journal of Abnormal Psychology*, 95, 274–281.

Pennebaker, J. W., & Francis, M. E. (1996). Cognitive, emotional, and language processes in disclosure. *Cognition and Emotion*, 10, 601–626.

Pennebaker, J. W., Francis, M. E., & Booth, R. J. (2001). Linguistic inquiry and word count (LIWC2001). Mahwah, NJ: Erlbaum Publishers.

Pennebaker, J. W., & Graybeal, A. (2001). Patterns of natural language use: Disclosure, personality, and social integration. *Current Directions in Psychological Science*, 10, 90–93.

Pennebaker, J. W., Kiecolt-Glaser, J., & Glaser, R. (1988). Disclosure of traumas and immune function: Health implications for psychotherapy. *Journal of Consulting and Clinical Psychology*, 56, 239–245.

Pennebaker, J. W., Mayne, T. J., & Francis, M. E. (1997). Linguistic predictors of adaptive bereavement. *Journal of Personality and Social Psychology*, 72, 863–871.

Pennebaker, J. W., Mehl, M. R., & Niederhoffer, K. (2003). Psychological aspects of natural language use: Our words, our selves. *Annual Review of Psychology*, 54, 547–577.

Petrie, K. P., Booth, R. J., & Pennebaker, J. W. (1998). The immunological effects of thought suppression. *Journal of Personality and Social Psychology*, 75, 1264–1272.

Pew Internet and American Life Project. (2003). Teenage Life Online: The rise of the instant-message generation and the Internet's impact on friendships and family relationships. Retrieved June 8, 2003, from http://www.pewinternet.org/reports.

Pierce, G. R., Sarason, B. R., & Sarason, I. G. (1992). General and specific support expectations and stress as predictors of perceived supportiveness: An experimental study. *Journal of Personality and Social Psychology*, 63, 297–307.

Richards, J. M., Beal, W. E., Seagal, J. D., & Pennebaker, J. W. (2000). Effects of disclosure of traumatic events and illness behavior among psychiatric prison inmates. *Journal of Abnormal Psychology*, 109,156–160.

Rimé, B. (1995). Mental rumination, social sharing, and the recovery from emotional exposure. In J. W. Pennebaker (Ed.), *Emotion, Disclosure, and Health* (pp. 271–291). Washington, DC: American Psychological Association.

Schoutrop, M. J. A., Lange, A., Brosschot, J., & Everaerd, W. (1997). Overcoming traumatic events by means of writing assignments. In A. Vingerhoets, F. van Bussel, & J. Boelhouwer (Eds.), *The (Non)expression of Emotions in Health and Disease* (pp. 279–289). Tilburg, The Netherlands: Tilburg University Press.

Slatcher, R. B., & Pennebaker, J. W. (2003). Modern Love: Language, Instant Messaging, and Romantic Relationships. Manuscript in preparation.

Sloan, D. M., & Marx, B.P. (2004). A closer examination of the structured written disclosure procedure. *Journal of Consulting and Clinical Psychology*, 72, 165–175.

Solano, L., Donati, V., Pecci, F., Persichetti, S., & Colaci, A. (2003). Post-operative course after papilloma resection: Effects of written disclosure of the experience in subjects with different alexithymia levels. *Psychosomatic Medicine*, 65, 477–484.

Spera, S. P., Buhrfeind, E. D., & Pennebaker, J. W. (1994). Expressive writing and coping with job loss. *Academy of Management Journal*, 37, 722–733.

Smyth, J. M. (1998). Written emotional expression: Effect sizes, outcome types, and moderating variables. *Journal of Consulting and Clinical Psychology*, 66, 174–184.

Smyth, J. M., Stone, A. A., Hurewitz, A., & Kaell, A. (1999). Effects of writing about stressful experiences on symptom reduction in patients with asthma or rheumatoid arthritis: A randomized trial. *Journal of the American Medical Association*, 14, 1304–1309.

Stanton, A. L., Danoff-Burg, S., Sworowski, L. A., Collins, C. A., Branstetter, A. D., Rodriguez-Hanley, A., Kirk, S. B., & Austenfield, J. L. (2002). Randomized, controlled trial of written emotional expression and benefit finding in breast cancer patients. *Journal of Clinical Oncology*, 20, 4160–4168.

Taylor, L., Wallander, J., Anderson, D., Beasley, P., & Brown, R. (2003). Improving chronic disease utilization, health status, and adjustment in adolescents and young adults with cystic fibrosis. *Journal of Clinical Psychology in Medical Settings*, 10, 9–160.

Traue, H. C., & Deighton, R. (1999). Inhibition, disclosure, and health: Don't simply slash the Gordian knot. *Advances in Mind-Body Medicine*, 15, 184–193.

Watson, D., & Clark, L. A. (1984). Negative affectivity: The disposition to experience aversive emotional states. *Psychological Bulletin*, 96, 465–490.

Wegner, D. M. (1994). Ironic processes of mental control. *Psychological Review*, 101, 34–52.

Weinberger, D., Schwartz, G. E., & Davidson, R. J. (1979). Low-anxious, high-anxious, and repressive coping styles: Psychometric patterns and behavioral and physiological responses to stress. *Journal of Abnormal Psychology*, 88, 369–380.

Wilmott, L., Harris, P., & Horne, R. (2003). The Effects of Written Emotional Disclosure Following First Myocardial Infarction. Manuscript in preparation.

16 Gender Differences in the Management of Work Stress: Preventing Distress and Savoring Eustress

Debra L. Nelson and Bret L. Simmons

CONTENTS

The role of gender in the stress process continues to be the subject of considerable research. There is a growing body of knowledge concerning women in the workplace and work-related stress (cf. Fielden & Cooper, 2002; Nelson & Burke, 2002). Writings and research on men's roles in relation to health are emerging as well (Burke, 2002; Burke & Nelson, 1998). Gender relates to the ways in which women and men are defined through cultural influences. The distinctions between sex and gender are often fuzzy, and this is reflected in the fact that the concepts are used interchangeably in some writings. The idea of gender is particularly important in stress research, because gender involves socially constructed roles that affect the expectations placed on men and women in both work and home lives. In Western

0-8493-1820-3/05/$0.00+$1.50

cultures, masculinity is associated with technical competence, rational decision making, emotional detachment, and aggressive behavior. Femininity, in contrast, is characterized by emotional expressivity, nurturance of others, passive communication, and an emphasis on relationships. These gender role expectations can place considerable stress on men and women.

In critically reviewing and integrating the literature on stress and gender differences, we concluded that two areas had received the lion's share of research attention. Several studies have focused on gender differences in stressors, with many of these studies identifying the unique stressors placed on women in the workplace. The other area that has been the subject of several studies is distress symptoms. These studies indicate that women and men might be prone to different dysfunctional consequences of stress.

Interestingly, we found one area of stress research that had received less attention in terms of gender differences. Although there are several studies that have examined differences in the ways women and men manage (or cope with) stress, these studies were more scattered and often lacked a coherent theoretical organizing scheme. In addition, the tone of the studies was often negative; that is, the studies emphasized dealing with distress and its negative effects. Our purpose in the current chapter is to critically review and integrate these studies using the framework of preventive stress management. We also propose a positive complement to the current preventive management framework, which we term savoring eustress.

We begin by briefly summarizing the literature on differences in stressors, or sources of stress. This review sets the stage for a possible explanation for gender differences in preventive management. Next, we briefly highlight the evidence for gender differences in distress symptoms. This section also provides a potential explanatory path for gender differences in the ways individuals manage stress.

We then present the preventive management philosophy and framework that serves as the overarching organizing scheme and theoretical backdrop for our critical review. Using this framework, we present the research evidence showing that women and men might manage stress differently in terms of three levels of stress management methods: primary-, secondary-, and tertiary-level prevention.

Our call for a more positive approach begins with a presentation of the concept of eustress, the positive, healthy response to stressors. Next, we introduce and develop the concept of savoring eustress as a positive complement to coping with distress. Finally, we present some unanswered questions for future researchers that we hope will serve to stimulate inquiry concerning the different methods women and men use in preventing or resolving distress and encouraging and savoring eustress.

GENDER DIFFERENCES IN STRESSORS

In studies examining which stressors are problematic for women or men, role stress has been a major theme. For women, the most prevalent role stressors are role conflict and role overload. Role conflict most often takes the form of conflicting expectations about the various roles of spouse, mother, and worker, among other roles (Frankenhauser, 1981). Role overload, a related stressor, stems from the sheer number of expectations of these multiple roles. Women also carry an average total weekly workload of 78 hours, whereas men's total weekly workload is 68 hours. Women's increased workload has effects on health, because epinephrine, cortisol, and other stress-related hormones tend to persist at high levels even after working hours (Lundberg & Frankenhauser, 1999).

Men's role stressors often take the form of gender role strain, or failure to fulfill male role expectations. Three types of gender role strain were identified by Pleck (1995). Discrepancy strain is experienced when a man cannot live up to the traditional masculine ideal. Trauma strain results from the inability to express emotion or engage in relationships. Dysfunctional strain occurs when men meet traditional masculine expectations, but display negative side effects of these expectations such as sexually harassing others or failing to fill the fatherly role. All three forms of gender role strain are proposed to be associated with the male socialization experience.

Women face many obstacles to achievement in the workplace, including the "glass ceiling," which is the invisible barrier holding women in lower-level jobs. In addition, the "maternal wall" is encountered by women who receive less desirable jobs or limited upward mobility once they have children (Williams, 1999). Another barrier to women's progress is their lack of access to developmental opportunities (e.g., challenging assignments, access to mentors) that might prepare them for upper-level positions (Nelson & Burke, 2000).

The jobs traditionally held by men carry stressors as well. These demands include long work hours, extensive travel, expectations of after-work socializing, corporate politics, and little time for family life (Alvesson & Billing, 1997). These job stressors are combined with the considerable confusion that surrounds men's roles in contemporary society. Allegations of reverse discrimination reflect this confusion. Men, in addition to the breadwinner role, are being called upon to take on more household and family responsibilities, and evidence shows that they are gradually doing so, but the total workload discrepancies between the genders remain intact (Bond et al., 1998).

Role-related stressors such as role overload, gender role stress, total workload, and career barriers are among the demands most investigated in terms of gender differences. There is some evidence for gender differences in stressors as a function of job characteristics. Many stressors reported more frequently by women (e.g., inadequate salary, personal insults, periods of inactivity) are associated with low-level, low-control jobs. It might be that it is the characteristics of the jobs that are typically held by women, and not gender per se, that produce stressors for women. As the number of women in the workforce continues to increase, equality in employment conditions (both good and bad) should lead to a reduction in variation between the sexes in experienced stressors (Jex, 1998). A study of male and female doctors in Scotland, for example, found that increased role complexity (home/work) was related to stress for both female and male doctors, which the researchers interpreted to suggest an increasing convergence in the occupational and domestic roles of male and female doctors (Swanson et al., 1998).

A second area of study within the stress process that has benefited from examinations of gender differences is that of distress symptoms, or the negative consequences of stress.

GENDER DIFFERENCES IN DISTRESS SYMPTOMS

There is also evidence that women and men manifest the negative consequences of stress in different ways. Epidemiological evidence indicates that although women report higher levels of distress, their symptoms tend to be less lethal than those reported by men and more often of a psychological or somatic nature (Matuszek et al., 1995). Women's distress symptoms often include headaches, heart palpitations, dizziness, shakiness, and insomnia and other sleep disturbances. Men's distress symptoms, such as cardiovascular diseases and injuries, tend to be lethal in nature. This can account for their lower life expectancy, approximately 8 years less than that of women.

The genders also differ in terms of behavioral symptoms of distress. Women are more likely to smoke and to use antidepressants, sleeping pills, and other prescription drugs than are men, and this is especially characteristic of female managers (Quick et al., 1997). In addition, stress-related eating disorders are more common among women. Men, however, tend to turn to alcohol more than do women, although alcohol abuse among women is on the rise (Harrison et al., 1989).

These findings must be tempered with the knowledge that women on the whole are more likely to recognize and report symptoms and to seek assistance in dealing with distress. This can be an explanatory factor pertaining to the differences in life expectancies between men and women.

The preceding brief discussions of gender differences in causes of stress and symptoms of distress represent the major themes that have been examined in studies of men's and women's experiences of stress. Before we turn to the issue of gender differences in managing stress, we present the preventive stress management model that forms the basis for our review.

THE PREVENTIVE MANAGEMENT PHILOSOPHY AND FRAMEWORK

One framework that has been advanced for categorizing stress management methods is preventive stress management, as originally presented by Quick and Quick (1984) and elaborated upon by Quick et al. (1997, 1998). These authors define preventive stress management as "an organizational philosophy and set of principles that employs specific methods for promoting individual and organizational health while preventing individual and organizational distress" (Quick et al., 1997, p. 149). In contrast to coping, preventive stress management encompasses a broader, more proactive approach to stressors. It also serves as a model for individual and organizational change, because it prescribes interventions for both individuals and organizations in order for each to become healthier under stress. In this chapter, we focus solely on the individual side of preventive management, as it is most applicable in the discussion of gender differences.

In addition to comprising a conceptual framework, preventive stress management constitutes a set of principles that serve as the core elements of the philosophy. Briefly, the principles are:

1. Individual and organizational health are interdependent.
2. Leaders have a responsibility for individual and organizational health.
3. Individual and organizational distress are not inevitable.
4. Each individual and organization reacts uniquely to stress.
5. Organizations are ever-changing, dynamic entities.

Although all of these principles are important, two in particular bear upon the question of gender differences in managing stress. The idea that individual distress is not inevitable is the key to the prevention approach. With its roots in medical and public health traditions, preventive management contains a set of techniques that are aimed at preventing (in addition to resolving) distress. While principle 5, as noted by Quick and Quick (1984), applies to organizations, the extension applicable here is that individuals are also ever changing. Principle 3 proposes that each individual reacts uniquely to stress. Taken together, these principles demonstrate that no single preventive management method can be prescribed for every stressor, every individual, or every situation.

Within the preventive management framework, stress is cast as a chronic health problem. Diseases follow an evolution from susceptibility to early disease to advanced or disabling disease. With heart disease, for example, individuals in the susceptibility stage are exposed to risks such as smoking or a sedentary lifestyle. In the early disease stage, the person might experience disease progression such as the formation of plaque within the arteries, but might experience only a few or no symptoms. In the advanced disease stage, the signs of heart disease, chest pains and ultimately heart attacks, might occur. In accordance with public health notions of prevention, there exist opportunities for intervention at each stage of the disease (stress) process, with the ultimate goal of slowing, stopping, or reversing the process. In preventive stress management, there are three levels. Primary prevention is aimed at eliminating or reducing the risk factors (stressors). It is the preferred level of intervention because it occurs before the onset of disease. Secondary prevention focuses on the individual's response to stress. It consists of methods such as relaxation and exercise that help individuals become more resilient. Tertiary prevention, mostly in the form of professional care, focuses on the symptoms of distress. The hierarchy of methods is important, with the recommendation that individuals concentrate on primary prevention, supplement with secondary prevention, and use tertiary methods as needed should distress symptoms arise.

Interestingly, it is the secondary and tertiary prevention methods that have been most widely prescribed and rigorously studied. Secondary (response-directed) methods such as relaxation training, spiritual activities, emotional outlets, exercise, and nutrition have also received attention in the media. Tertiary methods such as counseling, psychotherapy, and medical care are widely used. Yet it is the primary prevention methods that are touted to have the greatest payoff. Some of these methods focus on changing the stressor itself. Time management, delegation, planning, and changing the work environment all directly involve stressors. In addition, managing individuals' perceptions of stress constitutes a powerful primary prevention method. This can be accomplished through learned optimism, transformational coping, and changing type A behavior patterns.

It is worth noting that the literature on coping is complementary to, rather than in contrast to, preventive stress management. Folkman and Lazarus (1980), for example, have described coping as a cognitive and behavioral process of mastering, tolerating, and reducing both internal and external demands. Their work has centered around two forms of coping: problem focused and emotion focused. Problem-focused coping involves managing or changing the source of stress. As such, it is a form of primary prevention. Emotion-focused coping, involving the regulation of stress-related emotion, is one form of secondary prevention. The research on coping, therefore, can be subsumed within the overarching framework of preventive stress management.

In the next section, we focus on key methods at each level of prevention and review the evidence for gender differences in the use of these methods.

GENDER DIFFERENCES IN PREVENTIVE MANAGEMENT METHODS

The theory of preventive stress management proposes that individuals use a wide range of methods to deal with demands. Our review will follow the three-level model of primary, secondary, and tertiary stress management. Within each level, we will examine the evidence for gender differences in the use of specific prevention methods.

Primary Prevention Methods

Primary prevention methods have been divided into three broad categories: managing the stressor directly, managing perceptions of stressors, and managing one's lifestyle. Because this is the recommended starting point in the preventive stress management approach, we expected to find considerable research on gender differences in the use of these techniques.

Interestingly, there is little gender differences research on how men and women directly manage stressors. One line of research most applicable to the issue of directly managing stressors is that of problem-focused coping. Early research indicated that men were more likely to use coping strategies that directly altered a source of stress (Folkman & Lazarus, 1980). Subsequent research, however, showed that the sexes are equally likely to use problem-focused techniques, or that when education, occupation, and position are controlled for, gender differences are not found (Greenglass, 1988). Taking direct action to solve problems has also been considered in terms of affecting stressors. McDonald and Korabik (1991), for example, found that both male and female managers used direct action to cope with job stress. In a more recent study, Gianakos (2002) found that female adult working students were more likely to use direct action as a coping technique than were men. Greenglass (2002) noted that the type of coping used to deal with work stress often varies with the status, resources, and power tied to the individual's position in the organization, and that the social milieu in which a stressor is encountered must be a part of studies of gender differences and coping.

Quick et al. (1997) included social support as a method aimed at directly managing stressors because research indicates that it has a direct, positive effect on stressors. Social support can help individuals through suggestions from others on understanding and directly managing stressors. In addition, social support can help individuals reframe stressors such that they are less threatening. Studies demonstrate that women, more than men, tend to seek out advice, assistance, information, and emotional support from others in dealing with work stress (Greenglass et al., 1999; Greenglass, 2002). Women also provide more social support than do men (Liebler & Sandefur, 2002), and benefit more from the receipt of social support (Perrewe & Carlson, 2002). Research has sought to explain the efficacy of different types of support for men and women, and to explain the specific role of social support in the stress process. There is evidence, for example, that supervisory support at work is particularly helpful for women (Greenglass, 1993). Another study indicated that social support from coworkers was positively related to instrumental and preventive coping among women only (Greenglass, 2002).

There is mixed support for social support as a buffer, that is, that social support moderates the negative impact of work-related stressors (O'Driscoll, 2001). There is also evidence of a reverse buffering effect, such that certain forms of social support might negatively affect stress for certain individuals. MacEwen and Barling (1988) found that mothers who received more family support in dealing with interrole conflict experienced more negative changes in marital adjustment than those women who received low family support. The authors note that a possible explanation is that family support (emotional support) might not help directly change the stressor, especially if the source of stress is beyond the individual's control. A recent study suggests that gender role moderates the relationship between social support and strain such that more feminine individuals react more strongly and positively to social support than more masculine people do (Beehr et al., 2003).

Sometimes individuals cannot directly affect the source of stress; however, they can control their perceptions of the stressor. Methods suggested by Quick and Quick (1984) and elaborated upon by Quick et al. (1997) included learned optimism, transformational coping, and changing type A behavior patterns. Learned optimism, as articulated by Seligman (1990), enables individuals to live with hope and to view stressors as temporary and manageable. Transformational coping as a key ingredient in hardiness (Maddi, 1995) involves directly altering one's perception of a stressor by viewing it in a broad perspective, by believing that one can control the stressor and one's response, and by viewing stressors as challenges rather than threats. There is preliminary evidence that women are more likely to maintain positive attitudes throughout stressful situations, and this promotes the use of transformational coping (Lindquist et al., 1997). Type A behavior, as proposed by Friedman and Rosenman (1974), involves an action–emotion complex characterized by continuous, unsuccessful efforts to fight against real or imagined stressors. There is some evidence that type A behavior can be changed (cf. Roskies, 1987; Bennett et al., 1991), and because this change involves altering one's perception of stressors (often self-imposed stressors), Quick et al. (1997) consider this intervention a primary preventive management method.

Our literature review yielded few stress-related studies of gender differences in the use of the prevention methods that alter one's perception of a stressor. The question that arises is whether these techniques are amenable to gender differences, or whether there simply has been little investigation. Some research suggests that female managers have greater tendencies toward type A behavior than their male counterparts (Rees & Cooper, 1990). We found no studies, however, suggesting that either sex is more successful in changing type A behavior, or that one gender uses this as a strategy for managing stress to a greater extent than the other gender. A few studies on hardiness indicated no gender differences in hardiness among corporate, university, and military samples (Rosen et al., 1999; Soderstrom et al., 2000). Langan-Fox (2001) noted that few gender studies have investigated the role of personality within the career–personality–stress framework, and that optimism, hardiness, and type A behavior are prime targets for inclusion in such studies. With increased attention to mind–body interactions, we believe changing one's perceptions of stress to be powerful methods. More research is needed on gender differences in the use of these methods, the personality variables related to the methods, and the efficacy of these techniques for managing stress.

Lifestyle management is also considered to be primary prevention within the framework because it affects such stressors as work–home conflict, home–work conflict, and freedom from demands in either arena. The use of leisure time is particularly important to stress reduction, as is maintaining a balanced lifestyle. True leisure is the act of doing something fulfilling without having to strive for or reach a goal. There are gender differences in both the quantity and quality of leisure time. In the U.S., women experience less free time than do men, and it is of lesser quality. Men experience greater subjective benefit from their free time than do women. Women's leisure activities are often involved with contributing to family well-being, and these activities are not often seen as relaxing by women (Mattingly & Bianchi, 2003). A Scandinavian study's results echoed the U.S. findings, showing that Danish, Swedish, and Norwegian women all had less leisure time during weekdays than their male counterparts, and the presence of small children in the home increased the leisure time gap (Thrane, 2000).

In terms of primary preventive management methods, we need more gender differences research. We need to know more about how women and men directly manage stressors and manage their perception of stressors. The one area in which primary prevention research seems clear is that there is a leisure time gap in favor of men.

Secondary Prevention Methods

Secondary prevention methods are response directed and serve to dissipate the physical and psychological arousal that results when the stress response is activated. Among these methods are exercise, relaxation techniques, emotional outlets, and nutrition.

The role of exercise in recovery from the mind–body stress response is important in managing stress. Women report significantly less use of exercise and sports activities than men. This finding has been replicated across many samples. Nelson et al. (1989), in a study of human resource professionals, found that men reported significantly higher levels of exercise and sports activities such as racquet sports, running, swimming, weight lifting, and team sports. Fydenberg and Lewis (1993) found that male students used physical recreation to manage stress to a greater extent than female students did. In another study involving students, Friedman and Berger

(1991) found that jogging was related to greater mood improvement among both men and women who were scored high on a masculinity measure. In a study involving a national probability sample of U.S. households, Ross and Bird (1994) found that women were less likely to walk for exercise or to engage in more strenuous forms of exercise.

Among inventories measuring the reasons why people exercise, reducing stress is seldom included. Most often, these instruments include factors such as weight control, improved body image, or competitiveness. It is difficult, therefore, to ascertain whether men or women use exercise as a mechanism for controlling stress, although intuitively it makes sense. Some studies, however, have included distress or strain as outcome variables (cf. Nelson et al., 1989; Frydenberg & Lewis, 1993).

Another category of secondary prevention methods is relaxation techniques, aimed at achieving physical or mental relief from strain. Among these techniques are meditation, the relaxation response, biofeedback training, and progressive relaxation. There is considerable evidence of the efficacy of these methods in managing stress (cf. Benson & Stark, 1996). Kabat-Zinn et al. (1985), for example, reported improvements in chronic pain among patients trained in meditation, and Kindlon (1983) reported that students trained in meditiation showed significantly less test anxiety. Neither of these studies, however, found significant gender differences. Friedman and Berger (1991) found that among students trained in the relaxation response, women (independent of masculinity) and high masculinity men reported the greatest benefits. It appears that although both genders can benefit from relaxation techniques, gender role can be a moderator in the relationship between relaxation techniques and stress.

Emotional outlets such as talking things out or writing constitute another form of secondary prevention. Using emotional outlets can be distinguished from what is known as emotion-focused coping, which deals with the reactions to stressful events, and can include such things as self-blame and rumination. While some studies suggest that women engage more in emotion-focused coping (see Fielden & Cooper, 2002, for a discussion), other studies found no differences in such coping behaviors when women and men occupy similar jobs (Karambayya, 2002).

Emotional outlets, as preventive management techniques, are characterized by the healthy, constructive release of emotion. These include talking it out, or venting, and writing it out. Talking it out leads to catharsis, which initiates the recovery of the autonomic nervous system after the stress response (Gottleib, 1996). Women are more likely to endorse venting of emotions by talking with others as a prevention strategy (Torkelson & Nuhonen, 2003). This can be related to their greater reported use of social support mentioned earlier. There is considerable evidence for the benefits of writing letters, journals, or diaries to express emotions associated with stress. Pennebaker and his colleagues (1988) have demonstrated that writing about emotional trauma can positively affect the immune system and reduce health clinic visits associated with viral illnesses. Writing for as little as 15 minutes per day was associated with both mental and physical health, with equal benefits for men and women (Pennebaker & Seagel, 1999).

Nutrition, as a form of self-care, is particularly important during times of stress. Women are more likely than men to maintain healthy eating patterns under stress

(Nelson & Burke, 2000). In a large-scale study of government tax employees, men reported both higher scores for unhealthy eating habits and lower scores for healthy eating patterns than women, who reported healthier coping mechanisms in terms of nutrition.

In terms of secondary prevention, there do appear to be some gender differences. Men exercise more, but eat poorly. Women have a tendency to vent more or to talk out their stress with others. We need more research on gender differences in relaxation methods and in expressive writing as stress management methods.

Tertiary Prevention Methods

Healing the wounds of distress is the emphasis of tertiary prevention. These techniques involve professional care for distress symptoms. The care sought out can be psychological counseling and therapy or medical care. One of the more consistent findings in health and stress research is that women make more health care visits for psychological symptoms (Nelson & Burke, 2002). Women are higher users of medical services overall, and also of prescription drugs. Thus, we can say that women engage in tertiary prevention to a greater degree than do men. Researchers have begun to propose explanations for this gender difference. Women might be more willing to talk about symptoms, and to consider a broader range of symptoms, including psychological symptoms, as reasons to seek treatment. It might be more socially acceptable for women to report symptoms. Men are socialized to avoid asking for help and to ignore symptoms to get work done. Body-destroying attitudes and behaviors such as avoidance of asking for help, endurance of pain, symptom repression, and lack of self-care are characteristic of the masculine role (Burke, 2002). Alternatively, women might simply seek treatment more because of actual gender differences in symptom rates.

Several conclusions emerged from our review of gender differences in preventive management methods. First, despite the proposition that primary prevention is the first line of defense in stress management, gender differences in the primary methods are the ones least often investigated. Intuitively, it is appealing to think that changing the stressor itself or one's perception of it is the best way to manage stress; yet curiously, gender differences researchers have chosen to focus on the secondary and tertiary levels of prevention, which are in essence palliative or last-resort methods. Second, researchers have begun to move past simple gender differences in some cases to explore the reasons behind the differences. In terms of the finding that women are more prone to engage in help-seeking behavior (i.e., tertiary-level prevention), several explanations have been proposed. Finally, within the framework of preventive management, the research has focused exclusively on preventing or resolving distress. In the next section, we propose to accentuate the positive side of stress with a focus on eustress and savoring.

EUSTRESS: THE OTHER HALF OF THE STRESS PUZZLE

While the prevention of distress is the primary focus of the preventive stress management model, some have also suggested that there is also good stress, which Selye

(1976a, 1976b) termed *eustress*. Quick et al. (1997) associate eustress with healthy, positive outcomes. Positive appraisals of stressors "occur if the outcome of an encounter is construed as positive, that is, if it preserves or enhances well-being or promises to do so" (Lazarus & Folkman, 1984, p. 32). As indicators of the positive response to stressors resulting from positive appraisals, they suggest looking for the presence of positive or pleasurable psychological states and attitudes. A major issue in the study of eustress is to simultaneously establish the presence of both positive and negative psychological states, rather than merely inferring eustress by the absence of negative states. Instead of representing opposite ends of a single continuum, positive (eustress) and negative (distress) states can represent two distinct constructs, which would require separate multivariate indices for their measurement (Edwards & Cooper, 1988).

Consider the analogy of a bathtub to illustrate the point of thinking of eustress and distress as two distinct constructs. As a minimum, we are concerned about two things when we settle in for a bath — the level of water in the tub and the temperature of water in the tub. Essentially two things determine the level of water in the bathtub — the flow of water into the bathtub and the flow of water out of the bathtub over time. Likewise, the *simultaneous* flow of *both* hot and cold water into the bathtub determine the temperature of the water in the tub. If we liken the study of stress to the study of water in the bathtub, our current approach is like studying a bathtub with a single water faucet — cold water, representing distress. We know a lot about the sources of cold water, and we can tell individuals how to either decrease the flow of cold water into or increase the flow of cold water out of their bathtub. We also know quite a bit about the physiological, behavioral, and psychological consequences of sitting in a tub of cold water for a prolonged period. Our knowledge of cold water (distress) is important, but does not present a complete understanding of the water (stress) in the bathtub. A more complete model of stress would acknowledge that the bathtub does indeed have two faucets — hot and cold — and both are necessary to get the level and temperature of the water just right for a comfortable bath.

The strongest theoretical support for the concept of eustress can be found in the cognitive appraisal approach most commonly associated with the work of Richard Lazarus (1966). The essence of this approach to understanding stress is that people can have different responses to stressors they encounter depending on whether they appraise a relevant stressor as positive or negative. According to the cognitive appraisal approach, two individuals with significantly different perceptions of the same stressor (or a single individual with differing interpretations at different times) would respond differently. Likewise, two individuals with similar perceptions of the same (or different) stressors would experience similar responses (Roseman, 1984).

When a person encounters a stressor, she or he *evaluates* the encounter with respect to its significance for well-being. This evaluative process is the essence of cognitive appraisal. If a stressor is not appraised as irrelevant, Lazarus and Folkman (1984) assert that appraisals can be complex and mixed, depending on personal factors and the situational context. They essentially describe two types of appraisals and associated response patterns: positive and stressful.

Positive appraisals "occur if the outcome of an encounter is construed as positive, that is, if it preserves or enhances well-being or promises to do so" (Lazarus & Folkman, 1984, p. 32). As indicators of positive appraisals, they suggest looking for the presence of positive or pleasurable psychological states (e.g., exhilaration).

Stressful appraisals can also be thought of as negative appraisals. Negative appraisals include harm/loss, threat, and challenge. In *harm/loss*, some damage to the person has already occurred (e.g., injury, illness, loss of a loved one, damage to self-esteem). *Threat* involves harms or losses that have not yet occurred but are anticipated. *Challenge* appraisals occur if the outcome of an encounter holds the potential for gain or growth. As indicators of challenge appraisals, they suggest looking for some of the same positive or pleasurable psychological states they identify as indicators of the positive response (e.g., exhilaration).

Lazarus and Folkman (1984) do not view challenge and threat as poles of a single continuum. They believe that challenge and threat responses can occur simultaneously, as the result of the same stressor, and should be considered as separate but related constructs. While threat is clearly a negative appraisal, challenge is better thought of as a positive appraisal (they share the same indicators).

As such, the reasoning they apply to the distinction between challenge and threat to the higher levels of positive and negative responses can be extended. Accordingly, positive and negative responses can occur simultaneously, as a result of the same stressor, and should be considered separate but related constructs. Thus, for any given stressor, an individual can have *both* a degree of positive and a degree of negative response. This is consistent with Lazarus and Folkman's (1984) view that any psychophysiological theory of stress or emotion, which views the response as unidimensional disequilibrium or arousal, is untenable or at least grossly incomplete. They support this with research of emotions and autonomic nervous system activity (Elkman et al., 1983), as well as research of hormonal response to arousing conditions (Mason, 1974; Frankenhauser et al., 1978). The evidence is accumulating that our brains might indeed be wired to simultaneously experience positive and negative emotions separately (Davidson, 2000; Tomarken et al., 1992; Wheeler et al., 1993).

Rose's (1987) longitudinal study of air traffic controllers (ATCs) provides physiological evidence of the positive stress response. Over a 3-year period, the cortisol values of 201 men were measured every 20 minutes for 5 hours on three or more days and compared to both objective and subjective assessments of workload. Cortisol is a hormone secreted by the hypothalamic-pituitary-adrenal system that has been found to be responsive to a variety of different environmental challenges. Cortisol acts on a variety of the body's organs, but its primary effect is to increase the supply of glucose and fatty acids in the bloodstream. Cortisol can also have harmful effects on the body's digestion, immune response, and muscular-skeletal system (Quick et al., 1997).

While the increases in cortisol for all levels of workload were slight, the men who showed the highest increase in cortisol to increased work reported themselves as more satisfied and were regarded by peers as more competent. These high cortisol responders also showed less frequent illness than those with lower cortisol levels, who for any given level of work tended to have more minor health problems. Rose concludes "individuals who were busily engaged in work and who report a *challenge* but not a sense of being threatened or overwhelmed are better described as *engaged* rather than stressed and this appears to be a desirable state of affairs" (Rose, 1987, p. 145). Elsewhere, the happiness derived from engagement in mindful challenge has been termed *flow* (Csikszentmihalyi, 1990). In their review of Rose's study, Ganster and Schaubroek (1991) described the healthy state of physiological arousal experienced by the *engaged* workers as eustress.

SAVORING AS A COMPLEMENT TO PREVENTIVE MANAGEMENT AND COPING

The importance of eustress lies in its relationship to health and other positive outcomes. Engaging, challenging work can have positive health consequences for women. Similar to stress, health has also been viewed as a unidimensional construct representing the absence of the negative, that being disease. Yet health should be defined not only as the absence of illness, but also as the presence of a sense of purpose, quality connections with others, positive self-regard, and mastery (Ryff & Singer, 1998). Work in general and careers with no imposed limits on upper goals stand to provide a significant source of these aspects of health for women.

One of the most important questions that future research on eustress must address relates to the potential to *generate* the positive stress response. This is analogous to the extremely valuable work that has been done on preventive stress management, which is essentially focused on preventing the negative stress response (Quick et al., 1997). We hope that researchers will avoid the temptation to attempt to assign valence (i.e., positive and negative) to stressors as a way to prescribe formulas for eustress. That would be totally inconsistent with the theory of eustress presented here. The cognitive appraisal approach to stress requires that any assignment of valence be reserved for the stress response.

We believe that any model of eustress generation must recognize the individualistic nature of the endeavor that individuals must assume personal responsibility for. The concept of coping, finding ways to reduce the negative stress response or distress, is familiar. We suggest a new concept that we call savoring that does for eustress what coping does for distress. Savoring is recognizing and appreciating the positive response to demands at work and attempting to self-identify the sources that seem to most elicit the greatest sense of engagement and challenge.

Working women should be encouraged by the fact that despite the challenges, work can be a significant source of engagement, challenge, and health in their lives. Work, and for that matter life, will always be a mosaic of positive and negative experiences that are more than likely occurring simultaneously and interacting with each other in complex ways. In addition to valence, responses to work experiences differ with respect to their duration and intensity.

POTENTIAL GENDER DIFFERENCES IN EUSTRESS AND SAVORING

While Rose's (1987) work provides physiological evidence for eustress, it does not provide specific insight for women at work. Frankenhauser (1979, 1983, 1986) provided additional support for the concept that different psychological processes affect the physiological response pattern in different ways, and these response patterns were found to have slight gender differences. Through a series of experiments, she and her colleagues consistently found that two components of psychological arousal determined cortisol and catecholamine responses. The psychological state characterized by positive emotions was labeled *effort*, and the psychological state characterized by negative emotions was labeled *distress*. Indicators of effort were variables labeled *effort*, *tenseness*, and *concentration*, while indicators of distress were variables labeled *boredom*, *impatience*, *tiredness*, and *lack of interest* (Lundberg & Frankenhauser, 1980). Frankenhauser (1979) notes the general resemblance of these two factors and the cortisol factor and catecholamine factor reported by Ursin et al. (1978) in their study of parachute trainees.

Frankenhauser (1983) asserted that these findings support the notion that psychologically different conditions produce a selective response. In general, cortisol secretions were associated with the *negative* feelings of distress, and catecholamine secretions were associated with the *positive* feeling of effort. The general patterns of hormonal secretions were the same for males and females; however, there was a distinct sex difference in the magnitude of the response, with women reporting less intense effort and, accordingly, less of the catecholamines associated with positive emotions. Frankenhauser (1981) emphasized that "neurendocrine responses to the psychosocial environment are determined by the individual's cognitive appraisal of the situation and the emotional impact of the stimuli rather than by their objective characteristics" (p. 493).

This was confirmed in a study of positive and negative stress differences between male and female managers and clerical workers using several physiological indicators of stress. Positive stress was operationalized with self-report measures of engagement and ability to concentrate, and negative stress was indicated with time pressures and pressure by demands. This study found that both men and women experienced more positive stress than negative stress, but the positive stress levels were lower for women. Although the women in the study experienced a high degree of engagement and enjoyed their work, they had a harder time unwinding after work than did the men in the study.

A recent study of high-level white-collar male and female managers again found that both women and men at these high levels experienced their jobs as challenging and stimulating, although the situation was less favorable for women. Women experienced more distress as a result of their higher unpaid workload and commitments to home and family (Lundberg & Frankenhauser, 1999).

Hope has been identified as a potentially significant indicator of the eustress response (Simmons & Nelson, 2001). Some view hope as a positive emotion reflecting a degree of expected benefit resulting from an evaluation of a particular situation (Smith et al., 1993). Hope was defined as a cognitive set that is based on a sense of successful goal-directed determination and planning to meet goals (Snyder et al., 1996). As a belief that one has both the will and the way to accomplish one's goals, hope has also been suggested as an attribute of emotional intelligence (Huy, 1999). The state of hope thus provides a snapshot of a person's goal-directed thinking and engagement.

Gender differences in stated hope did not emerge in any of the studies conducted to develop and validate the scale used to measure it. The lack of gender differences for hope is consistent with findings of the scale for dispositional hope, which has been administered to thousands of men and women of different backgrounds, education, and occupations (Snyder, 1994). The positive spin on this finding is that men and women are equally hopeful.

Conversely, it might be that the goals toward which hope is applied are different for women and men (Snyder, 1994). Like a glass ceiling effect, women might not really expect to have many of life's goals, especially those associated with work, open to them. If women perceive that many work goals are beyond their reach, they might not even think of certain goals as being attainable. In effect, women might limit their goals to those left open to them. Thus, women might report high hope for the goals they believe they are allowed to have.

However, organizations now employ a significant number of women that have reached midlife and midcareer (Gordon & Whelan, 1998). Women at midcareer often have more positive models for thinking about success, career progression, and work and family responsibilities. Their desire for new challenges will likely find them directing their hope toward levels of career advancement that might have seemed unattainable when they first began their careers.

THE FUTURE

In this chapter, we have reviewed the research evidence for differences in the ways men and women preventively manage stress. We also presented eustress as the other, unexplored half of the stress experience, and introduced savoring eustress as a positive complement to coping with distress. The research on gender differences holds great promise for the future, because so many intriguing questions remain to be pursued.

Most studies of stress management methods have focused on the use of a single technique. In reality, individuals use a combination of prevention methods. Do the genders differ in terms of the combinations they choose? Are specific combinations of methods directed toward specific stressors? Future studies must acknowledge the complexity of the process of coping and examine a combination of methods. In addition, researchers need to examine preventive management methods within the context of the stress process, including both their antecedents (stressors, cognitive appraisal) and their consequences (distress, health). Recommending the inclusion of outcomes in prevention studies is essentially calling for more studies on the efficacy of the various preventive management methods.

Do men and women differ in their use of the three broad levels of preventive management methods? While we know that women tend to seek professional care (tertiary-level prevention) more readily than do men, this question remains unexplored for primary and secondary methods. Clearly, there is evidence, as we have critically reviewed earlier in the chapter, for gender differences in specific preventive management methods within each level. What we are calling for here is an examination of the levels themselves. Do women, for example, tend to use more primary (stressor-directed) prevention than men? Do men gravitate more toward secondary (response-focused) prevention?

In developing their theory of preventive stress management, Quick and Quick (1984) provided conceptual and evaluative research evidence for the individual preventive management techniques they included. Although evidence from studies of the various methods exists, no large-scale study has tested the basic premise of preventive management — specifically, that primary prevention is best, supplemented with secondary, with hopes of minimal use of tertiary. Evidence from public health supports the basic hierarchy, but it remains to be tested within the domain of stress. Consistent with the theme of this chapter, we also need to ascertain whether the model holds for women and men alike.

We have focused specifically on the individual side of preventive management. It is important to recognize, however, that the preventive management philosophy holds that both individuals and organizations have responsibilities for health. More research is warranted on gender differences related to the organizational side of preventive management. Are organizational stress management interventions directed most often toward men? Are women at a disadvantage, or vice versa? Given gender differences in stressors, the use of prevention methods, and distress symptoms, is it wise to target interventions toward specific sexes?

Another large and looming question is *why* women and men manage stress differently. Is it because of their exposure to different stressors? Is it because of the prevalence of different symptoms among the sexes? Are biologically based differences such as tend and befriend (Taylor et al., 2000) plausible explanatory factors? Do personality factors lead to the choice of specific prevention methods? Gender differences in personality can help us then study gender differences in preventive management. In addition to investigating differences, we need to study the explanations for these differences.

In addition, we strongly advocate the inclusion of eustress in future studies of work stress and preventive management. Failure to do so is to study only half of the complex fabric of the stress experience. We believe that eustress can be better conceptualized by identifying it as a positive aspect of the stress response itself rather than a positive effect of the stress response. We further assert that a more complex understanding is needed, one in which the presence or absence of the positive (eustress) as well as the presence or absence of the negative (distress) are necessary to fully appreciate the stress response and its effect on health and performance. Few, if any, demands are appraised as purely positive or purely negative. It is usually some combination of the two. For example, a survivor of downsizing can experience sadness and anxiety at the loss of respected coworkers and friends. Yet at the same time, he might feel energized and consider downsizing to be an opportunity for personal growth (Mishra & Spreitzer, 1998).

One way that leaders might generate eustress is by creating an environment at work that allows individuals to experience the eustress response. For example, consider the variable hope. The ability to generate hope among an organization's members might be particularly important during radical change efforts, which the nurses in our study were facing. When people believe that their actions will lead to positive results, they might be more willing to accept difficult and uncertain challenges. Managers can generate hope by establishing goals that are meaningful to all members, allocating the organizational resources necessary for individuals to excel at their jobs, and maintaining a frequent and inspirational dialogue with their employees.

Another initial step in this effort might be to identify which aspects of the work employees find most engaging and then, more importantly, identify *why* individuals find the work pleasurable and what managers can do to enhance the positive aspects of the work experience. Why do some individuals feel that work makes sense emotionally, that problems and demands are worth investing energy in, are worthy of commitment and *engagement*, and are challenges that are welcome? By doing so, managers can demonstrate that their *employees* are worth investing energy in, are worthy of commitment and engagement from managers, and that the challenges of improving the employees' work experience are welcome.

Finally, we believe that there must exist a complement to coping with distress such that rather than preventing or resolving the negative side of stress, individuals promote or prolong the positive side of stress. Savoring, in everyday parlance, means enjoying something with appreciation or dwelling on it with great delight. We believe that most individuals not only prefer eustress, but actually *savor*, or enjoy with appreciation, this positive response to aspects of demands they encounter at work. Athletes speak of being in the zone or at the top of their game; performing artists recognize a state of "flow" or complete immersion in the performance and attunement with the audience. Descriptions such as these are often accompanied by a desire to experience that positive, productive state more frequently, or for longer periods. Managers might facilitate savoring by exploring opportunities to improve policies, procedures, and the physical work environment in an effort to enhance employees' exposure to work that they find engaging and to eliminate potential impediments to eustress.

REFERENCES

Alvesson, M., & Billing, A. D. (1997). *Understanding Gender and Organizations*. London: Sage.

Beehr, T. A., Farmer, S. J., Glazer, S., Gudanowski, D. M., & Nair, V. N. (2003). The enigma of social support and occupational stress: Source congruence and gender role effects. *Journal of Occupational Health Psychology*, 8, 220–231.

Bennett, P., Wallace, L., Carroll, D., & Smith, N. (1991). Treating type A behaviours and mild hypertension in middle-aged men. *Journal of Psychosomatic Research*, 35, 209–223.

Benson, H., & Stark, M. (1996). *Timeless Healing: The Power and Biology of Belief*. New York: Scribner.

Bond, J. T., Galinsky, E., & Swanberg, J. E. (1998). *The 1997 National Study of the Changing Workforce*. New York: Families and Work Institute.

Burke, R. J. (2002). Men, masculinity and health. In D. L. Nelson & R. J. Burke (Eds.), *Gender, Work Stress and Health* (pp. 35–54). Washington, DC: American Psychological Association.

Burke, R. J., & Nelson, D. L. (1998). Organizational men: Masculinity and its discontents. *International Review of Industrial and Organizational Psychology*, 13, 225–271.

Csikszentmihalyi, M. (1990). *Flow: The Psychology of Optimal Experience.* New York: Harper & Row.

Davidson, R. J. (2000). Affective style, psychopathology, and resilience: Brain mechanisms and plasticity. *American Psychologist*, 55, 1196–1214.

Edwards, J. R., & Cooper, C. L. (1988). The impacts of positive psychological states on physical health: A review and theoretical framework. *Social Science Medicine*, 27, 1147–1459.

Elkman, P., Levenson, R. W., & Friesen, W. V. (1983). Autonomic nervous system activity distinguishes among emotions. *Science*, 221, 1208–1210.

Fielden, S. L., & Cooper, C. L. (2002). Managerial stress: Are women more at risk? In D. L. Nelson & R. J. Burke (Eds.), *Gender, Work Stress and Health* (pp. 19–34). Washington, DC: American Psychological Association.

Folkman, S., & Lazarus, R. (1980). An analysis of coping in a middle-aged community sample. *Journal of Health and Social Behavior*, 21, 219–239.

Frankenhauser, M. (1979). Psychobiological aspects of life stress. In S. Levine and H. Ursin (Eds.), *Coping and Health* (pp. 203–223). New York: Plenum Press.

Frankenhauser, M. (1981). Coping with stress at work. *International Journal of Health Services*, 11, 491–510.

Frankenhauser, M. (1983). The sympathetic-adrenal and pituitary-adrenal response to challenge: Comparison between the sexes. In T. M. Dembroski, T. H. Schmidt, & G. Blumchen (Eds.), *Biobehavioral Bases of Coronary Heart Disease* (pp. 91–105). New York: Karger.

Frankenhauser, M. (1986). A psychobiological framework for research on human stress and coping. In M. H. Appley & R. Trumbull (Eds.), *Dynamics of Stress: Physiological, Psychological, and Social Perspectives* (pp. 101–116). New York: Plenum Press.

Frankenhauser, M., Von Wright, M. R., Collins, A., Von Wright, J., Sedvall, G., and Swahn, C. G. (1978). Sex differences in psychoendocrine reactions to examination stress. *Psychosomatic Medicine*, 40, 334–343.

Friedman, E., & Berger, B. G. (1991). Gender roles, sport, and exercise. *Journal of Applied Sport Psychology*, 3, 61–86.

Friedman, M. D., & Rosenman, R. H. (1974). *Type A Behavior and Your Heart*. New York: Knopf.

Fydenberg, E., & Lewis, R. (1993). Boys play sports and girls turn to others: Age, gender and ethnicity as determinants of coping. *Journal of Adolescence*, 16, 252–266.

Ganster, D.C., & Schaubroeck, J. (1991). Work stress and employee health. *Journal of Management*, 17, 235–271.

Gianakos, I. (2002). Predictors of coping with work stress: The influences of sex, gender role, social desirability, and locus of control. *Sex Roles*, 46, 149–158.

Gordon, J.R., & Whelan, K.S. (1998). Successful professional women in midlife: How organizations can more effectively understand and respond to the challenges. *Academy of Management Executive*, 12, 8–24.

Gottlieb, B. H. (1996). Theories and practices of mobilizing support in stressful circumstances. In C. L. Cooper (Ed.), *Handbook of Stress, Medicine, and Health* (pp. 339–356). Boca Raton, FL: CRC Press.

Greenglass, E. R. (1988). Type A behavior and coping strategies in female and male supervisors. *Applied Psychology: An International Review*, 37, 271–288.

Greenglass, E. R. (1993). The contribution of social support to coping strategies. *Applied Psychology: An International Review*, 42, 323–340.

Greenglass, E. R. (2002). Work stress, coping, and social support: Implications for women's occupational well-being. In D. L. Nelson & R. J. Burke (Eds.), *Gender, Work Stress and Health* (pp. 85–96). Washington, DC: American Psychological Association.

Greenglass, E. R., Schwarzer, R., & Taubert, S. (1999). The proactive coping inventory (PCI): A multidimensional research instrument. Retrieved from http://userpage.fu-berlin.de/~health/greenpci.htm.

Harrison, J., Chin, J., & Ficarrotto, T. (1989). Warning: Masculinity may be dangerous to your health. In M. S. Kimmel & M. A. Messner (Eds.), *Men's Lives* (pp. 296–309). New York: Macmillan.

Huy, Q. N. (1999). Emotional capability, emotional intelligence, and radical change. *Academy of Management Review*, 24, 325–345.

Jex, S. M. (1998). *Stress and Job Performance*. Thousand Oaks, CA: Sage Publications.

Kabat-Zinn, J., Lipworth, L., & Bruney, R. (1985). The clinical use of mindfulness meditation for the self-regulation of chronic pain. *Journal of Behavioral Medicine*, 8, 163–190.

Karambayya, R. (2002). Women and corporate restructuring: Sources and consequences of stress. In D. L. Nelson & R. J. Burke (Eds.), *Gender, Work Stress and Health* (pp. 55–70). Washington, DC: American Psychological Association.

Kindlon, D. J. (1983). Comparison of use of meditation and rest in treatment of test anxiety. *Psychological Reports*, 53, 931–938.

Langan-Fox, J. (2001). Women's careers and occupational stress. In C. Cooper & I. Robertson (Eds.), *Well-Being in Organizations* (pp. 177–208). Chichester, England: John Wiley & Sons.

Lazarus, R. S. (1966). *Psychological Stress and the Coping Process*. New York: McGraw-Hill.

Lazarus, R. S., & Folkman, S. (1984). *Stress, Appraisal, and Coping*. New York: Springer Publishing Company.

Liebler, C. A., & Sandefur, G. D. (2002). Gender differences in the exchange of social support with friends, neighbors, and co-workers at midlife. *Social Science Research*, 31, 364.

Lindquist, T. L, Beilin, L. J., & Knuiman, M. W. (1997). Influence of lifestyle, coping, and job stress on blood pressure in men and women. *Hypertension*, 29, 1–7.

Lundberg, U., & Frankenhauser, M. (1980). Pituitary-adrenal and sympathetic-adrenal correlates of distress and effort. *Journal of Psychosomatic Research*, 24, 125–130.

Lundberg, U., & Frankenhauser, M. (1999). Stress and workload of men and women in high-ranking positions. *Journal of Occupational Health Psychology*, 4, 142–151.

MacEwen, K., & Barling, J. (1988). Interrole conflict, family support and marital adjustment of employed mothers: A short term longitudinal study. *Journal of Organizational Behavior*, 9, 241– 250.

Maddi, S. R. (1995). Workplace Hardiness for These Turbulent Times. Paper presented at the annual meeting of the Academy of Management, Vancouver, Canada.

Mason, J. W. (1974). Specificity in the organization response profiles. In P. Seeman & G. Brown (Eds.), *Frontiers in Neurology and Neuroscience Research*. Toronto: University of Toronto.

Mattingly, M. J., & Bianchi, S. M. (2003). Gender differences in the quantity and quality of free time: *Social Forces*, 81, 999–1030.

Matuszek, P. A. C., Nelson, D. L., & Quick, J. C. (1995). Gender differences in distress: Are we asking all the right questions? *Journal of Social Behavior and Personality*, 10, 99–120.

McDonald, L. M., & Korabik, K. (1991). Sources of stress and ways of coping among male and female managers. *Journal of Social Behavior and Personality*, 6, 185–198.

Mishra, A.K., & Spreitzer, G.M. 1998. Explaining how survivors respond to downsizing: The roles of trust, empowerment, justice, and work redesign. *Academy of Management Review*, 23, 567–588.

Nelson, D. L., & Burke, R. J. (2000). Women executives: Health, stress and success. *Academy of Management Executive*, 14, 107–121.

Nelson, D. L., & Burke, R. J. (2002). A framework for examining gender, work stress, and health. In D. L. Nelson & R. J. Burke (Eds.), *Gender, Work Stress and Health* (pp. 3–14). Washington, DC: American Psychological Association.

Nelson, D. L., Quick, J. C., & Hitt, M. A. (1989). Men and women of the personnel profession: Some similarities and differences in their stress. *Stress Medicine*, 5, 145–152.

O'Driscoll, M. P. (2001). The interface between job and off-job roles: Enhancement and conflict. In C. Cooper & I. Robertson, (Eds.), *Well-Being in Organizations* (pp. 149–176). Chichester, England: John Wiley & Sons.

Pennebaker, J. W., Kiecolt-Glaser, J. K., & Glaser, R. (1988). Disclosures of traumas and immune function: Health implications for psychotherapy. *Journal of Consulting and Clinical Psychology*, 56, 239–245.

Pennebaker, J. W., & Seagel, J. D. (1999). Forming a story: The health benefits of narrative. *Journal of Clinical Psychology*, 55, 1243.

Perrewe, P. L., & Carlson, D. S. (2002). Do men and women benefit from social support equally? Results from a field examination within the work and family context. In D. L. Nelson & R. J. Burke (Eds.), *Gender, Work Stress and Health* (pp. 101–114). Washington, DC: American Psychological Association.

Pleck, J. H. (1995). The gender role strain paradigm: An update. In R. F. Levant & W. S. Pollack (Eds.), *A New Psychology of Men* (pp. 11–32). New York: Basic Books.

Quick, J. C., & Quick, J. D. (1984). *Organizational Stress and Preventive Management*. New York: McGraw-Hill.

Quick, J. C., Quick, J. D., Nelson, D. L., & Hurrell, J. J., Jr. (1997). *Preventive Stress Management in Organizations*. Washington, DC: American Psychological Association.

Quick, J. D., Quick, J. C., & Nelson, D. L. (1998). The theory of preventive stress management in organizations. In C. Cooper (Ed.), *Theories of organizational Stress* (pp. 246–268). Oxford: Oxford University Press.

Rees, D., & Cooper, C. L. (1990). Occupational stress in health service workers in the UK. *Stress Medicine*, 8, 79–80.

Rose, R.M. (1987). Neuroendocrine effects of work stress. In J. C. Quick, R. S. Bhagal, J. E. Dalton, and J. D. Quick (Eds.), *Work Stress: Health Care Systems in the Workplace* (pp. 130–147). New York: Praeger.

Roseman, I.J. (1984). Cognitive determinants of emotion: A structural theory. In P. Shaver (Ed.), *Review of Personality and Social Psychology: Emotions, Relationships, and Health* (pp. 11–36). Beverly Hills, CA: Sage.

Rosen, L. N., Wright, K., Marlowe, D., Bartone, P., & Gifford, R. K. (1999). Gender differences in subjective distress attributable to anticipation of combat among U.S. Army soldiers deployed to the Persian Gulf during Operation Desert Storm. *Military Medicine*, 164, 753–757.

Roskies, E. (1987). *Stress Management for the Healthy Type A: Theory and Practice*. New York: Guilford Press.

Ross, C. E., & Bird, S. E. (1994). Sex stratification and healthy lifestyle: Consequences for men's and women's perceived health. *Journal of Health and Social Behavior*, 35, 161–178.

Ryff, C. D., & Singer, B. (1998). The contours of positive human health. *Psychological Inquiry*, 9, 1–28.

Seligman, M. E. P. (1990). *Learned Optimism*. New York: Knopf.

Selye, H. (1976a). *Stress in Health and Disease*. Boston: Butterworths.

Selye, H. (1976b). *The Stress of Life*, rev. ed. New York: McGraw-Hill.

Simmons, B. L., & Nelson, D. L. (2001). Eustress at work: The relationship between hope and health in hospital nurses. *Health Care Management Review*, 26, 7–18.

Smith, C. A., Haynes, K. N., Lazarus, R. S., & Pope, L. K. (1993). In search of the "hot" cognitions: Attributions, appraisals, and their relation to emotion. *Journal of Personality and Social Psychology*, 65, 916–929.

Snyder, C. R. (1994). *The Psychology of Hope: You Can Get There from Here*. New York: The Free Press.

Snyder, C. R., Sympson, S. C., Ybasco, F. C., Borders, T. F., Babyak, M. A., & Higgins, R. L. (1996). Development and validation of the state hope scale. *Journal of Personality and Social Psychology*, 70, 321–335.

Soderstrom, M., Dolbier, C., Leiferman, J., & Steinhardt, M. (2000). The relationship of hardiness, coping strategies, and perceived stress to symptoms of illness. *Journal of Behavioral Medicine*, 23, 311–328.

Swanson, V., Power, K. G., & Simpson, R. J. (1998). Occupational stress and family life: A comparison of male and female doctors. *Journal of Occupational and Organizational Psychology*, 71, 237–260.

Taylor, S., Klein, L., Lewis, B., Garung, R., Gruenewald, T., & Updegraff, J. (2000). Biobehavioral responses to stress in females: Tend and befriend, not fight or flight. *Psychological Review*, 107, 411–429.

Thrane, C. (2000). Men, women, and leisure time: Scandinavian evidence of gender inequality. *Leisure Sciences*, 22, 109–122.

Tomarken, A. J., Davidson, R. J., Wheeler, R. E., & Doss, R. C. (1992). Individual differences in anterior brain asymmetry and fundamental dimensions of emotion. *Journal of Personality and Social Psychology*, 62, 676–687.

Torkelson, E., & Nuhonen, T. (2003). Coping strategies and health symptoms among women and men in a downsizing organization. *Psychological Reports*, 92, 899–907.

Ursin, H., Baade, E., and Levine, S. (1978). *Psychobiology of Stress*. New York: Academic Press.

Wheeler, R. E., Davidson, R. J., & Tomarken, A. J. (1993). Frontal brain asymmetry and emotional reactivity: A biological substrate of affective style. *Psychophysiology*, 30, 82–89.

Williams, J. (1999). *Unbending Gender: Why Work and Family Conflict and What to Do about It*. New York: Oxford University Press.

17 Dealing with Stress: Families and Chronic Illness

David W. Kissane

CONTENTS

The family provides the most common source of support for the sick person, and even if the family is less than optimally supportive, it forms an influential background for any chronic illness. A web of reciprocal influences exists within the family as it strives to adapt to the needs of its ill member and the challenges that care provision brings. While acute illness might precipitate only a brief perturbation to the pattern of family life, chronic illness serves as both a cumulative stressor and a potential burden to all involved. How the family as a whole adapts to these circumstances ultimately influences the adjustment of the symptom bearer.

0-8493-1820-3/05/$0.00+$1.50

In this chapter, the nature of the family and patterns of family response to stress in the setting of chronic illness are considered, together with relevant extraneous influences. The relationship between family functioning and individual psychosocial morbidity is established to highlight the pertinence of adopting a family approach. Family-focused grief therapy is one possible intervention that seeks to optimize family functioning (Kissane & Bloch, 2002). Its themes and method of application are discussed alongside other models of family intervention employed to reduce the stress of chronic illness (Campbell & Patterson, 1995). Some challenges in working with complex families and the ethical dilemmas encountered conclude the discussion. The family is inextricably involved with chronic illness and therefore an appropriate component to consider in planning comprehensive care provision.

WHAT IS THE FAMILY?

While a family is conventionally defined by kinship, whether established by bloodlines or marriage, it can be a much more complex social structure than clinicians recognize in the clinical setting. The range of potential configurations is considerable — nuclear, extended, family of origin, adopted, blended, single parent, or gay — and illness is met within each and every of these configurations (Burguiere et al., 1996). Sociologists have noted the tension between sense of duty and emotional attachment within these relationships, with clear trends away from marriage as a property arrangement to those based on genuine romantic attraction (Giddens, 1998). The health care provider tends to bypass this complexity, simply accepting as family whoever the patient names as such. Indeed, rather than attending to structure, the functioning of the family as a dynamic and adaptive unit is more determinative of health and well-being.

Irrespective of the specific configuration of the kinship community, whenever illness occurs, any associated distress reverberates through the family, so that not only the index patient but also his or her partner, children, and a range of other relatives can be affected by the illness. In the setting of more serious and chronic illnesses like cancer, studies have shown that up to one third of spouses and one quarter of offspring carry significant psychosocial morbidity (Kissane et al., 1994). The related argument for adoption of a family-centered model of care is convincing.

PATTERNS OF FAMILY RESPONSE TO CHRONIC STRESS

Coping responses to the presence of a family member's chronic illness, whether diabetes, arthritis, respiratory, renal, cardiovascular, mental, or malignant disease, can be broadly conceptualized as adaptive or maladaptive. Emotional, cognitive, and behavioral features can be discerned within recognizable patterns of the family-as-a-whole response.

The common features of an adaptive family coping response involve members relating with openness and disclosing feelings honestly, sharing their distress, providing mutual support, and accepting both positive and negative feelings (Raphael, 1984). These families accommodate varied roles for their members flexibly, generating growth in teamwork and cohesion, while respecting differential rates of mourning. They tolerate both the challenges and burdens of illness and achieve creative outcomes for their membership over time.

In contrast, various maladaptive patterns of family response to chronic stress have been described. The key mechanisms that underpin such responses include avoidance, distortion, amplification, and prolongation. Let us briefly consider each pattern in turn.

Avoidant families are difficult to recruit into empirical studies, yet are common clinically, albeit retreating. They block the sharing of genuine feelings, stoic silence being their preferred modus operandi. They might intellectualize, find it hard to trust, or promote the keeping of a secret. If a more dominant member prevents others from sharing, the resultant repression might accentuate distress and prolong symptomatology (Bowlby-West, 1983; Kissane, 1994).

Distorting responses generate a range of strong emotions, wherein families blame, feel guilty, carry anger, or promulgate ambivalence. Sometimes idealization of the seriously ill person distorts through producing a reaction that clearly deviates from the expected and balanced response style. Nevertheless, negative reactions tend to dominate this distorting style. In the setting of chronic mental illness, for instance, families offering an excessively critical stance have been described as having "high expressed emotion," this being associated with a relapsing and chronic course of psychiatric disorder (Brown et al., 1972; Vaughn & Leff, 1976; Leff et al., 1989).

While similar in some respects to the intensity of distortion, amplification as a family response involves the distress being transmitted contagiously to others, often with disruption of cohesive bonds and the splitting of families (Lieberman & Black, 1982). Relationships thereafter fracture and disintegrate, with separation, rejection, and alienation. The conflict is very public, but clinical services struggle to contain such deep rifts.

Finally, prolongation reflects the propensity for the symptomatic to persist, sometimes untreated, with periodic exacerbations as recurring family dysfunction aggravates the wounds. Chronic depression or demoralization is a typical outcome from this sequence. In practice, various combinations of avoidance, distortion, amplification, and prolongation occur as families struggle inexorably with a chronic pattern of maladaptation.

Attention to such family styles highlights the relational approaches that families use to generate their responses. These have been summarized most succinctly as the communication of both thoughts and feelings, the capacity to tolerate difference through mutual respect, good problem solving and resolution of conflict, and cohesiveness represented by teamwork and mutual support (Kissane & Bloch, 2002). Within such modes of operating, the family structure and the specific roles of members can sometimes confound overall functioning, while acceptance of family norms, values, and rules can also influence the overall cohesion of the unit. The adaptive functioning of the family as a whole is nonetheless governed by its relational capacity, and attention to this feature of family life can have considerable utility clinically.

A synergy exists between these relational aspects of family functioning and developmental models of the individual as portrayed by psychoanalytic thinking

(Freud, 1917; Klein, 1940), attachment theory (Bowlby, 1969, 1988), and other notions of developmental psychology (Stern, 1985). Thus, the well-functioning family can provide the context for the development of secure attachments; the dysfunctional family can contribute to insecure attachments, whether avoidant, ambivalent, or disorganized (see, for instance, the writings of Ainsworth & Eichberg, 1991; Fonagy, 2001).

One insightful perspective on the dynamic processes of family reorganization in the setting of chronic illness (in this case, renal failure) was developed by Reiss and colleagues (Reiss, 1990; Reiss et al., 1993; Cole & Reiss, 1993; Weihs & Reiss, 2000). Within their model, change in the status and prognosis of the chronic illness shifts the family toward a disease-centered focus for a period, as the family responds to the demands of the disease and its treatment. An alliance builds with the medical team and family cohesiveness increases, until some new equilibrium is established as the illness trajectory fluctuates, permitting the family to move back and forth between a disease-centered and living-centered focus. These perturbations can repeat across the years until a more terminal phase of illness emerges, which again generates a disease-centered focus, albeit sometimes with some distancing of the patient from the rest of the family as the patient conserves energy in preparation for his or her death.

Such consideration of response patterns by families opens up the possibility of both classifying family types and responding with preventive and therapeutic interventions where needed. The goal herein is not to label families pejoratively (for, indeed, this would prove damaging), but to optimize their responses so that adaptive outcomes can be nurtured where needed. Moreover, this approach should lead health professionals to a greater emphasis on preventive rather than crisis-based interventions.

Family response patterns also point inherently to the functioning of the family as a unit. Like the physiology of the body, the dynamic operation of the family system merits study and understanding. The maladaptive family response is thus analogous to pathophysiology of the diseased body and ought to become the natural focus of clinical interventions that aim to improve the overall outcome for all concerned. However, before turning to such models of family-centered care, consideration of the myriad influences that can affect the functioning of the family as a whole is necessary, for these might need to be considered within the therapeutic model that is adopted.

FACTORS INFLUENCING THE FAMILY'S RESPONSE TO ILLNESS

Many confounding factors apply, for not only are the nature and course of illness as stressors relevant, but also who the family is through their membership and their sociodemographic and cultural setting. The life cycle of the family, its ethnicity, knowledge of disease, genetics, specific treatment and overall management, depth of supports, community resources, special skills, and mobility of members will influence both the resilience and vulnerability of the family in its response. Let us consider the major contributors here.

Life Cycle

Families move through their own developmental phases from courtship and the initiation of relationships, to reproduction when young children are reared, to the generativity of family membership who reach out to the broader community, through to sickness, aging, and neediness, when future generations are invited to take on the roles of nurturance and creativity while the health of senior family members deteriorates prior to their deaths (Carter & McGoldrick, 1980). Although a periodicity is evident when the natural order conforms to its anticipated pattern, in practice, disturbances of this natural order challenge families. When life-threatening illness arrives prematurely or chronic illness spoils the expected accomplishments of adult life, adjustment is inevitable (Rolland, 1984).

Thus, when illness occurs at an expected point in the family life cycle, its acceptance is easier intellectually than when it arrives out of sequence — illness is, of course, unwelcome emotionally at all points of the life cycle. Furthermore, untimely illness interferes with other tasks that might have been undertaken by a family at that stage (Walsh & McGoldrick, 1991a,b). Such timeliness of onset and the length of illness influence how the family perceives it as a stressor.

Nature, Course, and Meaning of the Illness

Chronic illness can bring vast variation in its challenge and potential burden to the patient, which in turn influences the carers and family members (Turk et al., 1985; Bloch et al., 1994). Support is provided under many guises — emotional, financial, social, and spiritual, to name a few. Ultimately, however, the meaning that the illness holds for the family is significant and can govern the family's response to care provision. The more dire and sinister the illness is perceived to be, the more likely the family will volunteer their assistance; au contraire, chronicity increases the likelihood of families overlooking the plight of the ill member and seeing any consequent disability or handicap as a nuisance that is best ignored.

Culture, Sick Role, and Illness Behavior

Not only does the local culture have a substantial impact on how the ill member behaves with respect to his or her illness, but it also guides the expectations and responses of the host family (Parsons, 1955). Much has been written about these concepts through the decades, but it was well illustrated by Engel's (1959) classic study of the pain-prone patient, in which childhood neglect occurred developmentally except for occasions when the child was ill or in pain. Health professionals need to understand these complex influences on the explanatory models of illness and the social and interpersonal behaviors that follow.

The Family's Needs and Resources

Single parents, migrant or refugee families, underserved communities, and the family's knowledge and utilization of resources will all influence the coping and adaptation of the family as a whole. Assessing unmet needs is a straightforward method of responding to families (Given & Given, 1996), but studies of family functioning have highlighted that dysfunctional families exhibit a reduced capacity to utilize community resources — their dysfunctionality interferes with their ability to accept help (Kissane et al., 1996a, 1996b).

Health and Well-Being of the Family

The well-functioning family who communicates their needs and concerns, consoles each other emotionally, provides mutual support and assistance, and responds to cumulative stressors with robustness contrasts readily with the maladaptive family, who lacks the wherewithal to adapt with such resilience. Health care providers do well therefore to concentrate their therapeutic energies on those at greater risk of a maladaptive outcome, in the process respecting the capacity of well-functioning families to rise successfully to the occasion (Kissane & Bloch, 2002).

THE RELATIONSHIP BETWEEN FAMILY FUNCTIONING AND INDIVIDUAL PSYCHOSOCIAL MORBIDITY

A cornerstone of the concept of working preventively with families is the positive association that has been demonstrated between family functioning and the presence of psychosocial morbidity among individual members of those families whose style of relating together is more dysfunctional. This principle was recognized initially in the families of patients with chronic schizophrenia, then in those with chronic depression and with a range of medically ill patients, including those receiving palliative care and becoming bereaved.

Mental illness casts family members into supportive roles and adds invariably a source of chronic stress and burden to the family. As mentioned, a sizeable body of research has demonstrated the relationship between the relapse of schizophrenia and the presence of a style of family functioning termed high expressed emotionality (Brown et al., 1972; Vaughn & Leff, 1976; Leff et al., 1989). In these families, members make a number of critical comments about each other and conflict is prominent. Not only is this family environment associated with an increased relapse of schizophrenia, but psychoeducational interventions have been shown to reduce this expressed emotionality, thus reducing the rate of relapse of schizophrenia. This work has subsequently been extended to instances of other chronic mental illnesses such as bipolar disorder, recurrent depression, and severe personality disorders.

The work of Keitner and colleagues demonstrated the contribution of family functioning in interacting with individual vulnerability in the generation and relapse of major depressive episodes (Keitner & Miller, 1990). Where depression proves to be relatively treatment resistant, attention to the family environment is wise, lest there be unrecognized perpetuating factors within these family relationships that could be ameliorated.

In the Melbourne family grief studies, the relationship between individuals developing complicated bereavement and the presence of dysfunctionality in their families was demonstrated. A cohort of 115 families was followed through palliative care and across 13 months of bereavement. Subscales of the Family Environment Scale (Moos & Moos, 1981), namely, cohesiveness, expressiveness, and conflict, were shown to be highly correlated with measures of distress, depression, and poor social functioning. The more dysfunctional the family, the greater the rate of individual psychosocial morbidity found among family members (Kissane et al., 1996b).

Using a cluster analytic method to explore patterns of family functioning, a classification emerged in these bereaved families that proved predictive of psychosocial morbidity. Two classes of family were well functioning and carried low rates of psychosocial morbidity: the first of these was termed *supportive* to reflect the good communication, cohesiveness, and the absence of conflict in these families; the second type was named *conflict resolving* because the presence of high cohesion and above-average expressiveness seemed to empower these families to tolerate a moderate level of conflict. By contrast, two classes were clearly dysfunctional: *hostile* families were characterized by high conflict and low cohesion; they appeared fractured and chaotic, even to the extent of members refusing to speak to each other for several years. The second dysfunctional class was termed *sullen* because of the muted anger and high rates of depression found amid their members — these families displayed the most intense levels of grief during bereavement. Interestingly, sullen families exercise highest control over family life, with greater rigidity and conformity to family expectations. Disagreements remain unresolved and anger simmers just beneath the surface. Both hostile and sullen types of families carry high rates of morbidity among their members. In between these dysfunctional and the better-functioning families lies a final class, named *intermediate*. These families are characterized by moderate cohesiveness, but also carry high rates of psychosocial morbidity.

This classification proved remarkably consistent across the period of advanced cancer commonly known as palliative care, as well as during the 13 months of bereavement. The clinical utility of the classification lies in its capacity to predict families at greatest risk of poor adaptation. This is achieved by screening for family functioning through completion of the Family Relationships Index, a 12-item, pencil-and paper, true-or-false questionnaire that can be readily administered to available family members as treatment is provided by an oncology program. Screening rules are outlined in our recent book (Kissane & Bloch, 2002).

Arising from these observational studies of families and their functioning came the empirically developed model of family-centered care, which we termed family-focused grief therapy (FFGT). Through the conduct of a randomized control trial of FFGT initially applied during palliative care and continued into bereavement, we came to treat a range of families experiencing concurrent life events such as chronic alcoholism and chronic physical disorders such as diabetes, familial polycystic renal disease, and somatization disorder, as well as families fractured by divorce and others with prominent cultural differences (Kissane et al., 2003). This clinical work provides provisional evidence for the broad application of a model of family intervention that seeks to improve family functioning during chronic illness, as well as in acute-on-chronic settings such as oncology.

FAMILY-FOCUSED GRIEF THERAPY

A focus on family functioning is central to our model of FFGT with the goal of optimizing this functioning as a pathway to relieve stress and improve psychological well-being. Key dimensions of functioning that are the focus of this model are the "three C's of family relationships": cohesion, communication, and conflict resolution. In an effort to nurture growth and avoid criticism, the strengths of each family are identified and affirmed as a means to harness appropriate change in family well-being.

The word *grief* in the model refers broadly to the adaptation that is necessary in circumstances of change. In the setting of illness, there is always some degree of loss, be it loss of health, disfigurement, infertility, handicap, and disability, or loss of dreams, employability, and financial security, or loss of confidence about one's future. Psychoanalytic theory has long recognized the importance of an ability to mourn such losses as essential to mature adaptation.

This time-limited FFGT model is divided into five stages: assessment, consensus over identified issues, focused treatment to relieve these concerns, consolidation of improved family functioning, and response prevention as part of termination. The number of sessions is therefore applied flexibly over several months, but typically involves four to eight family meetings. The family takes responsibility for considerable problem solving. The therapist's task is to sustain the family's orientation toward recognition of patterns of functioning and accepting responsibility for relevant change. A collaborative therapeutic alliance is central to the model.

Standard principles of family therapy incorporating the therapist's neutrality, the application of circular as well as linear questioning, the creation of hypotheses about family dynamics, and the identification of family strengths (highlighted realistically, lest these be seen as patronizing) are required when working with families with chronic illness. A number of illustrative questions for use by the therapist in garnering pertinent data from the family can be found in the book *Family Focused Grief Therapy*. At an appropriate point during assessment, the construction of a family genogram builds a three-generational picture of family relationships and patterns of family coping with loss, illness, or death. Such transgenerational understanding proves invaluable in recognizing the patterns of response adopted by the family as a whole.

COMMON THEMES THAT ARISE AS FAMILIES COPE WITH THE STRESS OF CHRONIC ILLNESS

Families spend time profitably considering as a group how they share the care provision of an ill family member. Practical help is of vital importance and the regular theme through which most discussion begins. Where the therapist can invite consideration of teamwork, the burden of care will fall less heavily on any individual member. Consideration can also be given to utilization of community resources, including use of respite, volunteers, home help, physical aides, and financial assistance.

The emotional response to suffering proves more challenging for families to share as a group. Yet this is the plight that people fear. Sharing distress creates a metaphorical "holding frame" through which the family becomes better able to contain its sense of vulnerability. When the value of the ill person can be given voice by the family, his or her sense of dignity is upheld. Moreover, whenever a threat of death prevails through more serious illness, open conversation about this does much in many cultures to alleviate unspoken fear. Should the cultural norm be to avoid mention of death per se, the commitment to hope within the tradition is still likely to prove very supportive.

Recognition of and appropriate treatment of clinical depression are vital to any chance of adaptive adjustment. This applies just as much to the family, for caregivers of seriously ill patients can become depressed in significant proportions. Depression can thus reverberate contagiously through the family group unless the distress is aired and symptoms considered thoughtfully. When the vegetative symptoms of depression might be confused with physical illness, Endicott (1984) proposed helpfully that attention be given to alternative symptoms like social withdrawal in place of insomnia, brooding or self-pity in place of fatigue, lack of responsivity or reactivity in place of poor concentration, and gloomy demeanor in place of appetite and weight loss. Most importantly, the efficacy of antidepressants combined with psychotherapy in treating depressed patients is well established (Wilson et al., 2000).

Frank disclosure of family members' reactions to illness can preempt abhorrence of bedsores, fungating wounds, smell, and bodily disfigurement. People can become stuck in awkwardness and allow the abject body to mar intimacy unless open discussion is fostered and the value of the ill person considered. FFGT seeks to nurture family intimacy. When death approaches, giving expression to good-byes is fostered. FFGT respects the role of cultural and religious practices as a background support to family members. The needs of all relatives remain important, including adolescents and younger children, as well as the very elderly.

THE ROLE OF DISCOVERING MEANING IN THE ILLNESS

A long literature (especially church literature) exists about the loss of meaning, spiritual torpor, acedia, or demoralization, as it has been variously termed throughout the centuries. This became focused within psychosomatic medicine through George Engel's "giving up–given up" syndrome (Engel, 1967), while Victor Frankl (1959, 1984) highlighted the importance of loss of meaning to coping whenever fate seems inescapable. Jerome Frank (1968, 1974) saw the maintenance of hope as vital to all forms of psychotherapy. During the 1990s, Susan Folkman reemphasized meaning as the source of positive affects among the carers of patients suffering from AIDS (Folkman, 1997, 2001; Folkman & Greer, 2000). She recognized meaning as a significant deficit from the original Lazarus and Folkman model of coping with stress. Clearly families also have a need to find meaning in the illness suffered by a family member. As a corollary, when families struggle and fail to perceive any meaning in illness, despair and demoralization are likely to follow for the group as a whole.

Meaning-centered therapies can be applied using a family model. Whether these take the form of Frankl's logotherapy, or make use of themes from interpersonal therapy (IPT), wherein change in role, grief work, and adaptation to transition are core features, the search for meaning becomes an important means of adjusting to the burdens and strains of illness. Therapists do well therefore to invite families to discuss what meaning an illness has for them, framing their questions to invite a search for positive sources of meaning alongside the more obvious negative consequences of the illness itself (Wright et al., 1996).

CHALLENGES AND PROBLEMS IN FAMILY WORK

A range of predictable challenges arise whenever therapists pursue family-centered care. These include engaging reluctant members to participate, setting realistic goals, working in the home, dealing constructively with conflict, coping with the uncertainty of prognosis, and sustaining progress over time.

Not all family members will want to take part in family meetings, or not all will be invited by the ill patient, despite the clinician's impression that this is going to occur. Active planning is therefore needed prior to any session, so that the invitation pathway is carefully considered, with the therapist reaching out to distant relatives as needed. Letters remain a powerful means of inviting interest in attendance. In the end, the therapist can only work with those willing to attend, and takes consolation in the power of systemic influence to reach less accessible family members over time.

Some problems are entrenched. Therapists need wisdom in not being drawn into the myth of becoming the family savior, especially when personality difficulties are long-standing and in need of comprehensive psychotherapy. Herein a pragmatic focus to family work is important. Referrals are appropriate for individual work, the family needing protection from becoming entangled in every crisis, lest it be distracted from its global objective of optimizing its functioning.

Home visits and the conduct of family meetings in the home are greatly appreciated and worthwhile, but the therapist needs to apply sensible caveats to recognize when this is unwise. Safety of the therapy is the therapist's remit, and unbridled family conflict, geographic disadvantage, and unsuitable environment are the noteworthy contraindications to home-based family meetings.

Uncertainty of prognosis might be based on the pathology of the particular illness, its potential response to treatment, and the range of therapies available at any time. Families get caught up in this uncertainty, which is ultimately existential, as the length of every life is indeed uncertain. Therapists will share this dilemma with the family. Modeling a means of open communication about such uncertainty, including communication with relevant health care providers, is important and aids the appropriate pacing of family work over time.

Through a further study of the fidelity of application of FFGT in a randomized controlled trial, Chan and colleagues (2003) identified both aspects of the process that therapists perform well and those they experience as more challenging. Therapists generally invite families to explore their style of communication, teamwork, conflict, and patterns of grief resolution fairly effectively. Indeed, families are helped greatly by simply having their grief named for what it is. On the other hand, therapists find it more difficult to construct a sensible summary of the family's concerns and feed this back to the family at the end of a standard session. In the FFGT integrity study, although therapists provided some direction to therapy in

75% of sessions, summaries of progress were only seen in 50%. Therapists need confidence in understanding what has emerged and experience in offering this insight back to the family group.

Therapists did not elicit family values, strengths, and beliefs in 58% of assessments. Some therapists neglect to emphasize the positive, while some families give little thought to a sense of tradition or family motto. Only 54% of therapists had developed a formalized treatment plan by the conclusion of the assessment phase of FFGT. A number of therapists deferred negotiation of this treatment plan until they had the opportunity to discuss the family in peer review supervision. In general, then, clinicians engaged in supervising therapists applying a model like FFGT need to ensure that sufficient attention is given to family strengths and to the formulation of an integrated understanding of the family's concerns, which can, in turn, be offered back to the family as a summary.

COMPLEX FAMILIES IN THE SETTING OF CHRONIC ILLNESS

Certain predictable events will add to the complexity involved in dealing with stress in the context of chronic illness. These include the occurrence of multiple serious physical illnesses within the same family, alcohol and other substance abuse, comorbid mental illness, and concurrent family problems as might occur with blended families, those adopting children, those with cultural diversity, and those facing the ultimate existential challenge — death and dying.

In these circumstances, the therapist cannot but attend to these concurrent issues, although attention to family functioning and its impact on these issues will enable greater insight into factors potentially perpetuating these problems. Wisdom dictates that the therapist not be too distracted by such issues, especially if long-standing. Tolerance of alcohol abuse is the leading example. Families will initially present this as unacceptable, yet when they can see the behavior as symptomatic of other concerns, they discover a way to focus on improving family functioning, with the concern over alcohol gradually fading from the scene.

When families are challenged with the unfairness of coincident multiple serious illnesses, their grief might be profound. The therapist contains such distress through genuine compassion and empathic support. Familial illness, when the genetics cause several members to be afflicted at the same time, calls for family support, even for well-functioning families, as the burden of such unfortunate circumstances can be great.

The prominent demands caused by chronic mental illness being superimposed on physical illness highlight the misfortune that befalls some within our community. Optimizing the use of resources becomes critical as families strive to find a transcendent means of coping with such cumulative stress. A search for meaning and a spiritual approach to coping can enhance family resilience.

As the life cycle unfolds, family problems left in abeyance at one stage might be revisited given more favorable circumstances. Thus, the concerns of children dating back to when their parents divorced might find a means of resolution when illness befalls their parents in later life. Such unfinished business becomes manageable with changed life circumstances, sometimes with blended families being able to achieve considerable maturity through openness to revisiting these issues. Invariably these problems have been relational, yet can be understood within a transgenerational pattern of behaving, such that blame is reduced and forgiveness promoted. Renewed understanding brings wisdom and tolerance to families in these circumstances.

Migration is so universal in this global world that its effects are easily overlooked at the family level. Yet tracing family patterns of coping across these generations brings increased understanding as different ethnic approaches are explored.

OTHER MODELS OF FAMILY INTERVENTION WITH THE CHRONICALLY ILL

The impact of the family has been noted on diabetic control in adolescents and insulin-dependent diabetics (Helz & Templeton, 1990; Wrigley & Mayou, 1991; Mengel et al., 1992), delay in responding to angina (Hackett & Cassem, 1969; Medalie & Goldbourt, 1976), adaptation to thalassemia (Georganda, 1988), compliance with dialysis (Reiss et al., 1986), chronic pain control (Turk et al., 1985; Kerns et al., 1990), and response to Huntington's disease (Kessler & Bloch, 1989). A number of models of family intervention with such chronically ill patients and their families have been described (McDaniel et al., 1997). Larberg and Cavallo (1984) reported on their pattern of intervening with families where a member suffered from multiple sclerosis, often a chronic relapsing or progressive disorder. They identified nodal points when the family's way of coping was disrupted and employed a needs-based approach to support these families.

Building on John Byng-Hall's (1988, 1991) notion of family scripts, in which there is transmission across generations of particular patterns of behaving in stressful circumstances, Steinglass and Horan (1988) developed a multigenerational model of intervening with multiple family groups. This approach has proven particularly useful with a variety of adolescent families and mental illness, and lends itself to application with families suffering from the same chronic illness. Sharing similar experiences and treatments with other families who have also lived through them promotes a sense of universality, that one is not alone with this plight and others have found the means to cope (Gonzalez et al., 1989). Multiple family groups prove cost-effective and link families socially to those living under similar circumstances.

John Rolland (1984, 1987, 1994) has applied a model of family therapy that comprehensively combines the family's response to illness with where they are located within the family life cycle. Acuteness of onset, rate of progression, predictability of outcome, and degree of incapacity all contribute to the family's response to the illness.

Psychoeducational models of family therapy have been well applied in settings of geriatric and cardiac illness. Dementia is a classical example generating a burden on families as carers, further problems arising among recent migrants, much younger partners, and recent second marriages (Brodaty & Hadzi-Pavlovic, 1990). Psychoeducational family interventions have been shown to potentially delay institutionalization (Greene & Monahan, 1987) and reduce stress (Brodaty & Gresham, 1989).

Cardiac rehabilitation programs have observed the contribution of promoting harmonious family relationships and strong social support to achieve improved physical health (Hanson et al., 1991; Worby et al., 1991). Attention to the family has also proved effective in education programs aiming to enhance patient compliance with medications. For instance, adherence to antihypertensive and other cardiac medications has been facilitated through family involvement, especially when the patient tries to deny the reality of his or her cardiac disease (Bar-On & Dreman, 1987). Similarly, Perlesz and colleagues (1992) applied a psychoeducational family model in the setting of a patient suffering traumatic brain damage.

Family therapy also has an identified place in the comprehensive management of chronic alcohol and other substance abuse (Bowen, 1974; Moos et al., 1982; Levine, 1985; Jacob, 1992). Stanton and colleagues (1982) achieved impressive results in a controlled study of family therapy compared with methadone maintenance programs, their study being subsequently replicated by others (Szapocznik & Kurtines, 1989). Alongside genetic factors, impoverished upbringing, and developmental conflicts, onset following traumatic loss events and habitual behavior patterns have all been implicated and need attention during therapies.

Problem solving has been applied in several models of family therapy. This overlaps with task-based approaches wherein a family might be invited to construct a novel solution to an identified problem. Families that work as a group and coordinate their response are found to be better functioning, in contrast with family members who decline to accept assistance from other relatives. David Reiss (1981) noted, however, that consensus-generating families run the risk of missing an optimal solution because of their dogged maintenance of a unified stance. In the Timberlawn or Beavers System model of family function (Lewis et al., 1976; Beavers & Hampson, 1990), prominent use is made of a family task and goal-directed negotiation, while monitoring family affect and style of relating. Although the initial approach differs, task- and solution-focused models achieve improved family functioning as an outcome, similar to FFGT.

ETHICAL ISSUES THAT ARISE IN FAMILY WORK

While never pathologizing the family is critical to avoid causing harm, the ethical issue par excellence that arises in family work is the problem of competing needs. Three competing assumptions come into view. Do the needs of the patient with the chronic illness prevail over those of the family? Or are all members equally relevant? Or does another, especially vulnerable, family member warrant particular attention? At times, pragmatism must prevail, but in general, one strives to meet the needs of all concerned. The better the functioning of any family, the smaller the number of ethical quandaries that seem to arise.

Family secrets present a classic challenge, one that places the therapist in a potentially invidious position. The FFGT model opts for honest communication, while respecting any individual's right to privacy. Truth becomes an issue when unsavory past events have occurred, or when the nature of a chronic illness (such as HIV-AIDS-related illness) has not been revealed to family members, or when changes in status of an illness occur — for instance, cancer recurrence or progression makes the disease potentially life threatening. Avoidance of truth telling is generally problematic and indicative of poor communication within the family, unless strong cultural grounds exist for not naming certain illnesses (Okamura et al., 1998). Should a family member insist on respect for privacy, this might need to be followed, but in general, the therapist asks the family to agree to always work in an open and trusting manner.

Whenever clinical services offer family work within a preventive framework of care provision, the principle of respect is an imperative, lest the therapist assumes a position of knowing best and seeking to impose an ideal, without necessarily appreciating all aspects of the particular family at hand (Aponte 1985; Walrond-Skinner & Watson 1987).

CONCLUSION

In this chapter, the family has been recognized as the most pertinent of social contexts in which chronic illness occurs and can be cared for. The functioning of the family as a dynamic group impacts the quality of life of its membership and becomes a potentially relevant factor perpetuating the illness. Interventions that focus on optimizing family functioning, whether through a model like FFGT, multiple family groups, or another form of problem-solving therapy, can do much to reduce family stress and improve the well-being of members. When clinical services can anticipate sequences within the cycle of chronic illness wherein a family intervention can be applied preventively, considerable morbidity can be reduced.

REFERENCES

Ainsworth, M., & Eichberg, C. (1991). Effects on infant-mother attachment of mother's unresolved loss of an attachment figure, or other traumatic experience. In C. Parkes, J. Stevenson-Hinde, & P. Marris (Eds.), *Attachment across the Life Cycle*. London: Routledge, 160–183.

Aponte, H.J. (1985). The negotiation of values in therapy. *Family Process*, 24, 323–338.

Bar-On, D., & Dreman, S. (1987). When spouses disagree: a predictor of cardiac rehabilitation. *Family Systems Medicine*, 5, 228–237.

Beavers, W.R., & Hampson, R.B. (1990). *Successful Families: Assessment and Intervention*. New York: Norton.

Bloch, S., Hafner, J., Harari, E., & Szmukler, G. (1994). *The Family in Clinical Psychiatry*. Oxford: Oxford University Press.

Bowen, M. (1974). Alcoholism viewed through family systems theory and family psychotherapy. *Annals of the New York Academy of Science*, 233, 115–122.

Bowlby, J. (1969). *Attachment and Loss*, Vol. 1, *Attachment*. New York: Basic Books.

Bowlby, J. (1988). *A Secure Base*. New York: Basic Books.

Bowlby-West, L. (1983). The impact of death on the family system. *Journal of Family Therapy*, 5, 279–294.

Brodaty, H., & Gresham, M. (1989). Effects of a training programme to reduce stress in carers of patients with dementia. *British Medical Journal*, 299, 1375–1379.

Brodaty, H., & Hadzi-Pavlovic, D. (1990). Psychosocial effects on carers of living with persons with dementia. *Australian and New Zealand Journal of Psychiatry*, 24, 351–361.

Brown, G., Birley, J., & Wing, J. (1972). Influence of family life on the course of schizophrenic disorders: a replication. *British Journal of Psychiatry*, 121, 241–258.

Burguiere, A., Klapisch-Zuber, C., Segalen, M., & Zonabend, F. (Eds.). (1996). *A History of Family*. Boston: Belknap Press of Harvard University.

Byng-Hall, J. (1988). Scripts and legends in families and family therapy. *Family Process*, 27, 167–180.

Byng-Hall, J. (1991). Family scripts and loss. In F. Walsh & M. McGoldrick (Eds.), *Living Beyond Loss: Death in the Family* (pp. 130–143). New York: Norton.

Campbell, T.L., & Patterson, J.M. (1995). The effectiveness of family interventions in the treatment of physical illness. *Journal of Marital and Family Therapy*, 21, 545–583.

Carter, E., & McGoldrick, M. (1980). *The Family Life Cycle: A Framework for Family Therapy*. New York: Gardner Press.

Chan, E., O'Neill, I., McKenzie, M., Love, A., & Kissane, D. (2004). What works for therapists conducting family meetings: treatment integrity in family focused grief therapy during palliative care and bereavement. *Journal of Pain and Symptom Management*, 27 (6), 502–512.

Cole, R.E., & Reiss, D. (1993). *How Do Families Cope with Chronic Illness?* Hillsdale, NJ: Lawrence Earlbaum.

Endicott, J. (1984). Measurement of depression in patients with cancer. *Cancer*, 53, 2243–2248.

Engel, G.L. (1959). Psychogenic pain and the 'pain prone' patient. *American Journal of Medicine*, 26, 899–918.

Engel, G.L. (1967). A psychological setting of somatic disease: the "giving up–given up complex." *Proceedings of Royal Society of Medicine*, 60, 553–555.

Folkman, S. (1997). Positive psychological states and coping with severe stress. *Social Science Medicine*, 45, 1207–1221.

Folkman, S. (2001). Revised coping theory and the process of bereavement. In M.S. Stroebe, R.O. Hansson, W. Stroebe, & H. Schut (Eds.), *Handbook of Bereavement Research: Consequences, Coping and Care* (pp. 563–584). Washington, DC: American Psychological Association.

Folkman, S., & Greer, S. (2000). Promoting psychological well-being in the face of serious illness: when theory, research and practice inform each other. *Psycho-oncology*, 9, 11–19.

Fonagy, P. (2001). *Attachment Theory and Psychoanalysis*. New York: Other Press.

Frank, J. (1968). The role of hope in psychotherapy. *International Journal of Psychiatry*, 5, 383–395.

Frank, J. (1974). The restoration of morale. *American Journal of Psychiatry*, 131, 271–274.

Frankl, V. (1959). *From Death Camp to Existentialism*. Boston: Beacon Press.

Frankl, V. (1984). *Man's Search for Meaning: An Introduction to Logotherapy*. New York: Simon & Schuster. (Original work published in 1946).

Freud, S. (1917). *Mourning and Melancholia*. London: Hogarth.

Georganda, E.T. (1988). Thalassemia and the adolescent: an investigation of chronic illness, individuals and systems. *Family Systems Medicine*, 6, 150–161.

Giddens, A. (1998). *Sociology*. Cambridge: Polity.

Given, B.A., & Given, C.W. (1996). Family caregivers' burden from cancer care. In R. McCorkle, M. Grant, M. Frank-Stromberg, & S.B. Baird (Eds.), *Cancer Nursing: A Comprehensive Textbook*. Philadelphia: Saunders.

Gonzalez, S., Steinglass, P., & Reiss, D. (1989). Putting the illness in its place: discussion groups for families with chronic medical illnesses. *Family Process*, 28, 69–87.

Greene, V.L., & Monahan, D.J. (1987). The effect on a professionally guided caregiver support and education group on institutionalization of care receivers. *The Gerontologist*, 27, 716–721.

Hackett, T.P., & Cassem, N.H. (1969). Factors contributing to delay in responding to signs and symptoms of acute myocardial infarction. *American Journal of Cardiology*, 24, 651–656.

Hanson, C.L., Klesger, R., & Ecki, L. (1991). Family relations, coping style and cardiovascular risk factors among children and their parents. *Family Systems Medicine*, 8, 387–398.

Helz, J.W., & Templeton, B. (1990). Evidence of the role of psychosocial factors in diabetes mellitus: a review. *American Journal of Psychiatry*, 147, 1275–1282.

Jacob, T. (1992). Family studies of alcoholism. *Journal of Family Psychology*, 5, 319–338.

Keitner, G.I., & Miller, I.W. (1990). Family functioning and major depression: an overview. *American Journal of Psychiatry*, 147, 1128–1137.

Kerns, R.D., Haythornthwaite, J., Southwick, S., & Giller, E.L. (1990). The role of marital interaction in chronic pain and depressive symptom severity. *Journal of Psychosomatic Research*, 34, 401–408.

Kessler, S., & Bloch, M. (1989). Social systems response to Huntington's disease. *Family Process*, 28, 59–68.

Kissane, D. (1994). Grief and the family. In S. Bloch, J. Hafner, E. Harari, & G. Szmukler (Eds.), *The Family in Clinical Psychiatry* (pp. 71–91). Oxford: Oxford University Press.

Kissane, D., Bloch, S., Burns, W., McKenzie, D., & Posterino, M. (1994). Psychological morbidity in the families of patients with cancer. *Psycho-oncology*, 3, 47–56.

Kissane, D., Bloch, S., Dowe, D., et al. (1996a). The Melbourne family grief study. 1. Perceptions of family functioning in bereavement. *American Journal of Psychiatry*, 153, 659–666.

Kissane, D., Bloch, S., Onghena, P., et al. (1996b). The Melbourne family grief study. 2. Psychosocial morbidity and grief in bereaved families. *American Journal of Psychiatry*, 153, 650–658.

Kissane, D.W., & Bloch, S. (2002). *Family Focused Grief Therapy*. Buckingham: Open University Press.

Kissane, D.W., McKenzie, M., McKenzie, D.P., Forbes, A., O'Neill, I., & Bloch, S. (2003). Psychosocial morbidity associated with patterns of family functioning in palliative care: baseline data from the Family Focused Grief Therapy controlled trial. *Palliative Medicine*, 17, 527–537.

Klein, M. (1940). Mourning and its relation to manic-depressive states. *International Journal of Psychoanalysis*, 21, 125–153.

Larberg, J., & Cavallo, P. (1984). The family reaction. In A.F. Simons (Ed.), *Multiple Sclerosis: Psychological and Social Aspects* (pp. 42–53). London: Heinemann.

Leff, J., Berkowitz, R., Shavit, N., et al. (1989). A trial of family therapy v. a relatives' group for schizophrenia. *British Journal of Psychiatry*, 154, 58–66.

Levine, B.L. (1985). Adolescent substance abuse: toward an integration of family systems and individual adaptation theories. *American Journal of Family Therapy*, 13, 3–16.

Lewis, J.M., Beavers, W.R., Gossett, J., et al. (1976). *No Single Thread. Psychological Health in Family Systems*. New York: Brunner/Mazel.

Lieberman, S., & Black, D. (1982). Loss, mourning and grief. In A. Bentovim, G. Barnes, & A. Cooklin (Eds.), *Family Therapy: Complementary Frameworks of Theory and Practice* (pp. 373–387). New York: Grune and Stratton.

McDaniel, S., Hepworth, J., & Doherty, W. (Eds.). (1997). *Stories of Medical Family Therapy.* New York: Basic Books.

Medalie, J., & Goldbourt, U. (1976). Angina pectoris in 10 thousand men. Psychosocial and other risk factors evidenced by a multivariate analysis of a five year incidence study. *American Journal of Medicine*, 60, 910–921.

Mengel, M.B., Blackett, P.R., Lawler, M.K., et al. (1992). Cardiovascular and neuroendocrine responsiveness in diabetic adolescents within a family context: association with poor diabetic control and dysfunctional family dynamics. *Family Systems Medicine*, 10, 5–33.

Moos, R., Finney, J., & Gamble, W. (1982). The process of recovery from alcoholism. II. Comparing spouses of alcoholic patients and matched community controls. *Journal of Studies on Alcohol*, 43, 888–909.

Moos, R.H., & Moos, B.S. (1981). *Family Environment Scale Manual*. Stanford: Consulting Psychologists Press.

Okamura, H., Uchitomi, Y., Sasako, M., Eguchi, K., & Kakizoe, T. (1998). Guidelines for telling the truth to cancer patients. *Japanese Journal of Clinical Oncology*, 28, 1–4.

Parsons, T. (1955). The American family: its relations to personality and to social structure. In T. Parsons & R. Bales (Eds.), *Family, Socialization and Interaction Process*. Glencoe, IL: Free Press.

Perlesz, A., Furlong, M., & McLachlan, D. (1992). Family work and acquired brain damage. *Australian and New Zealand Journal of Family Therapy*, 13, 145–153.

Raphael, B. (1984). *The Anatomy of Bereavement*. London: Hutchinson.

Reiss, D. (1981). *The Family's Construct of Reality.* Boston: Harvard University Press.

Reiss, D. (1990). Patient, family and staff responses to end-stage renal disease. *American Journal of Kidney Diseases*, 15, 194–200.

Reiss, D., Gonzalez, S., & Kramer, N. (1986). Family process, chronic illness and death. *Archives of General Psychiatry*, 43, 795–807.

Reiss, D., Steinglass, P., & Howe, G. (1993). The family's organization around illness. In R.E. Cole & D. Reiss (Eds.), *How Do Families Cope with Chronic Illness?* (pp. 173–213). Hillsdale, NJ: Erlbaum.

Rolland, J.S. (1984). Toward a psychosocial typology of a chronic and life-threatening illness. *Family Systems Medicine*, 2, 245–263.

Rolland, J.S. (1987). Chronic illness and the life-cycle: a conceptual framework. *Family Process*, 26, 203–221.

Rolland, J.S. (1994). *Families, Illness and Disability: An Integrative Treatment Model*. New York: Basic Books.

Stanton, M.D., Thomas, C., et al. (1982). *The Family Therapy of Drug Abuse and Addiction.* New York: Guilford Press.

Steinglass, P., & Horan, M.E. (1988). Families and chronic medical illness. In F. Walsh & C. Anderson (Eds.), *Chronic Disorders and the Family* (pp. 1127–1142). New York: Haworth Press.

Stern, D.N. (1985). *The Interpersonal World of the Infant: A View from Psychoanalysis and Developmental Psychology.* New York: Basic Books.

Szapocznik, J.I., & Kurtines, W.M. (Eds.). (1989). *Breakthroughs in the Family Therapy with Substance Abusing and Problem Youth.* New York: Springer.

Turk, D.C., Rudy, T.E., & Flor, H. (1985). Why a family perspective for pain? *International Journal of Family Therapy*, 7, (Suppl. 4), 223–234.

Vaughn, C., & Leff, J. (1976). The influence of family and social factors on the course of psychiatric illness: a comparison of schizophrenic and depressed neurotic patients. *British Journal of Psychiatry*, 129, 125–137.

Walrond-Skinner, S., & Watson, D. (1987). *Ethical Issues in Family Therapy.* London: Routledge and Kegan Paul.

Walsh, F., & McGoldrick, M. (Eds.). (1991a). *Living Beyond Loss: Death in the Family.* New York: Norton.

Walsh, F., & McGoldrick, M. (1991b). Loss and the family: a systemic perspective. In F. Walsh & M. McGoldrick (Eds.), *Living Beyond Loss: Death in the Family* (pp. 1–29). New York: Norton.

Weihs, K., & Reiss, D. (2000). Family reorganization in response to cancer: a developmental perspective. In L. Baider, C. Cooper, & A.K. De-Nour (Eds.), *Cancer and the Family* (pp. 17–39). Chichester, England: Wiley.

Wilson, K., Chochinov, H., de Faye, B., & Breitbart, W. (2000). Diagnosis and management of depression in palliative care. In H. Chochinov & W. Breitbart (Eds.), *Handbook of Psychiatry in Palliative Medicine* (pp. 25–49). Oxford: Oxford University Press.

Worby, C.M., Altrocchi, J., Veatch, T.L., & Crosby, R. (1991). Early identification of symptomatic post MI families. *Family Systems Medicine*, 9, 127–135.

Wright, L.M., Watson, W.L., & Bell, J.M. (1996). *Beliefs: The Heart of Healing in Families and Illness.* New York: Basic Books.

Wrigley, M., & Mayou, R. (1991). Psychosocial factors and admission for poor glycaemic control: a study of psychological and social factors in poorly-controlled insulin-dependent diabetic patients. *Journal of Psychosomatic Research*, 35, 335–343.

18 Dealing with Workplace Stress

Michiel Kompier

CONTENTS

0-8493-1820-3/05/$0.00+$1.50

INTRODUCTION

Work has a pivotal position in the life of many individuals. Therefore, this chapter focuses on the role of work in the development and prevention of stress-related ill health.

In his song "Factory," rock singer Bruce Springsteen paints a part of this picture as he tells us about his father: "Factory takes his hearing, factory gives him life, the working, just the working life." In this fine recording, Springsteen points at the dual character of work: the positive side (factory gives him life, maybe by providing pay, goods, companionship) and the negative side (it takes his hearing, probably due to exposure to high noise levels). Paid employment might well be a source of work pleasure, learning, and good performance, designed in a way that it preserves and stimulates (mental) health and job satisfaction. For many employees this is the case. On the other hand, work can pose too high demands or demands that are not well suited to the knowledge, skills, and abilities of the worker. Such improperly designed jobs can cause or contribute to stress. Stress is an individual, psychophysiological, and subjective state, characterized by the combination of high arousal and displeasure (Kristensen et al., 1998). The sensation of stress depends on the expected persistence, closeness, and lack of control of the situation (Greif, 1991). Generally speaking, stressful work refers to conditions where the demands on the worker exceed the worker's capacity to respond to them. In a process of chronic exposure and inadequate recovery, stress might lead to mental health problems and other ill health (Beehr, 1995; Kahn & Byosiere, 1992; Shirom, 2003).

In this chapter we will first step into theory, to find out which factors in work are major risk factors for stress and its consequences for ill health. We will look at differences and similarities in various important theoretical approaches. Following identification of such critical work features, we will investigate how prevalent these factors are among the working population, both in Europe and in the U.S. To further understand these outcomes and associated health consequences, we will take a closer look at today's working life, through the analysis of seven current trends in and around work and organizations that more or less shape these work characteristics. Next, we will discuss to what extent work stress can be regarded as an individual problem. Finally, the focus will be on the prevention of workplace stress.

There are four points that we would like to emphasize in advance: First, this chapter does not represent an exhaustive overview of the literature. Rather, it tries to put together theory and evidence from various related research fields, and to integrate along the greater lines (Semmer, 2003a). Thus, we will try to sketch the overall picture, while accepting that inevitably this will lead to the loss of detail and that this might lead to some oversimplifications.

Second, while in this chapter we will concentrate on the role of work and work characteristics in the causation or prevention of stress reactions, we need to bear in mind that the absence of work can also be of great importance in the occurrence of stress-related diseases (Price et al., 2002). In a way, as we will see, stress and unemployment are interrelated: the fear of becoming unemployed constitutes a major stress risk (see, for a meta-analyis and review, Sverke et al., 2002). Within the research field of unemployment, stress, and health there is ample evidence that "a good job" can be an important social determinant of good health, i.e., a salutogenic factor. It can be so because "decent work" contributes to goal and meaning in life, because it provides structure and content of the working day, week, year, and life, it stimulates identity and self-respect of the worker, and it provides social networks and material rewards (Levi, 2000).

Third, we will confine ourselves to those factors that are related to the job content, i.e., the job itself, including its functional and social contacts (psychosocial factors; Johnson & Johansson, 1991). It is important to note that poor physical working conditions and work and rest schedules (shift work) can adversely affect the experience of stress and the psychological and physical health of employees (Cox et al., 2000; Warr, 1992; Harma, 2003). Although we will touch on some ergonomic and working time questions, a thorough discussion of all these topics would go beyond the scope of this chapter.

Fourth, and related to this third point, in our discussion of the reduction of workplace stress we will concentrate on interventions that are directed at the job content and the work organization, i.e., measures at the organizational level. The reader should bear in mind that interventions can also be directed at the coping capacity of the employee (Kompier and Kristensen, 2001). For a comprehensive review of such individual-oriented stress management literature, consult Murphy (1996, 2003) and Van der Klink et al. (2001).

WHAT IS IT IN WORK THAT MAKES IT STRESSFUL?

The scientific literature provides a good basis for an answer to this question. As Cox and colleagues conclude in a recent review (2000, p. 10): "There is a wealth of scientific data on work stress, its causes and effects, and some of the mechanisms underpinning the relationships among these." Accordingly, stress research has provided us with good general models on the relations between work factors, personal characteristics, and short- and long-term consequences for the health and performance of individuals and organizations. Kompier (2003) discusses the seven most prominent theoretical approaches in the field of work and work design, stress, health and well-being, and job satisfaction. These theories are:

- Job characteristics model (Hackman & Oldham, 1975)
- Michigan organization stress model (Caplan et al., 1975; Kahn et al., 1964)
- Job demands–control model (Karasek, 1979, 1998)
- Sociotechnical approach (e.g., De Sitter, 1989; Cherns, 1987)
- Action–theoretical approach (Hacker, 1998; Frese & Zapf, 1994)
- Effort–reward imbalance model (Siegrist, 1996)
- Vitamin model (Warr, 1996)

This is not the place to study these models in detail. For a more thorough discussion of these theories, refer to Kompier (2003). Here it would suffice to say that these theories stem from different schools and research traditions, and that they refer to rather complex and dynamic relations between task characteristics, personal characteristics, and outcomes as fatigue, job satisfaction, health and well-being, sickness absenteeism, and turnover. In this field there are many methodological pitfalls (Frese, 1985; Kasl, 1978, 1987; Kompier & Kristensen, 2001; Kompier, 2002; Taris & Kompier, 2003). Furthermore, there are practical problems: it is difficult to perform well-designed studies in real companies (Griffiths, 1999; Kompier & Kristensen, 2000). Nevertheless, these theoretical approaches have stimulated a large body of empirical research. Most extensive studies have been performed around the job characteristics model, the Michigan organization stress model, and the job demands–control model. As a more general conclusion, it can be stated that substantial support has been found for all of these theories (Kompier, 2003).

There are some interesting differences between these theories. The first difference relates to the emphasis on either the subjective appraisal of the environment or the objective (or collective) environment, i.e., relatively irrespective of the individual evaluation. The first two models, job characteristics model and Michigan organization stress model, are more directed at the subjective individual and emphasize perceptions and cognitions. Four other models (job demands–control model, sociotechnical approach, action–theoretical approach, vitamin model) are more directed at the objective environment. As it emphasizes both extrinsic and intrinsic sources, the effort–reward imbalance model holds an in-between position. A second difference concerns the role that personality factors are assumed to play. Personality is primarily conceptualized as an independent variable in the job characteristics model, in the Michigan organization stress model, and in the effort–reward imbalance model. The job demands–control model and the action–theoretical approach emphasize the reverse relationship, in the sense that it is assumed that work enhances personality. These two models thus transform personality to (mainly) a dependent variable. The vitamin model tends to combine these two perspectives (bidirectional relations between work and personality), whereas in the sociotechnical approach the issue of individual differences is merely neglected. We will come back to this issue later. The third difference relates to either the presence or absence of detailed (re)design principles in the theory under study. Three of the seven theoretical approaches (job characteristics model, sociotechnical approach, and action–theoretical approach) have detailed various principles with respect to the design or redesign of work. Design principles can be derived from the other approaches, but detailed intervention strategies and theories are generally lacking (see below).

To identify critical job features — i.e., those factors in the psychosocial work environment that can either cause stress or promote motivation or learning — Table 18.1 presents a comparative overview of those work characteristics that are central in these seven approaches.

In spite of the aforementioned differences, it follows from Table 18.1 that there is a remarkable overlap between these approaches when it comes to identifying critical job features. These critical job characteristics are job demands (six of seven theories), autonomy (six of seven theories), and skill variety (six of seven theories). Other important psychosocial job characteristics are social support (or strongly related concepts) (four of seven theories), feedback (three), task identity (three), and job future ambiguity (or related constructs such as job insecurity, also part of three theories). Pay (money rewards, availability of money) as an aspect of terms of employment is an important factor in two theories.

TABLE 18.1
Critical Job Features in Seven Stress Theoretical Approaches

Work Characteristics	Job Characteristics Model	Michigan Organization Stress Model	Demands–Control Model	Sociotechnical Approach	Action–Theoretical Approach	Effort–Reward Imbalance Model	Vitamin Model
Skill variety	+	+	+	1	2		+
Task identity	+			1	2		
Task significance	+	+					+
Autonomy/control	+	+	+	+	+		+
Feedback	+				+		+
Job demands		+	+	+	+	+	3
Role conflict		+					3
Social support		+	+			+	+
Rewards						+	+
Job security		+				+	4
Role ambiguity		+					4
Physical security							4

Note: + = the current work characteristic plays a major role in the current theory; 1 = one construct (minimal division of labor) comprises both skill variety and task identity; 2 = one construct (completeness of action) comprises both skill variety and task identity; 3 = one construct (externally generated goals) comprises both job demands and role conflict; 4 = one construct (environmental clarity) comprises both career opportunities and role ambiguity.

These theories teach us that stress and motivation can be regarded as two sides of the same coin. If work provides the right mix of work characteristics — that is, high but not too high demands, skill variety, autonomy, social support and feedback, task identity, not too much job future ambiguity, and proper pay — work stimulates motivation and mental health as well as productive performance. As such, often healthy work is also productive work. When work does not provide a proper configuration of these work characteristics (e.g., too many demands, too little autonomy), it can provoke stress reactions.

Such critical job features can be conceptualized as risk factors, i.e., as characteristics of the psychosocial work environment that tend to elicit a certain type of reaction (stress reactions). This is a probabilistic, environmentally oriented concept of stressors (Semmer, 2003a) (see below).

PREVALENCE OF WORK STRESS: STRESS REACTIONS AND RISK FACTORS

How prevalent are these risk factors among the working population? And how many employees report stress reactions?

A recent picture of the prevalence of workplace stress reactions and of some major risk factors is provided by Merllié and Paoli (2001). This study among 21,500 European employees was performed by the European Foundation for the Improvement of Living and Working Conditions in Dublin. It shows that of these employees, 27% report that their health and safety are at risk because of their work. The most common work-related health problems are backache (33%), stress (28%), overall fatigue (23%), and neck and shoulders (23%). The same study showed that most European employees work at very high speed (56%) or under tight deadlines (60%) more than 25% of the time. These percentages are higher than those of 1990 (1990: high speed, 48%; tight deadlines, 50%) and 1995 (1995: high speed, 54%; tight deadlines, 56%) (Paoli, 1992, 1997). As most workers are nowadays employed in the service sector, this work pace is primarily dependent on direct demands from clients (67%) (1995: 65%) and colleagues (48%) (1995: 41%; 1990: figures not available). Of the employees who continuously work tight deadlines, 40% report stress and 42% report backache (against 20 and 27%, respectively, of the employees who never work under tight deadlines). Furthermore, 20% work 45 h in a week, the percentage being higher for self-employed persons.

From the same study it appears that large numbers of European employees have little job control and autonomy in their work: 36% have no choice over their order of tasks (1995: 36%), 29% have no choice over their pace of work (1995: 28%), and 30% have no choice over their methods of work (1995: 30%). These figures suggest an interesting pattern: psychological demands have increased without a comparable increase in autonomy (see also Landsbergis, 2003).

These risk factors in the psychosocial work environment are not evenly distributed in the working population. Certain occupational groups are at higher risks than other occupational groups. As a first illustration of this principle, Figure 18.1 shows

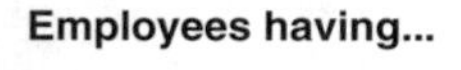

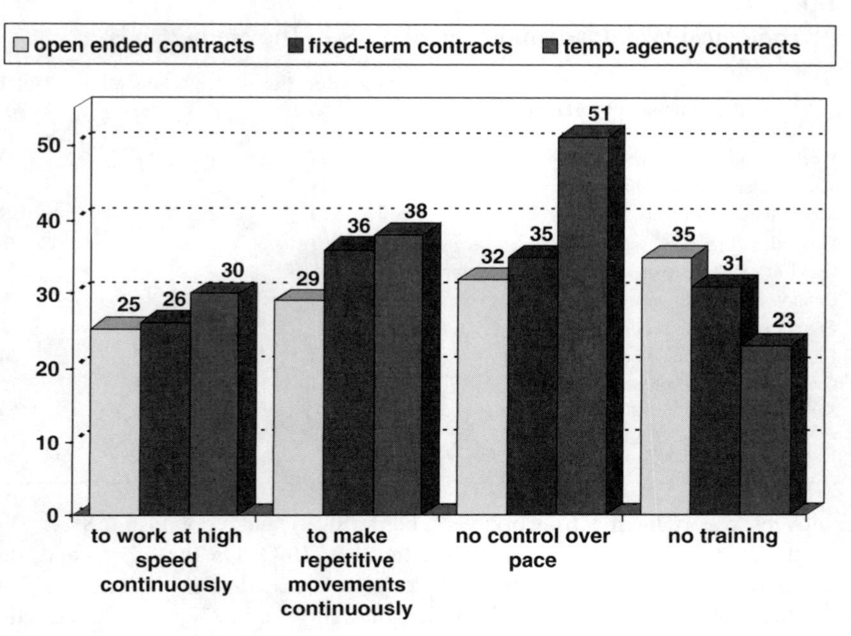

FIGURE 18.1 Employment status and psychosocial work environment among European workers. (Data from Merllié & Paoli, *Ten Years of Working Conditions in the European Union*, Dublin, European Foundation for the Improvement of Living and Working Conditions, 2001.)

that the psychosocial work environment is related to the employment status of the employee. Those who are employed by temporary agencies report the highest work speed, make the most frequent repetitive movements, have the least control over their work pace, and receive the least work-related training. As flexibilization is a major trend in modern working life (see below), these contingent workers seem to be a risk group for workplace stress.

The second illustration is based on a (yearly) study into the quality of working life that is performed by the Dutch Bureau of Statistics (CBS, 2002). The sample comprises 4,472 employees, of whom 1,071 have received basic education only and 374 have higher education (university).

It is shown in Table 18.2 that those employees with lower educational level work at a lower (though not necessarily low) work speed and report less time pressure, less learning opportunities, and less autonomy. Monotonous work is more common among lower-educated personnel.

Such figures do not only reflect European working life. Comparable figures are found in a representative sample of 3,000 American employees (Bond et al., 1998). Some of the 1997 figures could be compared to a comparable sample in 1977 (Table 18.3). The comparison applies to wage and salary workers only; it excludes self-employed, contract, or contingent workers. From Table 18.3 it appears that U.S.

TABLE 18.2
Psychological Workload among Employees in The Netherlands

Psychological Workload	Low Education (%)	High Education (%)	Total (%)
Work in high work pace	34	58	40
Work under high time pressure	25	53	35
Monotonous work	13	2	7
Possibility for developing	63	88	5
Good fit between work and experience/training	58	89	73
Cannot self-decide on work execution	42	14	29
Cannot self-decide on order of tasks	43	19	31
Cannot self-regulate work pace	38	32	34
Can self-think-up solutions	57	95	76
Sample	1071	374	4472

Data from CBS, 2002, *Statistisch Jaarboek 2002*, Voorburg/Heerlen, CBS, p. 212.

employees report having to work very hard (88%) and very fast (68%). These percentages are almost 20% higher than those of 1977. On the other hand, these U.S. workers do report high levels of job decision latitude and skill discretion. These percentages as well are importantly higher than those of 1977, though it might be that they are somewhat inflated because self-employed, contract, and contingent workers were not included in the sample (Landsbergis, 2003). From Figure 18.1 we learned that it is probable that those workers have less job control.

Also, burnout symptoms were investigated by Bond and coworkers (1998) (unfortunately no comparison to previous sample). Twenty-six percent felt emotionally drained from their work and 26% felt burned out and stressed by their work (often or very often during the last 3 months). One of three (36%) felt used up at the end of the workday, and 36% were tired when they got up in the morning and had to face another day on the job. This U.S. study also points at another prominent psychosocial risk factor: job insecurity and the risk of unemployment. Twenty-nine percent of the respondents found it somewhat or very likely that they would lose their current job in the next couple of years.

Bond and colleagues also asked questions with regard to work–home interaction, i.e., the way the work situation influences private life, and vice versa. Whereas 7% of the employees mentioned that family or personal life drained them of the energy they needed to do their job (often or very often), 28% reported no energy to do things with family or other important people in their lives because of their job (often or very often). This finding, which is quite robust in the literature (see Geurts & Demerouti, 2003, for an overview), suggests that the negative impact of work on one's private life is more powerful than the other way around (see below).

The picture that emerges from the Bond study is that of high psychological demands and high job control. Whereas recent theories such as the job demands–control model would predict average levels of health problems (Karasek

TABLE 18.3
Quality of the Psychosocial Work Environment in the U.S.

	1977	1997
My work requires that I work very fast	55%	68%
My job requires that I work very hard	70%	88%
I never seem to have enough time to get everything done on my job	40%	60%
I have the freedom to decide what I do on my job	56%	74%
I have a lot to say about what happens on my job	59%	71%
My job requires that I keep learning new things	82%	90%
My job requires that I be creative	59%	76%
My job lets me use my skills and abilities	76%	92%
How often during the past 3 months (often/very often):		
Emotionally drained from work		26%
Felt used up at the end of workday		36%
Tired when got up in morning and had to face another day on the job		36%
Felt burned out or stressed by work		26%
How likely to lose current job in next couple of years:		
Somewhat likely		20%
Very likely		9%
No energy to do things with family or other important people in because of job (often/very often)		28%
Family or personal life drain you of the energy you need to do your job (often/very often)		7%
The work that I do is meaningful to me		90%
General satisfaction with job:		
Very		47%
Somewhat		44%

Data from Bond et al., *The 1997 National Study of the Changing Workforce*, New York, Families and Work Institute, 1998.

& Theorell, 1990), the reported levels of burnout symptoms and fatigue are nevertheless quite high.

WHICH RECENT WORKPLACE DEVELOPMENTS ARE BEHIND THESE FIGURES?

With respect to critical job features, recent empirical studies point at high psychological demands, problems with job control (at least for certain occupational groups), and increased job insecurity. In addition, high levels of psychological stress reactions (e.g., fatigue, burnout symptoms) are reported. Which developments in the world of work and organizations are behind these figures, or to put it differently, which new systems of work organization have influenced these job characteristics? Over the last decades the world of work has undergone remarkable changes, and these changes have certainly influenced the psychosocial work environment and thereby affected stress at work. Seven major trends are outlined in the following subsections.

Increased Utilization of Information and Communication Technology

During the last 25 years we have witnessed the introduction of the personal computer, the laptop, the fax machine, the Internet, the intranet, mobile telephone, electronic-mail, I-mode, etc. As a consequence, nowadays everyone can be reached everywhere and instantly. As with all technology, instruments, and devices, the appropriateness of information and communication technology (ICT) depends largely on the way it is used (Hamborg & Greif, 2003). On the one hand, ICT can increase comfort, speed, and performance and thereby solve problems. On the other hand, ICT can contribute to an overflow of (often aversive) stimuli and thereby create new demands and problems. Let us consider two modes: mobile telephone and e-mail. Many companies have now provided their employees with mobile phones. Of course, mobile phones are handy, but often employees are expected to switch on these phones 24 hours a day, thus expanding the working day and diminishing the boundaries between work and home (see below). Potentially the availability of e-mail is a great gift; at low costs we can communicate with just about everyone. However, there is a flip side to this coin: because it is that easy to use (there is just no limit), everyone does indeed use it. It seems as if there is a kind of autonomous force behind these ICT applications. Because it is technically possible to have instant communication, we want (or even demand) instant communication. It is not unusual that to be sure that a message reaches the receiver, the sender simultaneously mails, calls, and faxes the same message.

Apart from this impatient information overflow, electronic mail certainly contributes negatively to the social intercourse between employees. In the "old days," when an employee or supervisor got upset, frustrated, or felt maltreated, he or she might have cursed in silence or sought some support from coworkers. Next, he or she considered which reaction was suited best. Such a reaction could be a letter. A draft letter was prepared, put aside for one day, adapted because the anger had become less intense, and then sent. Nowadays, when confronted with injustice, many employees send a furious e-mail reaction, instantly (and often with more than one spelling mistake). This might decrease their tension, but it often leads to a kind of escalation, because e-mail is not only an instantaneous but also an impersonal medium. It might cause people to write things that they would prefer not to mention face-to-face.

Rapid Expansion of the Service Sector

In most Western countries, the majority of employees work in the service sector, be it commercial (banking, insurance companies, hotel and catering industry, consultancy, etc.) or noncommercial (police, hospitals, prisons, schools, governmental institutions, etc.). For example, in the Netherlands, in 2000, this relates to 76% of all employees. The rise of the service sector is accompanied by a fall of industrial activity and agriculture. "Manufacturing jobs continue to decline, giving way to service and to knowledge work" (Sauter et al., 2002). As the service sector places the client in the middle, the rise of the service sector poses new or more intensified demands to workers: dealing with customers, clients, pupils, inmates, and patients. In this context, the concept of emotion work and emotional demands has been introduced in the literature (for an overview, see Zapf, 2002). Also, the concept of emotional dissonance has been introduced, as in the case of a flight attendant who has to wear a smile even if she does not feel like it. The client-centered nature of work can bring about pleasant as well as unpleasant encounters with clients. Examples of the latter have been labeled workplace violence. Violence at work can cause workplace trauma and anxiety disorders (Chappell & Di Martino, 2000; Leather et al., 1999).

Globalization of the Economy

Because of changing international and political conditions (e.g., the decline of the communist world) and the ICT developments, our world has been characterized as the "global village." Today's companies can compete all over the world. This provides new challenges (winning) as well as new threats (losing). International competition has increased. According to Cascio (1995), during the 1960s only 7% of the U.S. economy faced international competition, whereas in the 1980s this percentage had increased to 70%.

Changing Structure of the Workforce

In many countries the labor participation of women has increased. Whereas in the "early days" the segregation between workers and nonworkers paralleled gender segregation, nowadays women form a substantial part of the active working force. Consequently, the numbers of dual-earner couples and employed persons with caregiving responsibilities are rapidly growing (Geurts & Demerouti, 2003). Also, especially in the Western world, the level of education is increasing. New job starters are higher educated than the people that leave the labor force.

Changing Boundaries between Work and Home

As a consequence of the amount of dual-earning families, the availability of ICT, and the flexibilization of work (see below), the boundaries between work and nonwork (family) have changed. The traditional major segregation between the roles of workers and nonworkers has disappeared. No longer is work spatially, temporally, and socially distinct from nonwork. Because many physical and temporal limitations have been removed, many employees can perform their tasks outside the office. They can (tele)work at home instead of in the office, work at home during evenings or weekends, and even work in trains and boats and planes. A popular commercial advertisement (mobile telephone) in the Netherlands stipulates that "in a traffic jam, work just goes on." These developments have not remained unnoticed by researchers in occupational health psychology: a new body of knowledge has emerged on work–home interaction, that is, "a process whereby one's functioning (and behavior) in one domain is influenced by (quantitative and qualitative) demands from the other domain" (Geurts & Demerouti, 2003, pp. 288–289, also for an overview of theories and findings). Modern views acknowledge that the work and home domains can influence each other, both in positive and negative ways.

Creation of the 24-Hour Economy

A special type of flexibilization is the aspiration to produce or deliver services around the clock, i.e., nonstop, or at least more hours than when restricted to the traditional nine-to-five period. The 24-hour economy is only partially new: traditionally many employees work in shifts or at irregular times (in industry, transport, hotels, hospitals, fire brigades, etc.). Still, it is getting more and more normal to work irregular working hours.

Flexibilization and Utilization of New Production Concepts

Modern organizations have developed a range of new organizational practices that guide the aforementioned trends in work. Through these new production concepts, such organizations aim to survive and expand, and to cope successfully with changing circumstances. What these practices have in common is a greater emphasis on high performance and flexibility. Flexibilization refers to a more lenient, more versatile usage of employees and means, taking into account changing contextual demands (such as the demands for certain products). Flexibilization can be quantitative or qualitative in nature. Examples of the former are working overtime, part-time contracts, shift work, temporary contracts, working at home, or hiring workers from temporary employment agencies. According to various authors (Landsbergis, 2003; Spurgeon et al., 1997; Van der Hulst, 2003), there is an increase, not necessarily reflected in official statistics, of unpaid overtime worked by salaried workers to deal with excessive workloads. A recent study in the EU member states reports that about 13% of full-time employees work 51 or more hours a week (Bielenski et al., 2002). This number of hours exceeds the 48-hour maximum limit established by the European Directive on work time (European Council, 1993; Harma, 2003). In a thorough recent literature review, Van der Hulst (2003) shows that such long working hours are indeed associated with adverse health.

Examples of qualitative flexibilization are job rotation, multiskilling, and hiring freelancers and consultants. Often companies combine more than one of these types as they concentrate on their core business, introduce self-regulating teams, diminish the number of managerial levels (become flatter), emphasize total quality management, etc. One of the concepts is just-in-time management (supply control), and another is lean production: fewer employees, less machinery, less space, fewer supplies, and flexible, short delivery times and quality. According to the U.S. National Institute for Occupational Safety and Health (NIOSH) (Sauter et al., 2002), organizational practices have changed dramatically in the new economy. "To compete more effectively, many large companies have restructured themselves by downsizing their workforces and outsourcing all but core functions. At the same time, non-traditional employment practices that depend on temporary workers and contract labor have grown steadily" (Sauter et al., 2002, p. 1).

The above trends signify that modern employees, compared to workers of 20 years ago, increasingly work in offices (and less in industry or in agriculture), with information or clients (and less with tangible objects), and in teams (and less in isolation). The most striking development is the changing nature of work itself and its increased psychosocial workload. Largely, work has changed from physical to mental in nature. Today, for many employees, work poses primarily mental and emotional demands. Another development is that, through all these changes, job and work security decreased.

INDIVIDUAL DIFFERENCES

Thus far we have identified critical job features, studied their prevalence among the working population, and situated these factors in a broader context through the analysis of trends in and around organizations that more or less sculpture these job features. Our emphasis has merely been on the work context, whereas less attention was paid to the role of the individual employee. In this section, the focus is on the employee. There are several reasons why this is important. It is obvious that the pathway between the exposure to (combinations of) psychosocial work characteristics and health often goes via the individual appraisal of these characteristics. Stress reactions result from the individual's appraisal of a contextual factor. In addition, employees differ in the way they address stressful work factors (the concepts of active or passive coping).

So there is little doubt that stress is indeed an individual phenomenon. To illustrate the role of individual differences, there is the saying that "One man's meat is another man's poison." Indeed, there are large differences between people — differences in personality characteristics, experience, ambitions, and knowledge, skills, and abilities. There are also differences within people: the same "objective" task might be more demanding for someone when he is a freshman than — after a couple of years — when he has become a more experienced employee. Also, when fatigued, the same "objective" task demand is assessed as more demanding than when the employee is not fatigued.

Let us consider the examples of mountaineering and lion taming. It is true that some people are fond of climbing mountains or taming wild animals ("One man's meat is another man's poison"). We should, however, bear in mind that statistically these are minorities, and that for most persons these activities would be very stressful. The same reasoning applies to the psychosocial work environment. It is true that not all employees prefer skill variety, and it is true that there are people who prefer to work in splendid isolation. But we should not forget that most employees do like to use their skills and to communicate and cooperate with others. In this chapter we have therefore chosen a probabilistic conceptualization of stressors; i.e., certain work characteristics are defined as risk factors when they tend to elicit stress reactions in "most people most of the time, regardless of circumstances" (Sauter et al., 1998, pp. 34.2–34.3). In a similar vein, Cox et al. (2003) chose the term *psychosocial hazards*, which they define as "those aspects of the design and management of work, and its social and organizational contexts, that have the potential for causing psychological or physical harm" (p. 195). Please note, with Semmer (2003a), that such a probabilistic view "does not require that each and every individual will experience stress vis-à-vis a stressor — an argument which is often raised against an environmentally oriented concept of stressors" (p. 84).

This probabilistic conceptualization of factors in the psychosocial work environment (risk factors, stressors, psychosocial hazards) fits well in a broader occupational health perspective. It is in line with the conceptualization of other, more traditional risk factors in the workplace, such as noise, radiation, the lifting of heavy loads, working with chemical agents, or whole-body vibration. Employed workers mostly constitute a relatively healthy subset of the total population. Unless these doses are very high, not every employee will become deaf (noise) or develop musculoskeletal diseases (lifting) or ulcers (chemicals). Still, in certain exposure levels, these factors will cause or contribute to disease in most people most of the time.

We would like to finalize this section with two remarks. First, we feel that modern stress theory treats individual factors too much as independent or causal factors (i.e., as determinants of stress reactions) or as intervening factors (i.e., factors that strengthen or reduce the impact of psychosocial risk factors on stress reactions and ill health). There is surprisingly little theorizing on where these personality factors come from. Often one gets the idea that personality factors or someone's coping repertoire are just there. We feel that it is fruitful to think of personality factors also as an outcome variable, i.e., as a dependent variable. As is emphasized in two of the aforementioned theories (job demands–control model and action theory), one's personality is at least partly shaped by what we do, and for many people, what we do is, for a major part of the day, performing tasks at the workplace. Working people spend almost half of their nonsleeping hours at work. Therefore, their activities during these hours are of major importance to their health and personality (Levi, 2000). To give some examples, much studied and often conceptually related personal characteristics such as self-efficacy, hardiness, self-esteem, sense of coherence, and optimism are mostly defined as independent or intervening factors. In a recent overview, Semmer (2003a) has studied the role of the aforementioned personality characteristics to find evidence for a kind of stress resiliency. Looking "at the great lines," he concludes that those people are resilient who are more optimistic and trustful, tend to accept setbacks and failures as normal and not as indicators of their own incompetence, tend to see life as something that can be influenced and acted upon (internal locus of control) and see themselves as capable of doing so (self-efficacy), tend to see stressful events as a challenge, and show emotional stability and do not have a tendency to experience negative emotions (neuroticism) (Semmer, 2003a, p. 96). However, it also seems highly probable that, at least to some extent, such characteristics are an effect of working in stimulating and challenging working conditions (see, for example, Taris et al., 2003).

Related to this, we feel that too often occupational health psychologists tend to utilize too simple and too rigid schemata to understand the complex and dynamic relations between work characteristics, personal characteristics, work behavior, and health outcomes. Examples of these rigid schemata are A causes B or B causes A. What we should keep in mind is that in real life and within persons, these relations are very complex, that in the work–person–stress–health etiology there are many links and loops in the chain, and that various factors influence each other (and accordingly are influenced by other factors: bidirectionality or reverse causation). Such relations are dynamic and develop over time: variables in this process need to be conceptualized as independent and dependent variables, as well as intervening variables. Let us consider the example of social support, one of the critical job features in Table 18.1. This job feature is often treated as an independent variable (for example, low support from coworkers or supervisors can cause or contribute to stress reactions) or as a moderator (for example, high support can buffer the potential adverse effect of excessive job demands). Both paths are quite plausible, but this is only part of the puzzle. This factor itself might also be changed (i.e., conceptualized as a dependent variable), as in the case of an employee whose task demands were both high and varied, who originally received much support but as a consequence of the high demands started to make errors, failed on important assignments, and started to complain about his boss and his health. As a consequence, the employee was given less interesting tasks (change of job demands) and his colleagues did not ask him to join them for lunch anymore or make social talk with him. They even withheld information from this employee (change in social support). One of the challenges for occupational stress research is to try to unravel this knot, studying mechanisms, and to find out which paths are dominant (see Kompier, 2002; Taris & Kompier, 2003).

Second, we would like to warn against a tendency in modern stress research to overstretch the role of individual factors to the point "where stress is being reduced to nothing but a problem of idiosyncratic appraisals and coping styles, rendering such concepts as environmentally induced stress useless" (Semmer, 2003a, p. 84). In such a view, "every response is purely subjective" and "just as well could have been different." This bias to the individual bears the risk of reducing stress to an intrapsychic phenomenon, a phenomenon that in itself is not related to reality. Such a view unjustly draws away the attention from "collective" or "objective" stressors. Furthermore, it bears the risk of "blaming the victim." Of course, such a view also has consequences for the targets of intervention.

PREVENTION AND INTERVENTION

In this section we will first discuss international legislation regarding occupational stress. Next, we will introduce stress prevention and intervention principles on the organizational level. These principles follow from three of the theories that were mentioned above and from NIOSH. Finally, we will look at what these approaches have in common, and we will discuss some empirical studies that are based on the principles that were outlined before.

Legislation

Several European countries have introduced legislation with respect to the assessment and management of psychosocial factors at work. The European Framework Directive on health and safety at work (89/391/EEC; 1993), currently the major legal regulation on the quality of working life, provides the legal background for the assessment and management of psychosocial factors at work.

This framework states, among other things, that the employer:

> has a duty to ensure the safety and health of workers in every aspect related to the work, following general principles of prevention: avoiding risks; evaluating risks which cannot be avoided; combating the risks at the source; adapting the work to the individual, especially as regards the design of work places, the choice of work equipment and the choice of work and production methods, with a view, in particular, to alleviating monotonous work and work at a predetermined work rate and to reducing their effects on health; developing a coherent overall prevention policy which covers technology, organization of work, working conditions, social relationships and the influence of factors related to the working environment.

In 1999, the European Parliament formulated a comparable stand (European Parliament's Resolution A4-0050/99; February 25, 1999). It:

> considers that work must be adapted to people's abilities and needs and not vice-versa, and notes that by preventing a disparity from arising between the demands of work and the capacities of the workers, it is possible to retain employees until retirement age; considers that new technologies should be used in order to achieve these aims; draws attention to the problems resulting from a lack of autonomy at the workplace, monotonous and repetitive work and work with a narrow variety of content, all features which are typical of women's work in particular, and calls attention to be paid to the importance of ergonomics to the improvement of health and safety conditions at the workplace.

From this (inter)national legislation, two conclusions can be drawn: (1) its perspective on risk assessment and risk control fits well with this chapter's conceptualization of critical job features as risk factors or psychosocial hazards; and (2) according to these legal regulations, the preventive priority is to make the workplace less stressful by reducing or rooting out the risks (primary prevention; Cox et al., 2003; Levi, 2000).

Job Characteristics Model, Sociotechnical Approach, and Action–Theoretical Approach

Key elements for stress prevention can be selected from three of the seven theoretical approaches that were listed in Table 18.1: job characteristics model, sociotechnical approach, and action–theoretical approach. More than the four other theories, these three approaches have formulated pronounced design principles that we will briefly introduce.

Job Characteristics Model

Hackman and Oldham (1980) developed five principles with regard to the (re)design of tasks:

1. Combining tasks: job enlargement, by de-specializing a job and allowing individuals to do several different activities; the cycle time is enlarged.

Combining tasks is indicated in case of limited skill variety and low task identity.
2. The formation of natural work units, i.e., of those workers whose work is interrelated. Natural work groups are indicated in case of low task identity and low task significance.
3. The formation of a client-centered structure, i.e., enabling the worker to interact with the people who use or are affected by his or her work. Increasing client contacts is indicated when skill variety is low, when autonomy is limited, and when the worker receives little feedback from work.
4. Job enrichment, i.e., increasing the vertical loading of the job by allowing the worker more responsibility and discretion. Job enrichment is the remedy in case of limited autonomy.
5. Creating feedback channels: so that the employee receives more information from the work process. Open feedback channels are indicated in case feedback is low.

Sociotechnical Approach

The nucleus of modern sociotechnics is that insufficient job control is the most important stress risk, and that stress risks and opportunities for learning are dependent on the company's structure of the division of labor. Modern sociotechnics is a typical design theory. Cherns (1976, 1987) was one of the first who offered a set of principles of sociotechnical design. Against the background of the pioneering work of Cherns, Clegg (2000) formulated a set of sociotechnical principles to guide system design and some considerations of the role of these principles. The sociotechnical approach is very broad: it is directed at the integral reconstruction of the total production organization. There are two leading principles:

1. The minimal division of labor (no jobs that are fragmented or overspecialized) (Kuipers, 1989). This puts the theory in diametric opposition to the classical theory of Frederick Taylor (1911), with its vigorous division between mental work and manual work.
2. The building blocks of new organizations are working groups with an (semi)autonomous status.

Action–Theoretical Approach

Action theory promotes completeness of action (Hacker, 1998; Frese & Zapf, 1994). This implies that work is designed well when it provides opportunities to the worker to carry out all steps in the action process (goal setting, plan development, plan decision making, plan execution, monitoring and feedback processes) and when all levels of behavioral regulation (e.g., automatic and controlled information processing) are utilized.

According to action theory, the following principles are important for job design:

1. Work should allow employees to choose their own work strategy.
2. Work should encompass complete actions (see above).
3. Outside events that do not belong to the task (obstacles and interruptions often stemming from poor work organization) should be minimized.
4. People should be allowed to be active in their work.
5. People need control because control helps them to act more adequately, choosing appropriate strategies to deal with the situation.
6. Well-designed jobs need well-qualified workers.
7. Qualifications can only be upheld if work has a certain complexity.
8. Work should provide feedback.

Interventions according to NIOSH

Many stress researchers have provided categorizations of possible organization-directed interventions (e.g., Elkin & Rosch, 1990; Quick et al., 1997; Sauter et al., 1992; Cox et al., 2000). A well-balanced overview of "positive principles to guide the design of jobs in the interests of improving mental health" has been formulated by the NIOSH in its National Strategy for the Prevention of Work-Related Psychological Disorders (Sauter et al., 1992). Sauter and colleagues distinguish seven related recommendations:

1. Workload and work pace: Demands (both physical and mental) should be commensurate with the capabilities and resources of workers, avoiding underload as well as overload. Provisions should be made to allow recovery from demanding tasks or for increased job control under such circumstances. Increased control by the individual over the pace of work is one example of a positive step.
2. Work schedule: Work schedules should be compatible with demands and responsibilities outside the job. Recent trends toward flextime, a compressed workweek, and job sharing are positive steps. When schedules involve rotating shifts, the rate of rotation should be stable and predictable and should be in a forward (day-to-night) direction.
3. Work roles: Roles and responsibilities at work should be well defined. Job duties need to be clearly explained, and conflicts in terms of job expectations should be avoided.
4. Job future: Ambiguity should not exist in matters of job security and opportunities for career development. Employees need to be clearly informed of promotional opportunities and mechanisms for improving skills or professional growth within the organization, as well as impending organizational developments that might potentially affect their employment.
5. Social environment: Jobs should provide opportunities for personal interaction both for purposes of emotional support and for actual help as needed in accomplishing assigned tasks.
6. Job content: Jobs should be designed to provide meaning, stimulation, and an opportunity to use skills. Job rotation and increasing the scope of

work are examples of steps to improve narrow, fragmented work activities that fail to meet these criteria.

7. Participation and control: Individuals should be given the opportunity to have input on decisions or actions that affect their jobs and the performance of their tasks.

EXAMPLES OF EMPIRICAL STUDIES

A comparison of these overviews of preventative measures teaches us that some theories (job characteristics model, action theoretical approach) concentrate on the job content only, whereas other approaches (such as the sociotechnical approach) choose a broader range of interventions that also pertain to the broader context of the job itself. More importantly, as is the case with regard to the seven theoretical approaches presented in Table 18.1, such a comparison demonstrates a considerable consensus among various theoretical approaches when it comes to answering the question: How can workplace stress be reduced?

We will now report on some interesting empirical prevention and intervention studies that utilized one or more of the aforementioned measures. A recent overview of such intervention studies in the psychosocial work environment has been authored by Semmer (2003b). To categorize interventions according to their major focus, Semmer distinguishes between three types of interventions: (1) task and technical interventions, (2) improving role clarity and social relationships, and (3) more comprehensive multiple changes. We will use this categorization.

Task and Technical Interventions

This category of interventions comprises the redesign of task characteristics and changes in working conditions (ergonomics, time, and workload). Interesting research in this field stems from the Sheffield group and has been summarized by Parker et al. (1998). As Semmer (2003b) concludes, these Sheffield studies are noteworthy because (1) they contain data on important job features (e.g., demands, variety, control, role conflict), on self-reported health status, on stress reactions, and on job satisfaction, collected through standardized instruments; (2) these data are analyzed by appropriate statistical methods; and (3) the studies typically have a strong design. Also, the change process, for example, through increased participation, is being studied. One of the intervention studies took place in a department of a confectionary company that faced low morale problems, poor social relationships and communication, and high turnover (Wall & Clegg, 1981). Based on the job characteristics model, two changes were made: task identity (removing barriers in the production hall to make the whole production process visible) and autonomy (the group now decides on task allocation, rest breaks, production speed, etc.) were increased. Data were collected at three points of time — after 5 months and at 18 and 28 months — and positive changes were observed with regards to work motivation, work satisfaction, performance, and mental health. Long-term effects were the strongest. Unfortunately, the study lacked a control condition. To a certain degree, this constraint could be overcome through the systematic comparison of those work characteristics that were changed and those that had not been manipulated.

Several other cases deal with teamwork. Sprigg et al. (2000) reported that the introduction of team-based work led to the perception of better work characteristics, especially communication, influence over work, and cooperation, and job satisfaction increased, whereas stress reactions decreased. The latter effects were confined to a condition wherein task interdependence was high.

Kompier et al. (2000) selected, compared, and analyzed interventions and preventive actions that international bus companies have taken to decrease occupational stress and sickness absenteeism among bus drivers. These "natural experiments" comprised, inter alia, the introduction of team-based work and job rotation/enlargement/enrichment. Principles of worker participation were often followed. The variety in intervention programs, outcome measures, case evaluations, and methodological flaws makes it difficult to present a general picture of program effectiveness. However, analyses on more objective (sickness absenteeism, work disability, turnover) and subjective (subjective health status, work satisfaction, program satisfaction, perceived workload, work-related overcommitment) outcomes did point at positive effects.

It is true that in these studies there are various theoretical, practical, and methodological ambiguities. Still, looking at the greater lines, research in this area demonstrates that redesigning jobs through making them richer might well improve health and well-being and work satisfaction. Noteworthy is that meta-analyses by Fried and Ferris (1987) with respect to job satisfaction and by Beekun (1989) with respect to sickness absenteeism are in line with this conclusion. When it comes to changes in ergonomics, time regulations (e.g., break times), and workload, Semmer (2003b) deems a cautiously positive evaluation justified: these interventions do show potential for positive effects, although they do not guarantee them, and do not show much potential for negative effects.

Improving Role Clarity and Social Relationships

Many of the intervention projects in this field aim at the improvement of communication and feedback, cooperation, the reduction of conflict, and the clarification of roles and tasks. To give an example, two of the interventions among bus companies reported by Kompier et al. (2000) focused on improving communication and performance appraisal and feedback. Both reported a significant reduction in absenteeism. Again, summarizing the results of these and other social studies is not an easy task. There are some, but not very consistent, effects on absenteeism. There is a wide variety in designs, measures, time intervals, and outcome variables. Overall, with Semmer (2003b) we conclude that social interventions do have the potential for positive effects, but that there are not guaranteed effects. Most interestingly, the strength of the intervention and active participation might well be modifying variables.

More Comprehensive Multiple Changes

Kompier et al. (1998) and Kompier and Cooper (1999) have analyzed more comprehensive intervention programs, i.e., combinations of various measures.

An example of such an intervention program is reported by Lourijsen and coworkers (1999). The company under study is a Dutch hospital with circa 850 employees. The project lasted 4 years. Motives for the intervention project were high sickness absenteeism and problems in hiring new personnel. The project's initiative was taken by the hospital's management (top down). A steering committee was installed, there was some external consultancy, and there was active involvement from the employees (bottom up). The study included a control condition (a comparable hospital). First, a stress audit was made through interviews, checklists, a questionnaire, and an analysis of sickness absenteeism and turnover. Main risk factors were high psychosocial workload, interior climate, leadership style, physical workload, shift system, insufficient training, and career opportunities. For some of these factors, the total hospital was considered a risk group, and for others, only certain departments. Next, work-directed changes were chosen: changes in interior climate, working and resting times schedule, technical devices, reduction in physical workload, better work organization, and job enrichment.

Also, person-directed measures were chosen: better managerial information with regard to sickness absenteeism figures and better procedures with regard to sickness absenteeism, training for supervisors, better guidance in case of sickness, health promotional initiatives, and various trainings (for example, coping with aggression, individual stress management, alcohol, smoking). The implementation of these measures took place in various subprojects with a participative approach. The final responsibility for the implementation of these measures was by top management. Coordination took place via the steering committee, and the practical implementation was in subprojects by the line management in the departments. After the implementation, another round of data collection took place. A comparison of pretest and posttest yielded an improvement in working conditions, intensified attention for sick employees and for working conditions, and a better psychosocial work climate. When compared with the pretest, the control hospital scored better at some variables in the questionnaire (posttest). The absence percentage in the "experimental" hospital was significantly reduced from 8.9% in 1991 to 5.8% in 1994. This 1994 level was well below the average Dutch hospital level and below that of the control hospital. An analysis of costs and benefits yielded positive results: the benefits exceeded the costs, mainly due to the drop in sickness costs. There were several obstructing factors: for example, it was difficult to keep middle management and the employees involved over a longer period, there were differences in the steering committee, "everything took a lot of time," and it was difficult to assess objectively "which was a serious constraint and which was not." In addition, there were stimulating factors: the project's stepwise approach, the use of adequate instruments, a special information and discussion day for all employees, etc.

It is not easy to draw firm general conclusions from such comprehensive intervention projects. Evaluation of such projects reveals that stress prevention is no one-time event or merely a technical process. It is clear that it is not only *what* one does (content of the intervention), but also *how* (process factors). Still, it is strongly suggested in these studies that true prevention (i.e., preventive measures that are based on an adequate diagnosis identifying risk factors and risk groups, which theoretically and logically fit in with the problems, and which are introduced and implemented in a proper way) can be beneficial to both the employee and the organization.

EPILOGUE

In this chapter we have studied the role of the psychosocial work environment in the development and prevention of stress-related ill health. We have chosen a probabilistic conceptualization of factors in the psychosocial work environment (risk factors, stressors, psychosocial hazards) that fits well in a more general occupational health perspective. It was also emphasized that individual features are important in the complex and dynamic interplay between combinations of work characteristics, work behavior, and health outcomes.

To identify major risk factors for stress and its consequences for ill health, we have looked at differences and similarities in seven important theoretical approaches. These critical job features are job demands, autonomy, skill variety, and social support. Next, we investigated how prevalent these risk factors are in Europe and the U.S. As recent empirical studies point at high psychological demands, problems with job control, and increased job insecurity, it was concluded that these risk factors are common in modern work. Then, we analyzed which developments in the world of work are behind these empirical figures. Seven interrelated trends that more or less "sculpture" these job characteristics and thereby affect stress at the workplace have been distinguished.

Finally, we turned toward the issue of prevention. It was concluded that (1) according to international legislation, the preventive priority is to make the workplace less stressful by reducing or "rooting out" the risks; (2) there is considerable consensus among major theoretical approaches when it comes to answering the question, How can workplace stress be reduced?, i.e., through the redesign of work; and (3) empirical studies strongly suggest that true prevention can be beneficial to both the employee and the organization.

REFERENCES

Beehr, T.A. (1995). *Psychological Stress in the Workplace*. London: Routledge.

Beekun, R.I. (1989). Assessing the effectiveness of sociotechnical interventions: Antidote or fad? *Human Relations*, 10, 877–897.

Bielenski, H., Bolch, G. & Wagner, A. (2002). *Working Time Preferences in Sixteen European Countries*. Luxembourg: European Foundation for the Improvement of Living and Working Conditions.

Bond, T., Galinsky, E. & Swanberg, J.E. (1998). *The 1997 National Study of the Changing Workforce*. New York: Families and Work Institute.

Caplan, R., Cobb, S., French, J. & Harrison, R. (1975). *Job Demands and Worker Health, Main Effects and Occupational Differences*. Washington, DC: NIOSH.

Cascio, W. (1995). *Managing Human Resources: Productivity, Quality of Worklife, Profits*. New York: McGraw-Hill.

CBS (Dutch Bureau for Statistics). (2002). *Statistisch Jaarboek 2002* [*Yearbook Statistics 2002*]. Voorburg/Heerlen: CBS.

Chappell, D. & Di Martino, V. (2000). *Violence at Work*, 2nd ed. Geneva: International Labour Office.

Cherns, A.B. (1976). The principles of sociotechnical design. *Human Relations*, 29, 783–792.

Cherns, A.B. (1987). Principles of sociotechnical design revisited. *Human Relations*, 40, 153–162.

Clegg, C.W. (2000). Sociotechnical principles for system design. *Applied Ergonomics*, 31, 463–477.

Cox, T., Griffiths, A. & Gonzalez, R. (2000). *Research on Work-Related Stress*. Bilbao, Spain: European Agency for Safety and Health at Work.

Cox, T., Griffiths, A. & Randall, R. (2003). A risk management approach to the prevention of work stress. In Schabracq, M., Winnubst, J. & Cooper, C. (Eds.), *Handbook Work and Health Psychology.* Chichester, U.K.: Wiley, pp. 191–206.

De Sitter, L.U. (1989). Moderne sociotechniek [Modern sociotechnics]. *Gedrag en Organisatie*, 2, 222–251.

Elkin, A. & Rosch, P. (1990). Promoting mental health at the workplace: The prevention side of stress management. *Occupational Medicine: State of the Art Review*, 5, 739–754.

European Council. (1993). Concerning certain aspects of working time. *Official Journal European Communities*, L307, 18–24. (Council Directive 93/104/EC).

Frese, M. (1985). Stress at work and psychosomatic complaints: A causal interpretation. *Journal of Applied Psychology*, 70, 314–328.

Frese, M. & Zapf, D. (1994). Action as the core of work psychology: A German approach. In Triandis, H.C., Dunnette, M.D. & Hough, L.M. (Eds.), *Handbook of Industrial and Organizational Psychology*, 2nd ed., Vol. 4. Palo Alto, CA: Consulting Psychologists Press, pp. 271–340.

Fried, Y. & Ferris, G.R. (1987). The validity of the job characteristics model: A review and meta-analysis. *Personnel Psychology*, 40, 287–322.

Geurts, S. & Demerouti, E. (2003). Work/non-work interface: A review of theories and findings. In Schabracq, M., Winnubst, J. & Cooper, C., (Eds.), *Handbook Work and Health Psychology.* Chichester, U.K.: Wiley, pp. 279–312.

Greif, S. (1991). Stress in der Arbeit: Einfuhrung und Grundbegriffe. In Greif, S., Bamberg, E. & Semmer, N. (Eds.), *Psychicher Stress am Arbeitsplatz.* Gottingen: Hogrefe, pp. 1–28.

Griffiths, A. (1999). Organizational interventions: Facing the limits of the natural science paradigm. *Scandinavian Journal of Work, Environment and Health*, 25, 589–596.

Hacker, W. (1998). *Allgemeine Arbeits- und Ingenieurspsychologie*. Berlin: Deutscher Verlag der Wissenschaften.

Hackman, J.R. & Oldham, G.R. (1975). Development of the Job Diagnostic Survey. *Journal of Applied Psychology*, 60, 159–170.

Hackman, J.R. & Oldham, G.R. (1980). *Work Redesign*. Reading, MA: Addison-Wesley.

Hamborg, K.-C. & Greif, S. (2003). New technologies and stress. In Schabracq, M., Winnubst, J. & Cooper, C. (Eds.), *Handbook Work and Health Psychology.* Chichester, U.K.: Wiley, pp. 209–235.

Harma, M. (2003). Are long workhours a health risk? *Scandinavian Journal of Work, Environment and Health*, 29, 167–169.

Johnson, J.V. & Johansson, G. (Eds.). (1991). *The Psychosocial Work Environment: Work Organization, Democratization and Health*. Amityville, NY: Baywood.

Kahn, R.L. & Byosiere, P. (1992). Stress in organizations. In Dunnette, M.D. & Hough, L. (Eds.), *Handbook of Industrial and Organizational Psychology*, 2nd ed., Vol. 3. Palo Alto, CA: Consulting Psychologists Press, pp. 571–650.

Kahn, R.L., Wolfe, D., Quinn, R., Snoek, J. & Rosenthal, R. (1964). *Organizational Stress: Studies in Role Conflict and Ambiguity.* New York: Wiley.

Karasek, R.A. (1979). Job demands, job decision latitude, and mental strain: Implications for job redesign. *Administrative Science Quarterly*, 24, 285–308.

Karasek, R.A. (1998). Demand/control model: A social, emotional, and physiological approach to stress risk and active behaviour development. In Stellman, J. (Ed.), *Encyclopaedia of Occupational Health and Safety*. Geneva: International Labour Office, pp. 34.6–34.14.

Karasek, R.A. & Theorell, T. (1990). *Healthy Work: Stress, Productivity and the Reconstruction of Working Life*. New York: Basic Books.

Kasl, S.V. (1978). Epidemiological contributions to the study of work stress. In Cooper, C.L. & Payne, R. (Eds.), *Stress at Work*. New York: Wiley, pp. 3–48.

Kasl, S.V. (1987). Methodologies in stress and health: Past difficulties, present dilemmas, future directions. In Kasl, S.V. & Cooper, C.L. (Eds.), *Stress and Health: Issues in Research and Methodology*. Chichester, U.K.: John Wiley, pp. 307–318.

Kompier, M. (2002). The psychosocial work environment and health: What do we know and where should we go? *Scandinavian Journal of Work, Environment and Health*, 28, 1–4.

Kompier, M. (2003). Job design and well-being. In Schabracq, M., Winnubst, J. & Cooper, C. (Eds.), *Handbook Work and Health Psychology*. Chichester, U.K.: Wiley, pp. 429–454.

Kompier, M. & Cooper, C. (Eds.). (1999). *Preventing Stress, Improving Productivity: European Case Studies in the Workplace*. London: Routledge.

Kompier, M., Geurts, S., Grundemann, R., Vink, P. & Smulders, P. (1998). Cases in stress prevention: The success of a participative and stepwise approach. *Stress Medicine*, 14, 155–168.

Kompier, M.A.J. & Kristensen, T.S. (2001). Organizational work stress interventions in a theoretical, methodological and practical context. In Dunham, J. (Ed.), *Stress in the Workplace: Past, Present and Future*. London: Whurr, pp. 164–190.

Kompier, M., Van den Berg, A.-M., Aust, B. & Siegrist, J. (2000). Stress prevention in bus drivers: Evaluation of 13 natural experiments. *Journal of Occupational Health Psychology*, 5, 11–31.

Kristensen, T.S., Kornitzer, M. & Alfredson, L. (1998). *Social Factors, Work, Stress and Cardiovascular Disease Prevention in the European Union*. Brussels: The European Heart Network.

Kuipers, H. (1989). Zelforganisatie als ontwerpprincipe [Self organization as design principle]. *Gedrag en Organisatie*, 2, 199–201.

Landsbergis, P. (2003). The changing organization of work and the safety and health of working people: A commentary. *Journal of Occupational and Environmental Medicine*, 45, 61–72.

Leather, Ph., Brady, C., Lawrence, C., Beale, D. & Cox, T. (Eds.). (1999). *Work-Related Violence: Assessment and Intervention*. London: Routledge.

Levi, L. (2000). *Guidance on Work-Related Stress: Spice of Life or Kiss of Death?* Luxembourg: Office for Official Publications of the European Communities.

Lourijsen, E., Houtman, I., Kompier, M. & Grundemann, R. (1999). The Netherlands: A hospital, "healthy working for health." In Kompier, M. & Cooper, C. (Eds.), *Preventing Stress, Improving Productivity: European Case Studies in the Workplace*. London: Routledge, pp. 86–120.

Merllié, D. & Paoli, P. (2001). *Ten Years of Working Conditions in the European Union*. Dublin: European Foundation for the Improvement of Living and Working Conditions.

Murphy, L.R. (1996). Stress management in work settings: A critical review of the research literature. *American Journal of Health Promotion*, 11, 112–135.

Murphy, L.R. (2003). Stress management at work: Secondary prevention of stress. In Schabracq, M., Winnubst, J. & Cooper, C. (Eds.), *Handbook Work and Health Psychology.* Chichester, U.K.: Wiley, pp. 533–548.

Paoli, P. (1992). *First European Survey on the Work Environment 1991–1992*, Dublin: European Foundation for the Improvement of Living and Working Conditions.

Paoli, P. (1997). *Second European Survey on Working Conditions 1996.* Dublin: European Foundation for the Improvement of Living and Working Conditions.

Parker, S.K., Jackson, P.R., Sprigg, C.A. & Whybrow, A.C. (1998). *Organisational Interventions to Reduce the Impact of Poor Work Design*, HSE Contract Research Report 193/1998. Colegate, U.K.: Her Majesty's Stationary Office.

Price, R.H., Choi, J.N. & Vinokur, A. (2002). Links in the chain of adversity following job loss: How economic hardship and loss of personal control lead to depression, impaired functioning and poor health. *Journal of Occupational Health Psychology*, 7, 302–312.

Quick, J.C., Quick, J.D., Nelson, D.L. & Hurrell, J.J. (1997). *Preventive Stress Management in Organisations*. Washington, DC: American Psychological Association.

Sauter, S. et al. (NIOSH). (2002). *The Changing Organization of Work and the Safety and Health of Working People*. Cincinnati: NIOSH.

Sauter, S.L., Hurrell, J.J., Murphy, L.R. & Levi, L. (1998). Psychosocial and organizational factors. In Stellman, J. (Ed.), *Encyclopaedia of Occupational Health and Safety.* Geneva: International Labour Office, pp. 34.2–34.3.

Sauter, S.L., Murphy, L.R. & Hurrell, J.J., Jr. (1992). Prevention of work-related psychological disorders. A national strategy proposed by the National Institute for Occupational Safety and Health (NIOSH). In Keita, G.W. & Sauter, S.L. (Eds.), *Work and Well-Being: An Agenda for the 1990's*. Washington, DC: American Psychological Association.

Semmer, N.K. (2003a). Individual differences, work stress and health. In Schabracq, M., Winnubst, J. & Cooper, C. (Eds.), *Handbook Work and Health Psychology.* Chichester, U.K.: Wiley, pp. 84–120.

Semmer, N.K. (2003b). Job stress interventions and organization of work. In Quick, J.C. & Tetrick, L.E. (Eds.), *Handbook of Occupational Health Psychology.* Washington, DC: American Psychological Association, pp. 325–353.

Shirom, A. (2003). The effects of work stress on health. In Schabracq, M., Winnubst, J. & Cooper, C. (Eds.), *Handbook Work and Health Psychology.* Chichester, U.K.: Wiley, pp. 63–82.

Siegrist, J. (1996). Adverse health effects of high effort-low reward conditions at work. *Journal of Occupational Health Psychology*, 1, 27–43.

Sprigg, C.A., Jackson, P.R. & Parker, S.K. (2000). Production teamworking: The importance of interdependence and autonomy for employee strain and satisfaction. *Human Relations*, 53, 1519–1543.

Spurgeon, A., Harrington, J.M. & Cooper, C.L. (1997). Health and safety problems associated with long working hours: A review of the current position. *Occupational and Environmental Medicine*, 54, 367–375.

Sverke, M., Hellgren, J. & Naswall, K. (2002). No security: A meta-analysis and review of job insecurity and its consequences. *Journal of Occupational Health Psychology*, 7, 242–264.

Taris, T. & Kompier, M. (2003). Challenges in longitudinal designs in occupational health psychology. *Scandinavian Journal of Work, Environment and Health*, 29, 1–4.

Taris, T., Kompier, M., De Lange, A., Schaufeli, W. & Schreurs, P. (2003). Learning new behaviour patterns: A longitudinal test of Karasek's active learning hypothesis among Dutch teachers. *Work and Stress*, 17, 1–20.

Taylor, F.W. (1911). *Scientific Management*. New York: Harper & Brothers.

Van der Hulst, M. (2003). Long work hours and health. *Scandinavian Journal of Work, Environment and Health*, 29, 171–188.

Van der Klink, J.J.L., Blonk, R.W.B., Schene, A.H. & van Dijk, F.J.H. (2001). The benefits of interventions for work-related stress. *American Journal of Public Health*, 91, 270–276.

Wall, T.D. & Clegg, C.W. (1981). A longitudinal field study of group work redesign. *Journal of Occupational Behaviour*, 2, 31–49.

Warr, P.B. (1992). Job features and excessive stress. In Jenkins, R. & Coney, N. (Eds.), *Prevention of Mental Ill Health at Work*. London: HMSO.

Warr, P. (1996). Employee well-being. In Warr, P. (Ed.), *Psychology at Work*, 4th ed. London: Penguin Books, 224–253.

Zapf, D. (2002). Emotion work and psychological well-being. A review of the literature and some conceptual considerations. *Human Resource Management Review*, 12, 237–268.

19 The Many Faces of Control at Work

Kathryne E. Dupré, Julian Barling, and Manon Mireille LeBlanc

CONTENTS

> Jobs differ tremendously in the amount and type of control they allow employees. At one extreme is machine-paced factory work in which the employee must work at precisely determined times, performing specified tasks at the intervals determined by the machine. The classic "I Love Lucy" comedy sketch in a candy factory illustrates what happens when the employee cannot keep up with the assembly line, and shows Lucy frantically stuffing candy everywhere she can as she falls farther and farther behind. At the other extreme are the jobs of high-level management employees who are given assignments that can be done at any place, at any time, and in almost any manner they see fit. (Spector, 2002, p. 134)

Most people spend much of their lives involved in some sort of work. While there have always been many sources of work-related stress, work-related strain is reaching increasingly elevated levels (e.g., Cohen, 1997), with stress being identified as a major occupational health issue. One of the important steps in addressing any workplace health issue is to identify its sources (Cox & Cox, 1993). Although

0-8493-1820-3/05/$0.00+$1.50

research has identified numerous work-related stressors that ultimately result in various forms of strain (e.g., Pratt & Barling, 1988), the lack of job control has been identified by many as a very significant job stressor (Warr, 1987; Hepburn et al., 1997; Karasek, 1979; Karasek & Theorell, 1990; Parkes, 1989; Sauter et al., 1990) that warrants continued research and managerial attention (e.g., Spector, 2002). Correspondingly, over the last few decades there has been a continuous increase in research on the impact of control on a variety of work-related outcomes (e.g., Spector, 1986; Thompson, 1981). In this research, there is compelling evidence that control at work is a critical element in employees' health, well-being, and job-related activities (see, for example, Spector, 2002; Terry & Jimmieson, 1999).

In this chapter we address and underscore the importance of control at work. We review the existing empirical literature on relationships between forms of employee control at work and outcomes for employees and organizations, and highlight a number of the remaining questions and limitations that have been identified as important to this work. Of particular interest to us is the fact that research has focused predominantly on the consequences of either *having* or *not having* control at work, neglecting to thoroughly consider the importance or repercussions of *having lost* control or *feeling overcontrolled* at work. In this chapter we attempt to fill this void by including discussions of both losing control and feeling overcontrolled at work. We propose that future research should consider all of these forms of work control given their potential association with important individual and organizational outcomes. We begin with a brief discussion on the theoretical background and conceptualization of control at work.

THEORETICAL AND CONCEPTUAL DEVELOPMENT OF CONTROL AT WORK

Control has long been viewed as an essential and innate aspect of human nature (e.g., Miller, 1972; Skinner, 1995; White, 1959), and it is increasingly recognized as an important determinant of health and well-being (Miller, 1979; Thompson, 1981). Although it is possible to distinguish between objective and perceived control, in this chapter we focus on the perception of control, as this appears to have a stronger relationship with work-related outcomes (e.g., Ganster et al., 2001; Jimmieson & Terry, 1997; Spector, 2002). Perceived control is the belief in one's ability to influence outcomes: events are controllable when it is believed that one's actions affect outcomes, and events are uncontrollable when it is believed that nothing one does or can do will change what will occur (deCharms, 1968; Thompson, 1981).

Control at work focuses on job and organizational characteristics such as the extent to which employees perceive they are able to make decisions about their work (e.g., when and where to work, how to work, what type of tasks to do), and the extent to which there are opportunities for employees to use their skills and knowledge at work (e.g., Karasek & Theorell, 1990). In the work setting, control increases employees' beliefs that situations can be anticipated and managed. Although there are a multitude of workplace stressors (e.g., role conflict, role overload/underload, interpersonal relationships at work, technological advances, uncertainty; see Barling et al., in press), control has emerged as one of the most studied stressors at work, likely due to its strong association with a wide variety of outcomes (e.g., Ganster & Fusilier, 1989). A stressor refers to an objective characteristic or event in the environment and is something that has the potential to cause strain, which refers to both the short-term and long-term psychological, physical, behavioral, and physiological responses to stress (i.e., an individual's subjective experience of the particular stressor) (Jex & Beehr, 1991; Pratt & Barling, 1988). Not only has control been shown to act as a stressor with implications for subsequent strain, but it has also been found to act as a moderator to the stressor–strain relationship. Not all stressors lead to strain, and under some conditions (e.g., a lack of perceived job control), some stressors might be more closely linked with strain.

Although an employee can have control over any aspect of work (see, for example, Carayon & Zijlstra, 1999; Dwyer & Ganster, 1991; Ganster, 1988; Jackson et al., 1993), most research on work control focuses on control in terms of job characteristics. A wide variety of dimensions of job control have received attention across studies: for example, Hurrell and McLaney (1989) focused on task, decision, physical, and resource control; Wall et al. (1995) considered the importance of timing and method control; and Carayon and Zijlstra (1999) examined task, resource, and organizational control. Research on the topic of control at work continues to vary considerably in terms of what types of jobs are examined, the forms of control included, and the outcomes considered (Evans & Fischer, 1992). Jobs differ tremendously in the amount and type of control they allow employees, and there is no theory that defines the conceptual boundaries of the job control construct (Kasl, 1989; Sauter et al., 1989).

Many occupational health psychology theories suggest that stress-related outcomes can be improved by increasing employees' control over their work. Research is based on the assumption, and data indicating, that jobs that impose limits on control are associated with less favorable work outcomes. For example, the job characteristics model (Hackman & Oldham, 1975), action theory (Frese & Zapf, 1994), and job design theory (Carayon, 1993) of stress all propose that providing people with control over various aspects of their work will improve health-related outcomes. One of the most influential theories concerning job control is the demand–control model, first proposed by Karasek in 1979. Karasek's model focuses on organizational factors and has been the underlying theoretical basis for much research on job stress. According to his model, the influence of work demands (e.g., psychological stressors, such as a requirement for working fast and hard, having a great deal to do, or not having enough time) on health is moderated by the degree of control (i.e., "the working individual's potential control over his tasks and his conduct during the working day," p. 290). Karasek suggested that job demands were not in themselves harmful, but when combined with low employee control, these demands could affect employees' physical and mental health. The major prediction is that job strain, reflected in employees' mental and physical health problems, occurs when jobs are simultaneously high in demands and low in controllability.

The role of control in determining the effects of work stress in general, and the Karasek model in particular, has been the subject of much research (e.g., Bishop et al., 2003; Sauter et al., 1989). Although studies have shown that job demands can increase strain and strain-related outcomes, and that high job control can reduce these negative outcomes (Bosma et al., 1997; Johnson et al., 1996), empirical findings have not consistently supported a moderating pattern of influence between these variables (Carayon, 1993; de Rijk et al., 1998; Ganster & Fusilier, 1989; Jones & Fletcher, 1996; Landsbergis, 1988; Perrewe & Anthony, 1990; Sauter, 1989), whereas others have shown the predicted interaction (Fox et al., 1993; Parkes et al., 1994; Wall et al., 1996). To explain these discrepancies, methodological explanations relating to the conceptualization and measurement of job demands and job control have been proposed, as well as acknowledgment of the confounding effects of unmeasured third variables (e.g., socioeconomic status), the use of a varying range of measures of strain, and the differences in power when using alternative methods to test the model (Ganster, 1989; Karasek, 1979; Terry & Jimmieson, 1999; Wall et al., 1996). Additionally, many researchers have suggested that people adapt in different ways to the environment (Kristensen, 1995; Parkes, 1989; Warr, 1994) and that this can influence the nature of the demands–control relationship (Karasek, 1979; Parkes, 1990, 1994; Xie, 1996). Given the frequently contradictory findings, many researchers have expanded their focus to include other variables that might play important roles in the relationship between job control and various outcome variables, and these will be included in the following discussion. We now consider outcomes associated with different aspects of control at work, namely, having control at work, lacking control at work, losing control at work, and feeling overcontrolled at work.

HAVING CONTROL AT WORK

Generally speaking, control is associated with positive outcomes and a lack of control with more negative outcomes. As a result of such findings, in 1988 the National Institute for Occupational Safety and Health in the U.S. put forth a number of recommendations to manage stress at work, and among them was the recommendation that employees be given the opportunity to have input into decisions or actions that affect their jobs and performance. Although studies primarily examine the relationship between job control and individual-level outcome variables, it is important to keep in mind that control likely also has an indirect relationship with organizational-related outcomes through its individual-level impact. For example, when the health and well-being of employees are enhanced, organizational effectiveness will likely improve.

INDIVIDUAL HEALTH-RELATED OUTCOMES

Job control has been shown to relate to a number of important individual-level health outcomes. Numerous studies have shown that perceived job control protects employees against a wide variety of health ailments, including cardiovascular problems (Karasek et al., 1982), coronary heart disease (Karasek, 1990), medically certified sickness absences (Kivimäki et al., 1998), self-reported disease (Bosma et al., 1997), physiological and strain symptoms (Elovainio & Kivimäki, 1996; Jackson, 1983; Karasek, 1979, 1990; Steptoe et al., 1993; Theorell et al., 1990), emotional distress (Barnett & Brennan, 1995; Spector, 1986), and musculoskeletal problems (Bongers et al., 1993). Interestingly, some research suggests that job control can exert its effect on strain-related outcomes through justice evaluations (Elovainio et al., 2001). The ability to control particular aspects of the work environment can alter the perceived fairness of organizational-related variables (e.g., procedural justice) (see also Thibaut & Walker, 1975).

Various aspects of control have been related to individual health outcomes. For example, Fenwick and Tausig (2001) found that control over work scheduling had a positive effect on health outcomes. Van Yperen and Hagedoorn (2003) found that timing and method control reduced fatigue: in particular, as job demands increased, high job control was needed to limit fatigue. Bond and Bunce (2001) showed how by giving employees more discretion and choice in their work, a work reorganization intervention led to an increase in people's job control, and after a year, people's mental health improved, sickness absence rates improved, and self-rated job performance rose. Parker et al. (1997) demonstrated that increased role clarity and participation in decision making were associated with improved psychological health during a period of downsizing. They found a significant relationship between increases in control and job satisfaction 4 years after a strategic downsizing (in association with an empowerment initiative). Adams and Jex (1999) found that perceived control of time was related to health and job satisfaction. In addition, job control has been shown to have a positive impact on employees' family-related outcomes (e.g., Fenwick & Tausig, 2001). For example, in the study by Adams and Jex, perceived control was negatively related to work interfering with family and family interfering with work.

Although most research examining the impact of job control on work-related variables is cross-sectional, some recent longitudinal data exist that support the cross-sectional findings. For example, Dwyer and Fox (2000) found that job control predicted enhanced health over a 5-year period. Ganster et al. (2001) found that subjective and objective measures of workload demands interacted with personal control perceptions in predicting cumulative health care costs over a 5-year period. They found that high control at the beginning of their study predicted lower use of medical services over the following 5 years, as well as better mental health. In a 5-year follow-up study, Kivimäki et al. (1997) found that a high degree of job control predicted lower medically certified sickness absence in municipal workers. Nonetheless, other longitudinal research is not as supportive of this relationship. For example, Sargent and Terry (1998) found that task control, decision control, and work scheduling control had no long-term effect on depressive symptoms after controlling for initial levels of depression (see also Daniels & Guppy, 1994; Parkes, 1991; Parkes et al., 1994).

Individual Proactive and Learning-Related Outcomes

Until recently, researchers had not investigated proactive and learning-oriented outcomes of demand–control combinations (Theorell & Karasek, 1996). Considering a wider range of outcomes, beyond strain and strain-related variables, is consistent with the notion that mental health should not just be considered an absence of stress symptoms, but should also be viewed in terms of positive mental health indicators

(Warr, 1987, 1994). Correspondingly, an important outcome of job control is that it appears to improve individuals' ability to cope with various aspects of work, and in addition, it increases employees' effectiveness at work, both of which are critical for successful organizational functioning. One prediction from Karasek's (1979) model is that positive outcomes, such as motivation and learning, occur when an individual's job has high levels of both psychological demands and controllability.

A substantial amount of research has shown that control promotes individual outcomes such as organizational commitment, intrinsic motivation, and involvement (Spector, 1986). Parker and Sprigg (1999) found that higher job control (as well as low job demands and proactive personality) predicted employees' learning-related outcomes (i.e., sense of mastery, role breadth self-efficacy, and production ownership). Perceived control also seems to help employees minimize emotional reactions to job stressors, thus promoting a more constructive problem-focused coping strategy, rather than an alternate, and frequently more destructive, emotion-focused strategy (Latack, 1986; Spector, 2002). Job control not only results in employees having greater opportunity for solving and preventing problems (Jackson, 1989), but also potentially enhances employees' motivation to take ownership for a broad range of problems (Parker et al., 1997), promotes the development of knowledge needed to prevent faults (Wall et al., 1992), and has been associated with higher levels of "integrated understanding" (i.e., breadth of knowledge about the organization, such as understanding the bigger picture and knowing what other departments do) (Parker & Axtell, 2001, p. 1089). Research has further shown that enhanced job control (along with improved communication quality) predicted higher role breadth self-efficacy (i.e., employees' confidence that they can carry out a range of proactive, integrative, and interpersonal tasks) (Parker, 1998). Studies have also shown a link between job control and employee creativity (e.g., Oldham & Cummings, 1996), an outcome often cited as beneficial for both individuals and organizations.

Individual Work-Related Outcomes

Perceptions of workplace control are also related to a number of individual-level work-related variables (see Parker et al., 2003). Much research has demonstrated the relationship between control and a variety of work-related variables, including increased job satisfaction (Dwyer & Ganster, 1991; Greenberger et al., 1989; Krausz et al., 2000; McGilton & Pringle, 1999), increased organizational commitment (Barling & Kelloway, 1996; Krausz et al., 2000), decreased turnover intentions (Barling & Kelloway, 1996; Spector, 1986; Wall & Clegg, 1981), and increased employee attendance (Dwyer & Ganster, 1991; Smulders & Nijhuis, 1999; Spector, 1986). Of particular importance is a study by Yelin (1986) showing that with job control, employees with chronic illness are more likely to continue working, compared to employees with chronic illness but little job control.

Job control has also been shown to influence a number of safety-related variables that are vital to organizations. In a longitudinal study, Parker et al. (2001) found that job control was indirectly related to safety compliance via organizational commitment. Likewise, Simard and Marchand (1995) found that control positively influenced workgroups' propensity to take safety initiatives, and Geller et al. (1996)

argued that individuals' task control was positively related to proactive safety behaviors. Thus, it is apparent that having control at work has definite positive implications for the health and well-being of both employees and their organizations.

LACKING CONTROL AT WORK

> The man whose life is spent in performing a few simple operations, of which the effects are perhaps always the same, or very nearly the same, has no occasion to exert his understanding or to exercise his invention.... The torpor of his mind renders him not only incapable of relishing or bearing a part in any rational conversation, but of conceiving any generous, noble, or tender sentiment..." (Smith, 1937, p. 734–735).

In the same way that having control at work tends to relate to positive outcomes, feeling that one lacks control at work is associated with negative outcomes. Although the quotation above provides an excessively negative outlook on the experience of a lack of control at work, the bulk of the evidence does indicate a fairly consistent relationship between a lack of perceived job control and a variety of detrimental individual and organizational outcomes.

INDIVIDUAL HEALTH-RELATED OUTCOMES

As previously discussed, perceived job control is related to a number of individual health-related outcomes. Some research has focused on specifically examining the relationship between a lack of perceived job control and individual health-related outcomes (Sauter et al., 1990; Seligman, 1975; Terry & Jimmieson, 1999; Thompson, 1981; Wall et al., 1990; Warr, 1999). Over the past few decades, researchers have provided evidence that low levels of job control are related to negative stress-related outcomes (e.g., anxiety, absenteeism, physical complaints, illness, burnout, reduced performance; for reviews of the research, see Jex & Beehr, 1991; Sauter et al., 1989; Spector, 1986). The findings from these studies are quite compelling.

In 16 of 22 studies, Theorell and Karasek (1996) showed significant associations between high-demand–low-control jobs and cardiovascular disease or cardiovascular disease symptoms. For example, Bosma et al. (1998) found a link between a lack of job control (i.e., skill discretion and decision authority) and cardiovascular disease. In a 5-year follow-up study, these researchers found that both objective and subjective low control in the workplace predicted subsequent coronary heart disease among both men and women government employees. Another study found that high job demands and low decisional job control resulted in a higher heart rate and "pressure rate product" (i.e., an estimate of myocardial oxygen demand) among male patrol officers (Bishop et al., 2003). Landsbergis (1988) found that job dissatisfaction, depression, psychosomatic symptoms, and burnout are higher in jobs that combine high workload demands with low control (i.e., decision latitude). This association remained significant after controlling for age, sex, education, marital status, number of children, hours worked per week, and shift worked. Spector et al. (1988) found that low levels of perceived control were associated with anxiety, frustration, physical symptoms for the past 30 days, and doctor visits for the prior 3 months. McKnight and Glass (1995) showed that among nurses, perceptions of uncontrollability were directly associated with depression, emotional exhaustion, and perceived lack of accomplishment at work.

The findings above all demonstrate the negative effect that a lack of job control can have on individual health-related outcomes. In addition, a recent longitudinal study by Amick et al. (2002) has garnered considerable attention given its profound finding. Amick et al. (2002) followed workers in a 24-year study of 5000 households in the U.S. and found that working in low-control jobs (i.e., a lack of decision-making control over work performed on the job) for one's entire working life is associated with a 43% risk of premature death. One need not look much further than these longitudinal data to appreciate that research strongly suggests that a lack of control at work can have critical implications for individuals' health and well-being.

Individual Work-Related Outcomes

Perceptions of a lack of workplace control are also related to a number of individual-level work-related variables, including absence and turnover intentions (Spector, 1986). Additionally, just as enhancing perceptions of control appears to lead to faster learning and better task performance, reducing perceptions of control can lead to motivational and cognitive deficits (Seligman, 1975). The use of electronic performance monitoring is associated with lower feelings of control on the part of the employees who are being monitored in this fashion (Smith et al., 1992). In one study that examined the use of this type of monitoring, workers with complete control over monitoring felt more in control than workers with no control over monitoring. Of particular importance to this discussion is that those with control over monitoring also demonstrated superior task performance and higher task satisfaction (Stanton & Barnes-Farrell, 1996).

Although lacking control at work tends to be related to a number of detrimental individual and organizational outcomes, and having control at work tends to be related to a number of positive individual and organizational outcomes, there are boundary conditions that need to be understood to fully comprehend the potential impact of control on these outcomes.

BOUNDARY CONDITIONS RELATED TO CONTROL AT WORK

Despite the strong relationship between job control and many outcome variables, research clearly indicates that there are local or individual reactions to job control, particular situational variables, and differences in employees' desire for control that can alter these effects (e.g., Burger, 1989, 1995; Elovainio et al., 2000; McGilton & Pringle, 1999). For example, Elsass and Veiga (1997) found that although perceived control is inversely related to job strain, strain increases as the discrepancy between actual and desired levels of job control increases. Many people respond favorably to control, but for others it can exacerbate the detrimental effects of this form of stress.

There has been increasing attention devoted to how individual characteristics moderate responses to job control. In a number of studies, the moderating effect of job control is only evident for a subpopulation within the sample, for instance, for employees who are high in private self-consciousness (Kivimäki & Lindström, 1995), those with an internal locus of control (Daniels & Guppy, 1994), or those with an external locus of control (Parkes, 1991). This suggests that personality characteristics might in some cases determine whether employees benefit from high control in their jobs. Rodriguez et al. (2001) found that the stress-reducing effect of control is observed exclusively in employees with an internal locus of control. It has been suggested that locus of control is important because employees with an internal locus of control are likely to cope actively with job stress, whereas those with an external locus of control are likely to refrain from action, because they believe that changing the situation is beyond their ability (e.g., Parkes, 1989).

Hollmann et al. (2001) found that control over work method and timing had positive effects on musculoskeletal problems only when the physical workload was relatively light. These researchers suggest that the effects of high levels of physical workload on musculoskeletal symptoms are so strong that they override any buffering effect of control. Lee et al. (1990) found that people with high levels of type A behavior, who also have high perceived job control, perform better and have greater job satisfaction than those low in perceived control. Parker and Sprigg (1999) found that Karasek's (1979) demands–control interaction only applies to more proactive employees who are more likely to take advantage of higher job control and use it to manage job demands. These researchers argued that more passive employees likely do not take the opportunity to use job control when it is available.

Researchers acknowledge the important role of social support in the relationship between job control and outcome variables, and often suggest that strain is predicted by low job control, high job demands, and low work support (Dollard et al., 2000; Karasek & Theorell, 1990; Landsbergis et al., 1992; Leong et al., 1996; Noblet et al., 2001). In one study looking at the effects of a number of variables (i.e., job control, job demands, social support, balancing work and nonwork, length of working week, lack of resources to accomplish tasks, and constant pressure to perform to a high standard) on job satisfaction and psychological health, the combined influence of job control, job demands, and social support contributed 98% of the overall explained variance in job satisfaction and 90% of the overall explained variance in psychological health, of all of these variables (Noblet et al., 2001). In these studies, social or work-based support often moderates the effect of job demands and control on employee health (Johnson & Hall, 1988). Schaubroeck and Fink (1998), for example, showed that while supervisor consideration was positively related to performance outcomes when control was low, under high perceived control, consideration was negatively related to performance and extrarole behavior.

In a similar vein, an interesting finding appeared in a recent study by Arnold (2003). Although control over one's job choice is typically related to positive outcomes, including satisfaction, psychological well-being, and health (Isaksson & Johansson, 2000), Arnold found that reporting that one chose to be a sex worker moderated the relationship between occupational identification and well-being. In both "no choice" and "some choice" conditions for entering into sex work, when occupational identification was low, well-being was low. However, when perceived choice was low, and occupational identification was high, well-being was enhanced. Arnold suggests that if individuals perceive they have little or no choice about whether to work in a stigmatized role, then perhaps this protects their well-being by providing them more psychological protection against the idea that they have made a poor choice.

Finally, self-efficacy has been shown to moderate the relationship between job control and various outcome variables. Schaubroeck et al. (2001) found that high job control reduces the relationship between job demands and poor health among individuals with high self-efficacy. High job control exacerbated the association between job demands and poor health among individuals low on self-efficacy. Meanwhile, Schaubroeck and Merritt (1997) showed that among those low in self-efficacy, having perceived control can have adverse health consequences. In their study, high control combined with high job demands exerted negative health consequences for employees reporting lower self-efficacy. People who are not confident in various aspects of their jobs might be distressed by the greater responsibility of dealing with demands that stem from increased control.

LOSING CONTROL AT WORK

> We have discovered that many employees are using their e-mail and phones to communicate with outsiders — even, on occasion, for personal reasons. These communication tools are for business only. Therefore, effective today, we are deploying a new technology to block e-mails and phone calls to and from anyone other than company employees. (Houston, 2003, retrieved August 1, 2003, from http://asia.cnet.com/newstech/perspectives/0,39001148,39129192,00.htm)

While this is not an actual company memo, it refers to newly developed technology that does indeed have the potential to do what it purports to do. Tightening control over telephone calls, electronic messages, and other organization-related communication tools does occur, as does a reduction in employee job control in many other aspects of work. This is significant, because control that employees felt they had prior to the introduction of the technology is threatened or lost. Loss of control appears to be a particularly potent aspect of control, one that has many motivational, emotional, and cognitive consequences (e.g., Mineka, 1982; Mineka & Henderson, 1985; Wortman & Brehm, 1975), but one that has not been regularly considered in examinations of control at work. It appears that stronger consequences occur following a loss of control compared with a lack of control (Baum et al., 1992; Hanson et al., 1976), because original expectations of control have been shattered, leaving a greater sense of disappointment and apathy. Indeed, when examining control-related outcomes, many investigators have found that the most severe consequences occur following a loss of control (Baum et al., 1992; Hanson et al., 1976).

Wortman and Brehm (1975) proposed a reactance–learned helplessness theory to explain how individuals react to a perceived loss of control. The process of losing control is expected to follow a specific pattern such that reactance occurs followed by helplessness. They proposed that when threats are made to an individual's perception of control over an outcome, that person becomes angry and hostile, and actively attempts to maintain or regain control (e.g., Brehm, 1966, 1972). When individuals learn that their loss is unchangeable, they show low arousal and apathy, give up trying to regain control, and experience helplessness (Seligman, 1974, 1975). Research in naturalistic settings has confirmed this pattern of reaction to a loss of control (Baum et al., 1986; Heath & Davidson, 1988; Zippay, 1995). Of particular relevance is the study of people following the disaster at the Three Mile Island nuclear plant.

Baum et al. (1993) argue that events involving loss of control and violation of expectations for control have different effects than do events in which control was never expected. In early spring of 1979, an unprecedented accident occurred at the nuclear-generating facility at Three Mile Island in Pennsylvania when a reactor suddenly overheated (see Baum, 1990; Baum et al., 1983a, 1983b, 1993; Davidson et al., 1982). During the accident and emergency period, radiation was released and a variety of threats to life and health were reported in local and national media. Information provided by officials during this period was often confusing or contradictory, and after a series of reported dangers were aired, an evacuation advisory was issued for pregnant women and young children living near the reactor. Since the residents were given conflicting information by various authorities, the credibility of the information they received was reduced. Many residents felt they could not control events and also doubted others' (i.e., authorities) ability to do so (Baum et al., 1993). Some feared they had been exposed to radiation, and not only were they powerless to do anything to prevent exposure, but they were also unable to do anything to counteract the possible long-term consequences of that exposure. Estimates indicate that up to two thirds of the residents of a 5-mile ring around the reactor left their homes during the emergency. When residents returned to their homes, large amounts of radioactive gas remained in the reactor containment building and more than 400,000 gal of radioactive water was on the floor of the reactor building.

Evidence of long-term stress reactions has been reported among people living near the reactor at the nuclear-generating facility (Baum, 1990; Davidson & Baum, 1986). Several researchers found evidence of demoralization, symptom distress, and emotional upset among people living in the vicinity of the plant (see Baum, 1990). Residents who reported greater feelings of helplessness or less perceived control over their surroundings showed more signs of stress than did other individuals. Residents of the Three Mile Island area exhibited more symptoms of stress almost 18 months after the accident than did people living under different circumstances (e.g., residents of an area near an undamaged nuclear plant) (Baum et al., 1983b) and continued to report stress related to the accident 5 years later (Baum et al., 1993). Consider the following excerpt posted in the *Washington Post* reader forum 20 years after the incident:

> I lived near Three Mile Island and worked nights within the five mile radius while attending college. I will never forget how sunny it was that Wednesday morning when I innocently walked to my car and went home to sleep. When I got up that afternoon, I learned of the accident. Then on Friday, it worsened and I had just taken my car into

> the shop for repairs. I called a taxi, reclaimed my car, hastily packed some things, and left the area.
>
> The experience still makes me cry because of the intense emotions of fear and anger and confusion. The fact that radiation is invisible and odorless seemed to make it easy for some people to act as if it is also harmless. I still wonder about the health effects because the mean dose over the entire population is meaningless — what matters is the wind and if the radiation plume carrying the largest doses happened to be where you were those days.... I'll never be the same. (The Washington Post Company, 1999, para. 28)

The severity of the impact of this accident on residents living near the plant is clear in the words used in the quotation above. The chronic stress following an event such as this is likely related to the effect of losing control, such as the violation of expectations for regulating aspects of one's life normally under control (Baum et al., 1993). Data from studies at Three Mile Island in the wake of the nuclear accident suggested that loss of control, as well as the frequent experience of intrusive thoughts about the accident and its aftermath, were related to persistent stress (e.g., see Davidson et al., 1982). Residents living near Three Mile Island reported more control-related problems than did comparison subjects living more than 80 miles from the damaged power plant. In one study, for example, Three Mile Island residents performed more poorly on a behavioral task in terms of the number solved, attempts made, and time spent on the task than individuals living outside of Three Mile Island (Davidson et al., 1982). The events of the Three Mile Island disaster also made residents apprehensive of future accidents and the outcomes of those potential events.

An improved understanding of the loss of control at work is particularly important given that changes to the present state of work are likely to decrease employee job control. For example, Aronsson (1999) notes that work in the future will have greater mobility than it did in the late 1990s. Movement is expected between unemployment and employment, between full-time and part-time work, between occupations, between study and paid work, and between work and home. Associated with this might be increased perceptions of loss of control over work. Findings from a study by Karasek (1990) indicated that white-collar job changes often resulted in reduced job control, and that this was especially true for older workers and women. Moreover, technological changes to work, along with an increase in service and information work, can result in increased losses of job control for employees. For example, a study of clerical video display terminal operators demonstrated that they felt less control in their work than did their counterparts who did not use video display terminals (see Sauter et al., 1983; Smith et al., 1981).

Given that changes to the world of work appear to be occurring at an ever-increasing rate, understanding loss of control takes on paramount importance. Indeed, it has been suggested that reactions to one of the salient changes in today's workplace — the possibility of terrorism — might be explained by the loss of control (Inness & Barling, in press); whereas previously employees could feel assured of their security at work, there are now constant reminders of the potential for terrorist acts, and thus constant reminders of their loss of control.

FEELING OVERCONTROLLED AT WORK

In addition to having control at work, lacking control at work, and losing control at work, employees have the potential to feel overcontrolled at work. Researchers have begun to look at this aspect of control, and although there is scant research in comparison to the other forms of control at work, it appears to have the potential to profoundly affect both individuals and organizations.

Although employees might feel overcontrolled as a result of a number of work-related factors (e.g., coworkers, customers, and electronic systems), research to date has focused on perceptions of supervisory overcontrol, likely as a result of the power differential between supervisors and employees. Many supervisors can be overcontrolling, such as when they monitor their subordinates' personal and work behaviors too closely. While a certain level of supervisory control is appropriate, overcontrol can have deleterious effects on employees (Shirom et al., 2000), given that when employees lack a perception of personal control over certain elements of work, they often experience negative repercussions. Of prominent importance is that when employees feel overcontrolled by their supervisors, they might feel the need to restore the loss of balance in this relationship with their supervisors. Research has indicated that one way of accomplishing this is to strike back at the overcontrolling agent. Research findings indicate that feeling overcontrolled is associated with aggression against the overcontrolling agent (Dupré & Barling, 2004; Ehrensaft et al., 1999), as well as feelings of being treated unjustly by the overcontrolling individual (Dupré & Barling, 2004). In situations where individuals do not receive something to which they feel entitled (e.g., rewards), or are subject to something that they feel is inappropriate (e.g., unfair interpersonal treatment), a perception of injustice is likely to occur, probably because the experience of overcontrol causes the individual who feels overcontrolled to focus on the relationship and to feel that he or she has been treated inequitably (e.g., see Grote & Clark, 2001).

FUTURE RESEARCH

While a strong case can be made for the importance of a variety of aspects of job control, fundamental questions remain concerning the conceptualization and operationalization of the construct. There is a definite need for an improved understanding of job control, and how various aspects of job control affect subsequent outcomes.

Different dimensions of control do play different roles in influencing strain. For example, Carayon and Zijlstra (1999) found that high *task* control was related to *low* work pressure, whereas high *organization* control was related to *high* work pressure (both of these relationships were mediated by work pressure). Researchers need to take this into consideration in their research and attempt to delineate the predictors and outcomes associated with various forms of control at work. Another important point to consider and address in future research is that evidence suggests that aspects of control at work influence one another. For example, Jimmieson and Terry (1997, 1998, 1999) provided evidence that informational control might compensate for the negative impact of other forms of control. More recently, researchers have proposed a multidimensional conceptualization of control (Terry & Jimmieson,

1999). While some research has discussed different facets and levels of control (e.g., Sauter et al., 1989), very little empirical research has actually examined these different facets and levels (for an exception, see, for example, Troup & Dewe, 2002).

Because there are a number of aspects of control, it might be more useful to consider the factors that an individual strives to control, as well as the perceived degree of control over those factors, rather than focusing solely on whether an individual has control over a given situation in general. For example Dwyer and Fox (2000) found a moderating role for hostility in the link between job control and health care costs, but different results for job control when it came to cardiovascular health. Increased control resulted in reduced cardiovascular and respiratory health complaints among nurses, even for those with high hostility. The authors postulated that the discrepant results for job control when predicting different outcomes occurred because nurses have control over different aspects of their work. Control over work schedules and running stations, for example, might have more positive effects than control over other aspects of work such as increased decision-making control and accountability over patient care. In certain circumstances, and for particular employees, some aspects of control are likely more important than others. In a similar vein, it would be worthwhile for future research to continue to examine moderators that might influence the impact that various forms of job control have on individual and organizational outcomes.

Shapiro et al. (1987) noted the lack of uniform operational terminology in research on control and health, and suggested the need to more systematically address theoretical and conceptual aspects of the control construct. Some work has suggested that when job control is conceptualized and operationalized very specifically, inconsistent findings can be rectified. For example, Wall et al. (1996) used more focused measures of demands and control and found clear evidence that the elevation of risk with a demanding job appears only when demands occur in interaction with low control on the job. Parallel analyses using a measure of decision latitude (a general measure encompassing a wide range of job properties, including control, task variety, and learning opportunities) rather than job control did not show an equivalent effect. Likewise, in a review of 10 years of empirical research, Van der Doef and Maes (1999) found that the conceptualization of demands and control was a key factor in discriminating supportive from nonsupportive studies of the moderating influence of job control in the demand–control model. The conceptualization of control has varied across studies from very general to much more specific. As a result of the variation in the control construct, the existing literature might be underestimating both the role of job control as a moderator of job stressors and the direct impact that job control has on various outcome variables.

In part, some of the ambiguity about work and aspects of health arises because of the lack of rigorous studies. It remains a challenge to tie particular outcomes to particular work stressors, given the difficulty associated with choosing the appropriate temporal lag between the measurement of the stressor and the strain associated with it (Barling, 1990). As has been discussed, cross-sectional, self-report study designs predominate in the literature, and thus there is a definite need for additional longitudinal research in the domain of job control. In addition, it is also important to consider processes across levels of analysis. Multilevel processes are not well articulated or examined in the work stress literature (Bliese & Jex, 1999). An understanding of such processes would be useful to better understand the effects of work control. Jackson (1989) proposed an uncertainty framework for studies of job control that identifies the origins of, and responses to, uncertainty at different levels of analysis. In this model, individuals' feelings of control reflect their own job control as well as perceptions of control that derive from the larger systems in which individuals are embedded (e.g., departments' power within the organization). Of special interest are data suggesting that control is important not only for the well-being of workers, but also for the success of the organization. Karasek (1979) argued that increased control can reduce stress without threatening productivity, and research would benefit by furthering this argument.

We believe that it would be particularly worthwhile to focus more research attention on both losing control at work and feeling overcontrolled at work. Research on this topic focuses predominantly on being in control and, by extension, being out of control, but should be extended to consider losing control and being over-controlled. Of relevance here is the finding that job control has been shown to exert greater performance benefits in uncertain environments where flexible responses are required (e.g., Wall et al., 1990). Jackson (1989) made a similar argument in relation to health, proposing that control is important because, when faced with the stressor of uncertainty, people who feel in control will be more likely to use proactive problem solving rather than emotion-focused coping. In light of such suggestions, along with the fact that situations like these might at the same time result in a loss of control (as discussed above), it is imperative that research further investigate the notion of loss of job control to understand its implications for employees in a variety of current employment circumstances.

Advances in stress research in general and job control research in particular have been impeded by a lack of consensus among research findings. It is imperative that researchers strive to overcome the aforementioned limitations in future research. It has been said that the "challenge for the next decade of research is to identify the mechanisms that underpin the effects of work control" (Terry & Jimmieson, 1999, p. 137). Attaining this challenge would provide an enhanced understanding of the impact that job control has on both individual and organizational outcomes.

CONCLUSION

Control remains a fundamental aspect of work, and research highlights the importance of perceived work control for employee and organizational health and well-being. The issue of control at work has been, and continues to be, a common area of research. Given that many "employees have perceived a gradual loss of control over their work lives" (Sparks et al., 2001, p. 498), research on this important aspect of work needs to continue. Although much work has been guided by the notion that control exerts a positive effect across individuals, perceptions of job control can vary across individuals and situations in determining subsequent consequences. Future research in this area faces many challenges given that there are a number of issues that need to be considered to enhance the understanding of control at work. However, the considerable advances in research and understanding in recent years would suggest that the same will occur over the next few years, and it is likely that inconsistent findings will be clarified and that an improved integration of this literature is possible. The sense of personal control over various aspects of life has been a major focus of interest in understanding the stress process and in explicating the links among stressors, health, and well-being. A better understanding of how job control works in the stress process will most definitely contribute to a healthier and more productive workforce.

REFERENCES

Adams, G. A., & Jex, S. M. (1999). Relationships between time management, control, work-family conflict, and strain. *Journal of Occupational Health Psychology*, 4, 72–77.

Amick III, B. C., McDonough, P., Chang, H., Rogers, W. H., Duncan, G., & Pieper, C. (2002). The relationship between all-cause mortality and cumulative working life course psychosocial and physical exposures in the United States labor market from 1968–1992. *Psychosomatic Medicine*, 64, 370–381.

Arnold, K. A. (2003). Dirty Work and Well-Being. Unpublished doctoral dissertation, Queen's University, Kingston, Ontario, Canada.

Aronsson, G. (1999). Influence of worklife on public health. *Scandinavian Journal of Work, Environment and Health*, 25, 597–604.

Barling, J. (1990). *Employment, Stress And Family Functioning*. Toronto: Wiley.

Barling, J., & Kelloway, E. K. (1996). Job insecurity and health: The moderating role of workplace control. *Stress Medicine*, 12, 253–259.

Barling, J., Kelloway, E. K., & Frone, M. *Handbook of Work Stress*, Thousand Oaks, CA, Sage Publications, (in press).

Barnett, R. C., & Brennan, R. T. (1995). The relationship between job experiences and psychological distress: A structural equation approach. *Journal of Organizational Behavior*, 16, 259–276.

Baum, A. (1990). Stress, intrusive imagery, and chronic distress. *Health Psychology*, 9, 653–675.

Baum, A., Cohen, L., & Hall, M. (1993). Control and intrusive memories as possible determinants of chronic stress. *Psychosomatic Medicine*, 55, 274–286.

Baum, A., Fleming, R., & Davidson, L. M. (1983a). Natural disaster and technological catastrophe. *Environment and Behavior*, 15, 333–354.

Baum, A., Fleming, R., Israel, A., & O'Keefe, M. K. (1992). Symptoms of chronic stress following a natural disaster and discovery of a human-made hazard. *Environment and Behavior*, 24, 347–365.

Baum, A., Fleming, R., & Reddy, D. M. (1986). Unemployment stress: Loss of control, reactance and learned helplessness. *Social Science and Medicine*, 22, 509–516.

Baum, A., Gatchel, R. J., & Schaeffer, M. A. (1983b). Emotional, behavioral, and physiological effects of chronic stress at Three Mile Island. *Journal of Consulting and Clinical Psychology*, 51, 565–572.

Bishop, G. D., Enkelmann, H. C., Tong, E. M. W., Why, Y. P., Diong, S. M., Ang, J., & Khader, M. (2003). Job demands, decisional control, and cardiovascular responses. *Journal of Occupational Health Psychology*, 8, 146–156.

Bliese, P. D., & Jex, S. M. (1999). Incorporating multiple levels of analysis into occupational stress research. *Work and Stress*, 13, 1–6.

Bond, F. W., & Bunce, D. (2001). Job control mediates change in a work reorganization intervention for stress reduction. *Journal of Occupational Health Psychology*, 6, 290–302.

Bongers, P. M., de Winger, C. R., Kompier, M. A. J., & Hildebrandt, V. H. (1993). Psychosocial factors at work and musculoskeletal disease. *Scandinavian Journal of Work, Environment and Health*, 19, 297–312.

Bosma, H., Marmot, M. G., Hemingway, H., Nicholson, A. C., Brunner, E., & Stansfeld, S. A. (1997). Low job control and risk of coronary heart disease in the Whitehall II (prospective cohort) study. *British Medical Journal*, 314, 558–564.

Bosma, H., Stansfeld, S. A., & Marmot, M. G. (1998). Job control, personal characteristics and heart disease. *Journal of Occupational Health Psychology*, 3, 402–409.

Brehm, J. W. (1966). *A Theory of Psychological Reactance*. New York: Academic Press.

Brehm, J. (1972). Responses to ban of freedom: A theory of psychological reactance. Morrisville, NJ: General Learning Press.

Burger, J. M. (1989). Negative reactions to increases in perceived personal control. *Journal of Personality and Social Psychology*, 56, 246–256.

Burger, J. M. (1995). Need for control and self-esteem: Two routes to a high desire for control. In M. Kernis (Ed.), *Efficacy, Agency, and Self-Esteem* (pp. 217–233). New York: Plenum.

Carayon, P. (1993). A longitudinal test of Karasek's job strain model among office workers. *Work and Stress*, 10, 104–118.

Carayon, P., & Zijlstra, F. (1999). Relationship between job control, work pressure and strain: Studies in the USA and in the Netherlands. *Work and Stress*, 13, 32–48.

Cohen, A. (1997). Facing pressure. *Sales and Marketing Management*, 149, 30–38.

Cox, T., & Cox, S. (1993). Occupational health: Control and monitoring of psychosocial and organizational hazards at work. *Journal of the Royal Society of Health*, 113, 201–205.

Daniels, K., & Guppy, A. (1994). Occupational stress, social support, job control, and psychological well-being. *Human Relations*, 47, 1523–1544.

Davidson, L. M., & Baum, A. (1986). Chronic stress and posttraumatic stress disorders. *Journal of Consulting and Clinical Psychology*, 54, 303–308.

Davidson, L. M., Baum, A., & Collins, D. L. (1982). Stress and control-related problems at Three Mile Island. *Journal of Applied Social Psychology*, 12, 349–359.

deCharms, P. (1968). *Personal Causation*. New York: Academic Press.

de Rijk, A. E., Le Blanc, P. M., Schaufeli, W. B., & de Jonge, J. (1998). Active coping and need for control as moderators of the job demand-control model: Effects on burnout. *Journal of Occupational and Organizational Psychology*, 71, 1–18.

Dollard, M., Winefield, H., Winefield, A., & de Jonge, J. (2000). Psychosocial job strain and productivity in human service workers: A test of the demand-control-support model. *Journal of Occupational and Organizational Psychology*, 73, 501ñ510.

Dupré, K. E., & Barling, J. (2004). The Prediction and Prevention of Workplace Aggression. Manuscript submitted for publication.

Dwyer, D. J., & Fox, M. L. (2000). The moderating role of hostility in the relationship between job characteristics and health. *Academy of Management Journal*, 43, 1086–1096.

Dwyer, D. J., & Ganster, D. C. (1991). The effects of job demands and control on employee attendance and satisfaction. *Journal of Organizational Behavior*, 12, 595–608.

Ehrensaft, M. K., Langhinrichsen-Rohling, J., Heyman, R. E., O'Leary, K. D., & Lawrence, E. (1999). Feeling controlled in marriage: A phenomenon specific to physically aggressive couples? *Journal of Family Psychology*, 13, 20–32.

Elovainio, M., & Kivimäki, M. (1996). Occupational stresses, goal clarity, control, and strain among nurses in the Finnish health care system. *Research in Nursing and Health*, 19, 517–524.

Elovainio, M., Kivimäki, M., & Helkama, K. (2001). Organizational justice evaluations, job control, and occupational strain. *Journal of Applied Psychology*, 86, 418–424.

Elovainio, M., Kivimäki, M., Steen, N., & Kalliomäki-Levanto, T. (2000). Organizational and individual factors affecting mental health and job satisfaction: A multilevel analysis of job control and personality. *Journal of Applied Psychology*, 5, 269–277.

Elsass, P. M., & Veiga, J. F. (1997). Job control and job strain: A test of three models. *Journal of Occupational Health Psychology*, 2, 195–211.

Evans, B. K., & Fischer, D. G. (1992). A hierarchical model of participatory decision-making, job autonomy, and perceived control. *Human Relations*, 45, 1169–1189.

Fenwick, R., & Tausig, M. (2001). Scheduling stress: Family and health outcomes of shift work and schedule control. *The American Behavioral Scientist*, 44, 1179–1198.

Fox, M. L., Dwyer, D. J., & Ganster, D. C. (1993). Effects of stressful job demands and control on physiological and attitudinal outcomes in a hospital setting. *Academy of Management Journal*, 36, 289–318.

Frese, M., & Zapf, D. (1994). Action as the core of work psychology: A German approach. In H. C. Triandis, M. D. Dunnette, & L. M. Hough (Eds.), *Handbook of Industrial and Organizational Psychology*, 2nd ed., Vol. 4 (pp. 271–340). Palo Alto, CA: Consulting Psychologists Press.

Ganster, D. C. (1988). Improving measures of work control in occupational stress research. In J. J. Hurrell, Jr., L. R. Murphy, S. L. Sauter, & C. L. Cooper (Eds.), *Occupational Stress: Issues and Developments in Research* (pp. 88–99). New York: Taylor & Francis.

Ganster, D. C. (1989). Worker control and well-being: A review of research in the workplace. In S. L. Sauter, J. J. Hurrell, Jr., & C. L. Cooper (Eds), *Job Control and Worker Health* (pp. 3–23). Chichester, U.K.: Wiley.

Ganster, D. C., Fox, M. L., & Dwyer, D. J. (2001). Explaining employees' health care costs: A prospective examination of stressful job demands, personal control, and physiological reactivity. *Journal of Applied Psychology*, 86, 954–964.

Ganster, D. C., & Fusilier, M. R. (1989). Control in the workplace. In C. L. Cooper & I. T. Robertson (Eds.), *International Review of Industrial and Organizational Psychology*, Vol. 4 (pp. 235–280). Chichester, U.K.: Wiley.

Geller, E. S., Roberts, D. S., & Gilmore, M. R. (1996). Predicting propensity to actively care for occupational safety. *Journal of Safety Research*, 27, 1–8.

Greenberger, D. B., Strasser, S., Cummings, L. L., & Dunham, R. B. (1989). The impact of personal control on performance and satisfaction. *Organizational Behavior and Human Decision Processes*, 43, 29–51.

Grote, N. K., & Clark, M. S. (2001). Perceiving unfairness in the family: Cause or consequence of marital distress? *Journal of Personality and Social Psychology*, 80, 281–293.

Hackman, J. R., & Oldham, G. R. (1975). Development of the Job Diagnostic Survey. *Journal of Applied Psychology*, 60, 159–170.

Hanson, J. P., Larsen, M., & Snowden, C. T. (1976). The effects of control over high intensity noise on plasma cortisol levels in rhesus monkeys. *Behavioral Biology*, 16, 333–340.

Heath, L., & Davidson, L. (1988). Dealing with the threat of rape: Reactance or learned helplessness? *Journal of Applied Social Psychology*, 18, 1334–1351.

Hepburn, C. G., Loughlin, C. A., & Barling, J. (1997). Coping with chronic work stress. In B. Gottlieb (Ed.), *Coping and Health in Organizations* (pp. 343–366). London: Taylor & Francis.

Hollmann, S., Heuer, H., & Schmidt, K. (2001). Control at work: A generalized resource factor for the prevention of musculoskeletal symptoms? *Work and Stress*, 15, 29–39.

Houston, P. (2003, May 6). Boss, Don't Take Away My IM. In CNETAsia. Retrieved August 1, 2003, from http://asia.cnet.com/newstech/perspectives/0,39001148,39129192,00.htm.

Hurrell, J. J., Jr., & McLaney, M. A. (1989). Control, job demands, and job satisfaction. In S. L. Sauter, J. J. Hurrell, Jr., & C. L. Cooper (Eds.), *Job Control and Worker Health* (pp. 97–103). Chichester, U.K.: Wiley.

Inness, M., & Barling, J. Terrorism. In J. Barline, E.K. Kelloway, and M.R. Frone, *Handbook of Work Stress*, Thousand Oaks, CA: Sage Publications (In press).

Isaksson, K., & Johansson, G. (2000). Adaptation to continued work and early retirement following downsizing: Long-term effects and gender differences. *Journal of Occupational and Organizational Psychology*, 73, 241–256.

Jackson, P. R., Wall, T. D., Martin, R., & Davids, K. (1993). New measures of job control, cognitive demand, and production responsibility. *Journal of Applied Psychology*, 78, 753–762.

Jackson, S. E. (1983). Participation in decision making as a strategy for reducing job-related strain. *Journal of Applied Psychology*, 68, 3–19.

Jackson, S. E. (1989). Does job control control job stress? In S. L. Sauter, J. J. Hurrell, Jr., & C. L. Cooper (Eds.), *Job Control and Worker Health* (pp. 25–53). Chichester, U.K.: Wiley.

Jex, S. M., & Beehr, T. A. (1991). Emerging theoretical and methodological issues in the study of work-related stress. In G. R. Ferris & K. M. Rowland (Eds.), *Research in Personnel and Human Resources Management*, Vol. 9 (pp. 311–365). Greenwich, CT: JAI Press.

Jimmieson, N. L., & Terry, D. J. (1997). Responses to an in-basket activity: The role of work stress, work control, and task information on adjustment. *Journal of Occupational Health Psychology*, 2, 72–83.

Jimmieson, N. L., & Terry, D. J. (1998). An experimental study of the effects of work stress, work control, and task information on adjustment. *Applied Psychology: An International Review*, 47, 343–369.

Jimmieson, N. L., & Terry, D. J. (1999). The moderating role of task characteristics in determining responses to a stressful work simulation. *Journal of Organizational Behavior*, 20, 709–736.

Johnson, J. V., & Hall, E. M. (1988). Job strain, workplace social support, and cardiovascular disease: A cross-sectional study of a random sample of the Swedish working population. *American Journal of Public Health*, 78, 1336–1342.

Johnson, J. V., Stewart, W., Hall, E. M., Fedlund, P., & Theorell, T. (1996). Long-term psychosocial work environment and cardiovascular mortality among Swedish men. *American Journal of Public Health*, 86, 324–331.

Jones, F., & Fletcher, B. C. (1996). Job control and health. In M. Schabracq, J. A. M. Winnubst, & C. L. Cooper (Eds.), *Handbook of Work and Health Psychology* (pp. 33–50). Chichester, U.K.: Wiley.

Karasek, R. A. (1979). Job demands, job decision latitude, and mental strain: Implications for job redesign. *Administrative Science Quarterly*, 24, 258–308.

Karasek, R. A. (1990). Lower health risk with increase job control among white collar workers. *Journal of Organizational Behavior*, 11, 171–185.

Karasek, R. A., Russell, R., & Theorell, T. G. (1982). Physiology of stress and regeneration in job related cardiovascular illness. *Journal of Human Stress*, 3, 29–42.

Karasek, R. A., & Theorell, T. (1990). *Healthy Work-Stress, Productivity and the Reconstruction of Working Life*. New York: Basic Books.

Kasl, S. V. (1989). An epidemiological perspective on the role of control in health. In S. L. Sauter, J. J. Hurrell, Jr., & C. L. Cooper (Eds.), *Job Control and Work Health* (pp. 161–190). Chichester, U.K.: Wiley.

Kivimäki, M., & Lindström, K. (1995). Effects of private self-consciousness and control on the occupational stress-strain relationship. *Stress Medicine*, 11, 7–16.

Kivimäki, M., Vahtera, J., Koskenvuo, M., Uutela, A., & Pentti, J. (1998). How hostile individuals respond to stressful changes in work life: Testing a psychosocial vulnerability model. *Psychological Medicine*, 28, 903–913.

Kivimäki, M., Vahtera, J., Thomson, L., Griffiths, A., Cox, T., & Pentti, J. (1997). Psychosocial factors predicting employee sickness absence during economic decline. *Journal of Applied Psychology*, 82, 858–872.

Krausz, M., Sagie, A., & Bidermann, Y. (2000). Actual and preferred work schedules and scheduling control as determinants of job-related attitudes. *Journal of Vocational Behavior*, 56, 1–11.

Kristensen, T. S. (1995). The demand-control-support model: Methodological challenges for future research. *Stress Medicine*, 11, 17–26.

Landsbergis, P. A. (1988). Occupational stress among health care workers: A test of the job demands-control model. *Journal of Organizational Behavior*, 9, 217–239.

Landsbergis, P. A., Schnall, P. L., Deitz, D., Freidman, R., & Pickering, T. (1992). The patterning of psychological attributes and distress by 'job strain' and social support in a sample of working men. *Journal of Behavioral Medicine*, 15, 379–405.

Latack, J. C. (1986). Coping with job stress: Measures and future directions for scale development. *Journal of Applied Psychology*, 71, 377–385.

Lee, C., Ashford, S. J., & Bobko, P. (1990). Interactive effects of "type A" behavior and perceived control on worker performance, job satisfaction, and somatic complaints. *Academy of Management Journal*, 33, 870–881.

Leong, C. S., Furnham, A., & Cooper, C. L. (1996). The moderating effect of organisational commitment on the occupational stress outcome relationship. *Human Relations*, 49, 1345–1354.

McGilton, K. S., & Pringle, D. M. (1999). The effects of perceived and preferred control on nurses' job satisfaction in long term care environments. *Research in Nursing and Health*, 22, 251–261.

McKnight, J. D., & Glass, D. C. (1995). Perceptions of control, burnout, and depressive symptomology: A replication and extension. *Journal of Consulting and Clinical Psychology*, 63, 490–494.

Miller, J. G. (1972). Living systems: The organization. *Behavioral Science*, 17, 1–182.

Miller, S. M. (1979). Controllability and human stress: Method, evidence, theory. *Behavior Research and Therapy*, 17, 287–304.

Mineka, S. (1982). Depression and helplessness in primates. In H. E. Fitzgerald, J. A. Mullins, & P. Gage (Eds.), *Child Nurturance Series*, Vol. 3, *Studies of Development in Nonhuman Primates*. New York: Plenum.

Mineka, S., & Hendersen, R. W. (1985). Controllability and predictability in acquired motivation. *Annual Review of Psychology*, 36, 495–529.

National Institute for Occupational Safety and Health. (1988). Proposed national strategies for the prevention of leading work-related diseases and injuries. In Psychological Disorders, (DHHS [NIOSH] Publication No. 89-13). Washington, D.C.: U.S. Department of Health and Human Services.

Noblet, A., Rodwell, J., & McWilliams, J. (2001). The job strain model is enough for managers: No augmentation needed. *Journal of Managerial Psychology*, 16, 635–649.

Oldham, G. R., & Cummings, A. (1996). Employee creativity: Personal and contextual factors at work. *Academy of Management Journal*, 39, 607–634.

Parker, S. K. (1998). Enhancing role breadth self-efficacy: The role of job enrichment and other organizational interventions. *Journal of Applied Psychology*, 83, 835–852.

Parker, S. K., & Axtell, C. M. (2001). Seeing another point of view: Antecedents and outcomes of employee perspective taking. *Academy of Management Journal*, 44, 1085–1100.

Parker, S. K., Axtell, C. M., & Turner, N. (2001). Designing a safer workplace: Importance of job autonomy, communication quality, and supportive supervisors. *Journal of Occupational Health Psychology*, 6, 211–228.

Parker, S. K., Chmiel, N., & Wall, T. D. (1997). Work characteristics and employee well-being with a context of strategic downsizing. *Journal of Occupational Health Psychology*, 2, 289–303.

Parker, S. K., & Sprigg, C. A. (1999). Minimizing strain and maximizing learning: The role of job demands, job control, and proactive personality. *Journal of Applied Psychology*, 84, 925–939.

Parker, S. K., Turner, N., & Griffin, M. A. (2003). Designing healthy work. In D. A. Hofmann & L. E. Tetrick (Eds.), *Health and Safety in Organizations: A Multilevel Perspective* (pp. 91–130). San Francisco: Jossey-Bass.

Parker, S. K., Wall, T. D., & Jackson, P. R. (1997). "That's not my job": Developing flexible employee work orientations. *Academy of Management Journal*, 40, 899–929.

Parkes, K. R. (1989). Personal control in an occupational context. In A. Steptoe & A. Appels (Eds.), *Stress, Personal Control, and Health* (pp. 21–47). Chichester, U.K.: Wiley.

Parkes, K. R. (1990). Coping, negative affect and the work environment: Additive and interactive predictors of mental health. *Journal of Applied Psychology*, 75, 399–409.

Parkes, K. R. (1991). Locus of control as a moderator: An explanation for additive versus interactive findings in the demand-discretion model of work stress? *British Journal of Psychology*, 82, 291–312.

Parkes, K. R. (1994). Personality and coping as moderators of work stress processes: Models, methods, and measures. *Work and Stress*, 8, 110–129.

Parkes, K. R., Mendham, C. A., & von Rabenau, C. (1994). Social support and the demand-discretion model of job stress: Tests of additive and interactive effects in two samples. *Journal of Vocational Behavior*, 44, 91–113.

Perrewe, P. L., & Anthony, W. P. (1990). Stress in a steel pipe mill: The impact of job demands, personal control, and employee age on somatic complaints. *Journal of Social Behavior and Personality*, 5, 77–90.

Pratt, L. I., & Barling, J. (1988). Differentiating between daily events, acute and chronic stressors: A framework and its implications. In J. J. Hurrell, Jr., L. R. Murphy, S. L. Sauter, & C. L. Cooper (Eds.), *Occupational Stress: Issues and Development in Research* (pp. 41–51). London: Taylor & Francis.

Rodríguez, I., Bravo, M. J., & Schaufeli, W. (2001). The demands-control-support model, locus of control and job dissatisfaction: A longitudinal study. *Work and Stress*, 15, 97–114.

Sargent, L. D., & Terry, D. J. (1998). The effects of work control and job demands on employee adjustment and work performance. *Journal of Occupational and Organizational Psychology*, 71, 219–236.

Sauter, S. L. (1989). Moderating effects of job control on health complaints in office work. In S. L. Sauter, J. J. Hurrell, Jr., & C. L. Cooper (Eds.), *Job Control and Worker Health* (pp. 91–96). New York: Wiley.

Sauter, S. L., Gottlieb, M. A., Jones, K. C., Dodson, V. N., & Rohrer, K. M. (1983). Job and health implications of VDT use: Initial results of the Wisconsin-NIOSH study. *Communications of the Association for Computing Machinery*, 26, 284–294.

Sauter, S. L., Hurrell, J. J., Jr., & Cooper, C. L. (Eds.). (1989). *Job Control and Worker Health*. New York: Wiley.

Sauter, S. L., Murphy, L. R., & Hurrell, J. J., Jr. (1990). Prevention of work-related psychological disorders. *American Psychologist*, 45, 1146–1158.

Schaubroeck, J., & Fink, L. S. (1998). Facilitating and inhibiting effects of job control and social support on stress outcomes and role behavior: A contingency model. *Journal of Organizational Behavior*, 19, 167–195.

Schaubroeck, J., Jones, J. R., & Xie, J. L. (2001). Individual differences in utilizing control to cope with job demands: Effects on susceptibility to infectious disease. *Journal of Applied Psychology*, 86, 265–278.

Schaubroeck, J., & Merritt, D. E. (1997). Divergent effects of job control on coping with work stressors: The key role of self-efficacy. *Academy of Management Journal*, 40, 738–754.

Seligman, M. E. P. (1974). Depression and learned helplessness. In R. J. Friedman & M. M. Katz (Eds.), *The Psychology of Depression: Contemporary Theory and Research* (pp. 83–113). Washington, DC: Winston-Wiley.

Seligman, M. E. P. (1975). *Helplessness*. San Francisco: Freeman.

Shapiro, D. H., Jr., Evans, G. W., & Shapiro, J. (1987). Human control. *Science*, 238, 260.

Shirom, A., Melamed, S., & Nir-Dotan, M. (2000). The relationships among objective and subjective environmental stress levels and serum uric acid: The moderating effects of perceived control. *Journal of Occupational Health Psychology*, 5, 374–386.

Simard, M., & Marchand, A. (1995). A multilevel analysis of organizational factors related to the taking of initiative by work groups. *Safety Science*, 21, 113–129.

Skinner, E. A. (1995). *Perceived Control, Motivation, and Coping*. Newbury Park, CA: Sage Publications.

Smith, A. (1937). *An Inquiry into the Nature and Causes of the Wealth of Nations*, New York: Modern Library.

Smith, M. J., Carayon, P., Sanders, K. J., Lim, S., & LeGrande, D. (1992). Employee stress and health complaints in jobs with and without electronic performance monitoring. *Applied Ergonomics*, 1, 17–28.

Smith, M. J., Cohen, B. G. F., Stammerjohn, L. W., & Happ, A. (1981). An investigation of health complaints and job stress in video display operations. *Human Factors*, 23, 387–400.

Smulders, P. G. W., & Nijhuis, F. J. N. (1999). The job demands-job control model and absence behaviour: Results of a 3-year longitudinal study. *Work and Stress*, 13, 115–131.

Sparks, K., Faragher, B., & Cooper, C. L. (2001). Well-being and occupational health in the 21st century workplace. *Journal of Occupational and Organizational Psychology*, 74, 489–509.

Spector, P. E. (1986). Perceived control by employees: A meta-analysis of studies concerning autonomy and participation at work. *Human Relations*, 39, 1005–1016.

Spector, P. E. (2002). Employee control and occupational stress. *Current Directions in Psychological Science*, 11, 133–136.

Spector, P. E., Dwyer, D. J., & Jex, S. M. (1988). Relation of job stressors to affective, health, and performance outcomes: A comparison of multiple data sources. *Journal of Applied Psychology,* 73, 11–19.

Stanton, J. M., & Barnes-Farrell, J. L. (1996). Effects of electronic performance monitoring on personal control, task satisfaction, and task performance. *Journal of Applied Psychology,* 81, 738–745.

Steptoe, A., Fieldman, G., Evans, O., & Perry, L. (1993). Control over work pace, job strain and cardiovascular responses in middle-aged men. *Journal of Hypertension, 11,* 751–759.

Terry, D. J., & Jimmieson, N. L. (1999). Work control and employee well-being: A decade review. In C. L. Cooper & I. T. Robertson (Eds.), *International Review of Industrial and Organizational Psychology 1999* (pp. 95–148). Chichester, U.K.: John Wiley.

Theorell, T. G., & Karasek, R. A. (1996). Current issues relating psychosocial job strain and cardiovascular disease research. *Journal of Occupational Health Psychology,* 1, 9–26.

Theorell, T. G., Karasek, R. A., & Eneroth, P. (1990). Job strain variations in relation to plasma testosterone fluctuations in working men: A longitudinal study. *European Journal of Internal Medicine,* 227, 31–36.

Thibaut, J., & Walker, L. (1975). *Procedural Justice: A Psychological Analysis.* Hillsdale, NJ: Erlbaum.

Thompson, S. C. (1981). Will it hurt less if I control it? A complex answer to a simple question. *Psychological Bulletin,* 90, 89–101.

Troup, C., & Dewe, P. (2002). Exploring the nature of control and its role in the appraisal of workplace stress. *Work and Stress,* 16, 335–355.

Van der Doef, M., & Maes, S. (1999). The job demand-control (-support) model and psychological well-being: A review of 20 years of empirical research. *Work and Stress,* 13, 87–114.

Van Yperen, N. W., & Hagedoorn, M. (2003). Do high job demands increase intrinsic motivation or fatigue or both? The role of job control and job social support. *Academy of Management Journal,* 46, 339–348.

Wall, T. D., & Clegg, C. W. (1981). A longitudinal study of group work redesign. *Journal of Occupational Behavior,* 2, 31–49.

Wall, T. D., Corbett, M. J., Martin, R., Clegg, C. W., & Jackson, P. R. (1990). Advanced manufacturing technology, work design, and performance: A change study. *Journal of Applied Psychology,* 75, 691–697.

Wall, T. D., Jackson, P. R., & Davids, K. (1992). Operator work design and robotics system performance: A serendipitous field study. *Journal of Applied Psychology,* 77, 353–362.

Wall, T. T., Jackson, P. R., & Mullarkey, S. (1995). Further evidence on some new measures of job control, cognitive demand and production responsibility. *Journal of Organizational Behavior,* 15, 431–455.

Wall, T. D., Jackson, P. R., Mullarkey, S., & Parker, S. K. (1996). The demands-control model of job strain: A more specific test. *Journal of Occupational and Organizational Psychology,* 69, 153–166.

Warr, P. B. (1987). *Work, Unemployment, and Mental Health.* Oxford: Clarendon Press.

Warr, P. B. (1994). A conceptual framework for the study of work and mental health. *Work and Stress,* 8, 84–97.

Warr, P. B. (1999). Well-being in the workplace. In D. Kahneman, E. Diener, & N. Schwarz (Eds.), *Well-Being: The Foundations of Hedonic Psychology* (pp. 392–412). New York: Russell Sage Foundation.

The Washington Post Company. (1999). Reader Forum: Remembering Three Mile Island Twenty Years Later. Message posted to http://discuss.washingtonpost.com/wp-srv/zforum/99/tmi_forum.htm. Retrieved August 1, 2003.

White, R. W. (1959). Motivation reconsidered: The concept of competence. *Psychological Review*, 66, 297–333.

Wortman, C., & Brehm, J. C. (1975). Responses to uncontrollable outcomes: An integration of reactance theory and the learned helplessness model. In L. Berkowitz (Ed.), *Advances in Experimental Social Psychology* (pp. 278–336). New York: Academic Press.

Xie, J. L. (1996). Karasek's model in the People's Republic of China: Effects of job demands, control, and individual differences. *Academy of Management Journal*, 39, 1594–1618.

Yelin, E. H. (1986). The myth of malingering: Why individuals withdraw from work in the presence of illness. *Milbank Quarterly*, 64, 622–649.

Zippay, A. (1995). Tracing behavioral changes among discouraged workers: What happens to the work ethic? *Psychological Reports*, 76, 531–543.

Index

A

B

C

D

E

F

G

H

I

J

L

M

N

O

P

Q

R

S

T

U

V

W

Y